The Way It Was

To Robert Putnam —
Who was not so far behind m
Barney Oul
August 1992

Also by George Crile, Jr., M.D.

HOSPITAL CARE OF THE SURGICAL PATIENT
(with Frank Shively)
Springfield, Ill., and Baltimore, Md.: Charles C. Thomas, 1943

PRACTICAL ASPECTS OF THYROID DISEASE
Philadelphia and London: W. B. Saunders, 1949

TREASURE DIVING HOLIDAYS
(with Jane Crile)
New York: Viking Press, 1954. London: Collins, 1954

CANCER AND COMMON SENSE
New York: Viking Press, 1955. London: Robert Hale Ltd., 1957

MORE THAN BOOTY
(with Jane Crile)
New York: McGraw Hill, 1965

A BIOLOGICAL CONSIDERATION
OF THE TREATMENT OF BREAST CANCER
Springfield, Ill.: Charles C. Thomas, 1967

A NATURALISTIC VIEW OF MAN
New York and Cleveland: World Publishing, 1969

ABOVE AND BELOW:
A JOURNEY THROUGH OUR NATIONAL UNDERWATER PARKS
(with Helga Sandburg)
New York: McGraw Hill, 1969

TO ACT AS A UNIT:
THE STORY OF THE CLEVELAND CLINIC
(with A. T. Bunts)
Cleveland: Cleveland Clinic, 1971

WHAT WOMEN SHOULD KNOW
ABOUT THE BREAST CANCER CONTROVERSY
New York: Macmillan, 1973

SURGERY: YOUR CHOICES, YOUR ALTERNATIVES
New York: Delacorte Press, 1978

THE CRILE CORNBALL COLLECTION
Privately printed, 1980

THE
WAY
IT
WAS

Sex, Surgery,

Treasure, and Travel,

1907–1987

GEORGE CRILE, Jr., M.D.

THE KENT STATE UNIVERSITY PRESS

Kent, Ohio, and London, England

Library of Congress Catalog Card Number 92-2971

ISBN 0-87338-465-2

Manufactured in the United States of America

Library of Congress Cataloging-in-Publication Data

Crile, George, 1907–

The way it was: sex, surgery, treasure, and travel, 1907–1987/

George Crile, Jr.

p.   cm.

Includes index.

ISBN 0-87338-465-2 (alk. paper) ∞

1. Crile, George, 1907– . 2. Surgeons—Ohio—Biography.

I. Title.

RD27.35.C75A3 1992

617′.092—dc20

[B]   92-2971

British Library Cataloging-in-Publication data are available.

*Gratefully I dedicate this book
to the memory of*
MY MOTHER,
*whose flawless files contained
all the letters, photos, and memorabilia
that have made it possible for me to recount
the days of my youth.*

Contents

1

Reminiscences of Childhood

T HE CLEVELAND presented in the first half of this story was a growing, thriving industrial center that was the largest city between New York and Chicago and the fifth largest in the country. Industry was centered here because it was in Cleveland that the rail lines from the Pennsylvania coal mines met the iron ore that came down the lakes from Minnesota. The wealth and the generosity of the early industrialists promoted the growth of Cleveland's schools, universities, theaters, and museums and made Cleveland one of the cultural centers of the country.

My father, George Crile, Sr., also played a role in the city's history. Before he founded the Cleveland Clinic, he was the chief of Surgery at Western Reserve University. During his career he was president of the American College of Surgeons, author of twenty-four books on surgery, research, and philosophy, and a recognized medical leader, both in this country and abroad. Patients came to him from all over the world.

My mother Grace was the daughter of John Harris McBride, of Scotch-Irish ancestry, who operated the huge Root and McBride Wholesale Dry Goods Company in what is now called the Warehouse District of Cleveland. The McBrides' sons went to Yale and their daughters to the best finishing schools. It was into this family that my father married and in 1907 that I was born. My sister Margaret (Peg) was six years older and my sister Elizabeth (Elo) was four years older than I. Six years later I would have a younger brother, Robert (Bob).

We lived in a house on Euclid Avenue at East Sixty-third Street—then a residential part of Cleveland. My grandfather McBride's house was next door to us and behind it was a barn that contained dilapidated buggies, a one-horse open shay, and an ancient closed-in, two-passenger electric car. Grandmother's chauffeur lived a block away, with a more modern car. Behind the barn there was a chicken coop and behind it about six acres of pasture in which two cows and sometimes a horse would graze. My rabbit hutch, where I raised Belgian hares and learned about sex, was between our own house and the pasture. Alice Page Cleveland, who was my age, lived just over the fence from the rabbit hutch and frequently would join me in observation of the activities of its inhabitants.

On Sundays, my mother would join her mother and her devout Aunt Ella in attending services at the Episcopal church twenty blocks west of us. Dr. Walter Breed, a stately figure, preached the sermons and read the Gospel. I have no recollection as to whether or not my father attended these services, but I am quite sure he didn't make a habit of it. He had left his religion on the farm when he went to medical school. I enjoyed the church because I saw lots of people and there was Sunday school and that was fun. Also I always liked the sound of the Bible readings and the resonance of the bishop's voice as it echoed in the vaults and arches of the cathedral. It was cool there, too.

After church there was Sunday dinner, often provided by one of the family's chickens, and in the afternoons sometimes there was tennis, for we had a court next to the pasture. In winter there was skating because we froze the tennis court into a hockey rink. But this era was coming to an end. Seventy years ago the industries of Cleveland were expanding, the city's population was growing (nearly three-quarters of the population was of foreign origin), and those who could afford it were leaving the old residential areas and moving to the suburbs. By the time I was nine, we had bought a couple of hundred acres of woodland twenty-five miles from Cleveland, where we had a camp with tents to sleep in and a shack to cook in and a pasture and a barn for riding horses. From that time on our Sundays were spent in the country, where my father passed on to us all that he had learned on his father's farm about the earth and its creatures and all that he had learned about horseback riding when he was a brigade surgeon in the Spanish-American War. There too, under the guidance of my ex-schoolteacher governess (Miss Marguerite Hall) I collected and classified all sorts of insects and butterflies. At that time, with the marvelous facility of the young to learn new words, I was able to rattle off the six-syllable scientific names of a dozen or more species of lepidoptera.

Inevitably, in connection with my "scientific collections," there arose questions about the origins of life and about birth, metamorphosis and death. My father always answered in terms of science, never resorting to an explanation that involved the supernatural. My mother, now weaned away from her early beliefs, supported my father's views so that I was never so much as exposed to the idea that there could be any explanation of life except in terms of science. For example, my mother recorded in her biography that when I was seven years old my grandfather died. The news was broken to me gently in terms of falling leaves returning to dust. "I know," I am alleged to have said. "He went back to his chemicals."

One of the most important influences on the minds of the Crile children was my father's "weasel stories" which were based on the adventures of a family of weasels that bore our names. The stories were told at breakfast every morning. No child was ever late. The best part of the weasel stories was that they were science fiction, used by my father to explain to us all sorts of fundamental principles. They always ended with a question of how would the weasels get out of some impossible situation. If none of us could dream up a means of escape the poor weasel had to remain in its fix until the next morning. If a solution was suggested, the story would go on until another hopeless situation arose.

So dependent did we become on the weasel stories that my father would sometimes, when he was away, send installments of them by telegram:

Day letter. The Western Union Telegraph Company, Baltimore, MD. 2/19/13. Elo & Barney Crile. Animals are scrambling out of hibernation. Fierce wolf rushed at weasels. Weasels scrambled up what they thought was tree but to their horror they found they were on an elephant's back. Elephant angry. Pack of fierce wolves surround elephant. Weasels in panic. Tomorrow something will happen.

> Dada.

And the following day:

Sharp claws of weasels tickled the elephant's back. Elephant decided to lie down among the wolves and roll over to scratch his back. Wolves with mouths wide open said now we will catch the weasels. Just as elephant started to lie down something extraordinary happened. Will tell tomorrow.

> Dada.

3

Sadly, there is no record of how the weasels escaped. The telegrams were sent to Elo and me when dad was at a meeting in Baltimore and we were in Lakeside Hospital after having our tonsils and adenoids removed, which at that time was a binding medical ritual. Mother wrote that both Elo and I anticipated the event so eagerly that we had to flip a coin to determine who would have the pleasure of being operated on first.

In addition to the weasel stories, my father would give each of us a problem to solve—usually a naturalistic one like "Why does a chicken run ahead of a car, dodging from side to side?" The answer was that its chief enemies had been hawks and foxes which it evaded by dodging. Unfamiliar with the danger of being run over, the chicken used the only escape tactics that were built into it. Incidentally, it is interesting that chickens no longer do this as much as they used to. The champion dodgers all got run over with the result that the dodging genes were bred out.

Long before I entered school my father would ask me grave questions such as, "Why does only the male sheep have horns whereas both cows and bulls have horns?" After long study and discussion my written answer, preserved by my mother, was as follows:

> The rison why only the mail sheep have horns and the mail and femail cows have hirns is this. Mail sheep have many wives and fight off all such as lions, tigers, wolves and other mail sheep. If they wives' husband is cilled by a other sheep, they all follow the sheep that wins the mail cown only have one wife at a time so they are more intifedgel [individual]. Meanwhile if her husband is cilled she does not always marry the cown that cills him, and sometimes is left to gard her baby alone. So she would develop horns.

I don't know whether this was accepted, spelling and all, but soon after there came another answer to a sex-based problem:

> II The rooster has a coam [comb] because the bigger it is the more the femail likes him.
>
> IV The rooster does not lay eggs because the mail has to fertilize them.

A reward of a dollar, big money in those days, was always offered for the correct answer to each question. Sometimes the answer would come to one of us right away. Sometimes it wouldn't come until finally, after a month or more of daily help and hints, one of us would guess it. When the right answer was given, no reward would be paid

4

until the child had written out the answer. What could constitute better training for organizing thoughts? My father would have made the world's greatest schoolteacher if he had persisted in that, his earliest profession.

In the spring of 1913, when I was seven, Mother learned from a shocked friend that I had told her child, "I don't believe in Fairies or Santa Claus or God." Later Mother asked me if I had made such a statement and recorded my reply:

He seemed to realize he was to be reprimanded and blushingly with a big swallow he said "Yes." I asked him why he said so, and he said, "Because I don't believe in them." I said, "But Barney why did you say you don't believe in God?" "Because he isn't a man," was the reply. I said, "Do you believe in Jesus?" "Oh yes," came promptly; "He was a man." "Do you believe in Mahomet and in Buddah?" I asked. "Yes, they both were men." I let it go, feeling his point was well taken—that he could not grasp the spiritual.

Nor have I been able to ever since!

Later that year my brother Bob was born. I was at the Winous Point Duck Shooting Club with Miss Hall and my sisters when I received a letter from my father:

Aug. 19, 1913

Dear Barney,

Little brother is wondering what big brother looks like and I know he wants to see him. He expects much from his big brother Barney. He expects Barney will help him to play, to learn about animals and plants, will protect him against enemies. If big brother Barney does that then little brother will give loyalty and assistance and affection to his big brother.

But we have not named him yet. What do Elo and you suggest for a name? I miss you very much. Remembrance to Miss Hall and much love from

Dada

In 1915 we moved to a Cleveland Heights mansion with eighteen bedrooms. The chauffeur and his wife and children lived above the garage in a separate house a hundred yards away. In the summers two gardeners came every day to tend the grounds and in winter to shovel the snow and stoke the enormous coal furnaces that heated the house. There was a cook, a kitchen maid, a butler, a downstairs maid, and two upstairs maids who lived in one wing of the U-shaped

Italian-style, three-story mansion, and there was a governess, formerly a schoolteacher, who was like a member of the family. The butler, whose name was Snuddin, had a bedroom and bath in the basement, next door to a large room, a whole end of which was occupied by a huge noisy machine that stood at least six feet high and worked around the clock to make a couple of quarts of ice cubes. It was the marvel of its time. There were also, of course, a couple of laundresses who came three days a week and a sewing lady who came quite regularly. My mother, whose job it was to run this vast enterprise, did it largely through a secretary, Miss Maloney, who came five days a week. Today, this period has to me a dream-like quality, reminiscent of the lives of the little princes that are described in fairy tales.

In August 1914, when World War I broke out, my father—who never was one to let a war be fought without him and who in the Spanish-American War had been a member of Cleveland's Troop A Cavalry Regiment—had a long talk with his friend, Myron T. Herrick, the ambassador to France. They decided that father and a few others would volunteer for service in what was known as "The American Ambulance." "For me," father wrote in his autobiography, "America entered the First World War when the Germans nearly reached Paris, in 1914, and the Honorable Myron T. Herrick decided to remain when other ambassadors left." Through arrangements made by Herrick with the French government, my father and the American Ambulance Unit were established in a high school building at Neuilly-sur-Seine.

My father was fifty years old and had four children, the youngest only one year old. He sailed to France on the *Lusitania* in December 1914 and stayed for three months, close to the front, where he was able to see and treat and learn about the casualties of war. This was invaluable, because later, when the United States would enter the war, he would be able to give advice to Dr. William C. Gorgas, the U.S. Army surgeon general.

My admiration for my father is boundless, but I still cannot understand the motivation that drove him at this time to leave his wife and children and his enormous surgical practice and sail back and forth across the submarine-haunted seas. It was not long after he crossed that the *Lusitania* was torpedoed, we entered the war, and he headed the "Lakeside Hospital Unit," the first American army unit to land on French soil.

At the age of ten, and like my father, deeply impressed by the war, I took my first step into the fine art of poetry. It was published on the first page of the sixth grade yearbook of University School.

Do You Think I Am Too Young?

Once I saw some bluebells
Dancing in the sunlight
I thought that they were angels
They were so blue and bright.
They seemed to say, "Go to war
"Why do you stay here any more?"
So I thought I was a slacker
Not to go and fight
And help with Vimy Height.
But at tea when I nibbled my cracker
I thought I was too young
For of years I've only ten,
And not yet do I rank among men;
But as time rolls along,
And I grow strong,
I won't want to stay home any more,
I'll want to go to war.

My memory of school is blurred. I don't remember learning anything at all. Part of that was because when I was about six years old, I
was sent with my governess, Miss Hall, to Atlantic City for six
months. I had had swollen glands in my neck, and my father, sensi-
tized by the death of two of his sisters from bovine tuberculosis,
thought that I must be getting it too. Strange, in retrospect, that so
knowledgeable a physician should have elected to send me to the seashore for the treatment of this nonexistent disease. It has often made
me wonder what silly things we still are advising our children and
grandchildren to do, and how absurd our treatment of them will
sound when our children and grandchildren are our ages.

Although the seashore probably had no effect on whatever it was
that was wrong with my glands, the six months with the learned Miss
Hall had an enormous effect on my life. I was supposed to rest a lot
and stay in bed part of the time. I learned to expect the tide to come in,
and I watched the waves break down my sand castles, and I saw the
crabs and fishlets as they played in the surf. All that long winter, Miss
Hall read to me tirelessly from the classics. She taught me to read and
to write and something about numbers, so that by the time I was
seven and supposed to enter the second grade, I was doing fourth
grade work. This was a disaster for me, because my father and mother
were great friends of Mrs. Lyman, the principal of Laurel, Cleveland's
leading girls' school. Mrs. Lyman agreed to "take me at Laurel for

7

grading" which meant putting me in classes composed entirely of huge women who were three years older and twice as big as I. They were also very strong and very mean and took out on me all the repressed malice that they felt from time to time toward fathers and older brothers. There was one other boy in these classes—Allen Thomas, who was my age but much smaller and frailer. The girls tortured and teased him as much as they did me. I was never happier than when Mrs. Lyman said I could go into the fourth grade of University School, where the boys were not only smaller than girls of the same age but also were only two years older than I.

My handwriting always was bad, but my marks in the early years of school were good, although never excellent. In 1915, aged eight, while I was in the fourth grade of Laurel School and because of my long and close association with Miss Hall, I could keep up with the girls— intellectually: Reading A, Spelling B +, Arithmetic A, Penmanship B–, Language A, German B–, French A +, Application A, Times absent 1. Signed, *Nannette B. Lips.*

I still have a vivid recollection of Miss Lips—a charming and sympathetic and intellectually stimulating woman, probably in her midforties. It is interesting that my A + was in French, which came naturally to me. This was because before we moved to Cleveland Heights, we lived almost next door to a French woman, Madame Klein, who made her living by teaching French conversation in the Berlitz style—she would not tolerate a word of English. From the age of about four until we moved away, I spoke French every day with Madame Klein and she read aloud to me—mainly the tales of the Three Musketeers.

German was the opposite. World War I came along, and we were living in the mansion in Cleveland Heights. James Kilmurray, the chauffeur, was Scotch and the woman my mother had employed to teach me piano was German. "She is a spy," James would whisper to me, "be careful—do not stay with her alone." This terror of the German lady carried over to my school so that I was repelled by the familiar guttural sound of the language. That is why I had the B– in German.

My two older sisters, my younger brother and I, and all of our rich friends were driven by chauffeurs. We went to private schools and dancing schools and later to all the debutante parties. It was a miracle that we survived and grew up to be relatively stable people. Most of our friends didn't.

The thing that saved me from the disaster of being spoiled by riches was that my father had been born in southern Ohio and had paid his way through medical school by working on the family farm and by teaching in country schools. He never had lost his respect for the land, and in hope of instilling the same respect in me, in the summer of 1919, when I was eleven, he sent me to work on his brother's farm in Chili, Ohio, for bed, board, and ten cents a week. It was on Uncle Alec's farm that summer that I picked up an incurable habit that sometimes has been an asset and at other times has gotten me into trouble. I refer to having a fixed belief that the way most things are done is unnecessarily complicated and time-consuming. As a result I have always had an overpowering urge to cut corners and simplify. It started like this.

The ten cents a week that I earned was for setting up corn. My seventeen-year-old cousin, George Crile, would run the horse-drawn cultivator round and round the gently sloping hill on which the young corn was growing, the cultivator's metal blades turning over the earth to kill the weeds. The trouble was that sometimes a big clod of earth would fall on a delicate three-inch corn sprout and bury it. My job was to set up the bent or buried corn plants. Round and round the field we went, and as the sun grew hotter I dreamed, each time we went by it, of the bend in the creek where the swimming hole was—how cool and clear the water would be. Then I had an idea. I could run down to the pool, take a swim and run back to catch the cultivator on the next round. By working fast, back and forth between rows, I could straighten up the corn just as thoroughly as I could by following slowly behind the plow.

The first time I tried the new system, my cousin hardly noticed that I had left. By the time he really understood what was going on, I was swimming two-thirds of the time and setting up three rows at a time.

"You can't do that," George told me firmly.

"Why not?" I asked.

"That's not the way you set up corn. You're supposed to follow the plow and do it right, one row at a time."

"But I'm doing it right."

We had come to an impasse. At lunch we consulted my uncle. After he had walked the field, and found the corn properly set up, I was allowed to spend two-thirds of my work time in swimming. I've been finding shortcuts ever since. That is why I don't believe an authority who says a complex operation is necessary. He has to give me a good reason why a simpler one wouldn't work as well. But on the negative side, my ability to find shortcuts in my chores in house or garden has, on occasion, led to such outbursts of rage that the stability of a marriage was threatened.

Another lesson I learned in my childhood is still vivid. I was ten or eleven years old and playing tennis with my older sister Elizabeth. Each of us had won two points.

"Deuce," I yelled.

"No, it's 30 all," she said.

"Deuce," I yelled back.

"Thirty all," she screamed.

"It's the same," I told her. "Deuce and 30 all are the same. Either way the next one to win two straight points wins the game."

"But you've only got two points. It's 30 all."

"Deuce," I said.

My sister left the court weeping and appealed to my mother—a well-trained, skillful tennis player. My mother was gentle but firm. "I see what you mean," she said, "but it's still 30 all."

The matter was never satisfactorily resolved between me and the female members of the family, but when I put the question to my father, who had never had time to play tennis, he said, "What's the difference?"

As time went by, I noticed that many wars were waged over the meaning of meaningless words.

At University School I was a sissy. I had two sisters, a mother, a governess, a household full of maids, and all but one of my classmates at Laurel had been girls. I knew nothing about men or boys or sports, other than tennis. Moreover, my mother dressed me as an English boarding school boy with stiff collars, full ties, and the whole Little-Lord-Fauntleroy outfit. The boys mussed me up and wrote on my collar and teased me continually. I assumed that this was the way school was and never related my troubles to my family, until finally the governess or someone reported to my mother the way my clothes and collars looked. Mother questioned me, and I told her. She consulted with my father. As usual my father had a complete and perfect solution. "He's big enough. If we teach him, he'll be able to defend himself. We'll have him take boxing lessons."

So three times a week after school the chauffeur drove me to the gymnasium, where a private instructor taught me the art of self-defense.

A few months passed, and with the encouragement of my instructor, I had become quite confident. A group of us were standing outside the main school building waiting to be picked up and taken home when the boy named Simon, who had for so long been bullying me, started to knock me around again. I hit him back and, using my newly learned technique, beat him up. The audience looked on, astonished. That was the first and last fist fight I was ever engaged in.

I was growing fast, and there were early signs of sexual maturity. Although I was still signed up for tennis as my official sport, there were some compulsory athletics in which I engaged. Exactly how I got involved in it I can't remember, but one day I was playing football. There in front of me was a big flabby boy who threatened to tackle our ball carrier. I took him out—threw my body across him, knocking him down—and out. He lay there, gasping, for a couple of minutes. I hadn't meant to do anything like that, but suddenly I felt my power. Although two years younger than most of these boys, physically, I was at least the equal of most of them. That was the end of my career on the tennis courts and the beginning of my interest in football. By my sophomore year, I was playing end on the class team and the head coach had told me that next year I'd be on the varsity. That was an honor beyond belief because in those days, before the huge public high schools had effective athletic programs, the private schools—with their football fields, stadiums, and coaches—were apt to have the best teams and to furnish the Ivy League colleges with their best players.

To my intense disappointment, I was not to play on the University School team. My parents had decided to send me away to a "prep school." I don't think this was my father's idea, because I was doing well enough in school and was getting into no trouble at home. My mother, however, was a McBride brought up in the old English tradition of finishing schools for girls and prep schools for boys. Later she would arrange for my younger brother to go away to school starting in the seventh grade. In any event, off I went to Hotchkiss School in Lakeville, Connecticut, where boys from all over the country came to prepare themselves for the Ivy League colleges.

Prep school was not my first experience in being away from home and family. In the summers, since the age of eight, I had gone to our country place, the Knob, to vacation for a week or two with my father's very intellectual secretary and editor, Miss Amy Rowland, and her companion, Miss White, a kindergarten teacher. There I spent pleasant days roaming the summer woods with my BB gun and spent much energy in making a series of dams and lakes on the hillside where a clear spring, lined with white quartz pebbles, bubbled up from the black soil.

There also, while my father was still away in World War I, my manual training teacher, Doc Rollinson, ran a summer camp. Doc was an extraordinary man whom I have never forgotten. One of the wise men who had founded and endowed University School had made a provision that there would be a compulsory course—manual training. Doc was the teacher. A very old man, he seemed, for he had a grey hair or two. He was ruddy-faced, stout, and hearty. Every boy was his friend. In his course, no one ever had a mark lower than an A. He knew each of us by name and he knew all of our failings.

It was a miracle that Doc Rollinson was able to see us through without injuries. No school today would dare expose its students to the risks that confronted us in that great workshop. As I remember, the room was about the size of a football field. (I am sure that it was only a quarter of that, but still it was an enormous area.) It was filled with overhead swirling belts that powered lathes and saws and punch machines which might have been the envy of Warner and Swasey. As a ten-year-old, I entered the area with the reverence with which one might enter a cathedral. But, instead of the resonance of the music of an organ there was the rumbling belts and the cacophony of the hammers on metal and the screeching of the lathes. It was impressive. To each of us a task was assigned.

Doc Rollinson was a genius. There was a limited number of lathes, buzz saws, and chain saws, and also a limited amount of wood to make things from. He distributed everything equally and impartially. He told me that I had to make a footstool. It was up to me to conceive the design, fabricate, smooth, stain, shellac, and polish this product. It took me a year, but I did it. I can still remember the workbench at which I sawed and planed and nailed and painted and polished the dark walnut wood of that stool. I remember the pride and satisfaction of the day when I presented it to my politely appreciative parents. For years it was displayed in all its glory in the living room of our home. From time to time I stroked it—soft as the fur of a cat.

It was not the satisfaction of creating a footstool that makes me remember this period of my life. It is the memory of that vast room full of what today would be considered dangerous moving belts and machinery. All of this was supervised not by a Ph.D. in manual training, but by a teacher who liked to work with his hands, to take children to summer camps, and to dive off springboards so high that none of us dared follow.

In the summer camp we lived in tents pitched in the wooded summit of our East Knob of Little Mountain—the second highest spot in northern Ohio. On the edge of a seventy-foot cliff, we could stand and look down on sandstone conglomerates forty-feet high studded with quartz pebbles that once were on the beach of a sea and then were dropped here by a glacier. In the distance, with no sign of habitation between, was Lake Erie—bright and blue. Each day we walked a mile and a half to swim in the pond of a neighbor who had dammed up a creek to make a lake and built a high-diving platform and even a sort of roller coaster on the hillside, down which, at breathtaking speed, one could slide into the water on coasting toboggans.

Every morning two of us would be delegated to walk three miles to another neighbor who had a dairy farm and to return with buckets of milk and cream. There were rockets and firecrackers set off on the hilltop on the Fourth of July, and I remember, to my shame, that a friend and I walked a mile one night (with no permission from Doc Rollinson) to shoot a Roman candle into the open window of a people-filled church and then flee away into the forest and the night. And then there was rock climbing and cliff climbing and exploring the caves.

Little Mountain and its Knobs are of glacial origin. Once they were the shore of an ocean or vast lake. The glacier, or some tremor of the earth's crust, left a number of deep cracks in the sandstone, some of them a hundred feet deep and only three or four feet wide. Some of these are still open as precipitous clefts a quarter of a mile long, eighty feet deep and twenty feet wide. Others, the narrower ones, as a result of the growth of tree roots and vegetation, have been roofed over to form caves. In most of these streams of water flow, ice cold from the springs, and it was these caves that all of us loved to explore, wading knee-deep, our breath frosty when we came to the occasional patch of sunlight. We didn't use flashlights. We just clung to the walls and felt our way through, and all the while we reassured one another by asking if it was in this cave that the bottomless pit had been found. There were nighttime explorations too. We would watch the sunset. As darkness fell, we would leave the campfire and walk the long mile to the top of Little Mountain where, half a century before, a stylish summer resort had flourished.

There were two large tinderbox, yellow-painted wooden hotels each of which must have had a hundred rooms, and there were many small and large summer cabins—all of them empty. There were tennis courts, grown up in weeds, disrepaired riding horse stables, and overgrown horseback trails along the cliffs and down to the chasms and caves that once made Little Mountain so famous. In one of these, known as the Devil's Kitchen, there were carved in the sandstone walls a thousand or more graffiti, many of them dating back to the 1870s.

In the last three decades of the nineteenth century, Little Mountain had been a popular resort, fed by the roaring red interurban trolleys that ran along Euclid from Cleveland to Painesville. Stop 61 was the

Little Mountain Road where guests were met by horses and buggies sent from the Little Mountain Hotels. What happened to the resort I never knew. Perhaps the advent of the motorcar made it easier to go farther afield so that Little Mountain was bypassed. Perhaps golf and swimming surpassed horseback riding and trail walking as outdoor sports. In any event the hotels and cabins were closed and crumbling. No one lived there except a caretaker. We used to sneak by him to run down to the hotels and throw stones through what windows were left intact and then run home.

Then we heard about the murder in room 113. We had to investigate. It was a moonlit night but ghostly dark beneath the towering hemlocks and pines that stood by the hotel. We tiptoed up to a broken window and climbed through. With flashlights we explored the long bare corridor, looking for room 113. The floorboards creaked and our footsteps echoed. "It's supposed to be at the end of the corridor," my companion whispered to me. We opened the door, gently, tentatively, and the beam of our flashlight explored the empty room. The walls were bare. There wasn't a table or chair. Suddenly an owl hooted outside the window. We looked up and then on the ceiling we saw it. The great red stain that they told us was the blood of the victim. In the pale light of the torch the stain seemed to be spreading and we thought we could see the blood dripping from it. We turned and ran down the corridor and all the way home. "It was just the way they told us it would be," we told our friends. "There was this great stain of blood from the woman who had had her heart cut out by the pruning shears!"

We had two superb summers at Doc Rollinson's camp, and in spite of the fact that we were given great responsibility in a relatively primitive setting, there were no injuries, no child abuse, and so far as I know no real sins were committed. I do, however, remember receiving some enlightening education from a boy a year older than most of us, who sat on the edge of the cliff and gave us explicit instructions in masturbation. Try as we would, we were unable to emulate him.

After my father returned from World War I, our longtime carpenter friend, Tom Shelton, built us a cabin on top of the Knob. There were wooden frames on which army surplus tents were stretched to shelter our beds. By then, we had an icehouse filled with sawdust, under which the blocks of ice, cut in our pond, were buried. There was a kerosene stove and a stable of horses and a groom and Jack Kilmurray and his wife Mary Bell, who kept house and cooked for us. The Knob got so civilized that every Sunday we would go riding and pick peaches from the orchards we now owned and bring them home and have Mary Bell crush them up so that we could put them in the freezing can and beat them into the world's most delicious ice cream.

Then my family decided to send me off to a real camp—Keewaydin, a boy's camp on an island—three hundred miles north of Toronto on Lake Timagami. There were a dozen or more boys from University School on the train with me who went to Toronto and then on north to Timagami Station. There we would be met by the *Timagami Belle*—a huge (for an inland lake) triple-decker steamship reminiscent of those on the Mississippi. Two hundred or more boys had come north on the train from Toronto, and all of us and our pack bags were somehow stowed away in the *Belle*. The steam whistle blew, the paddle wheels turned, and we left the dock for the twenty-mile cruise up the narrow, winding waterways of Timagami to the island where the tents and cabins of the camp were ready for us.

I am eternally grateful to my parents and to the directors of Keewaydin Camp for making it possible for me to see a side of life that otherwise I would never have gotten to know. There were three divisions of Keewaydin—Manitou for small boys up to about twelve, Waubeno for adolescents up to about fifteen, and Timagami for the older boys. Each of them was divided into sections of about a dozen boys, and each section had a native guide and a staff man—usually a teacher but sometimes a college or graduate student taking a free vacation in the wilderness. There were several additional assistant staff men for the younger boys.

Very little time was spent in the base camp, but when we were there something was always going on—water sports, campfire songs and talks, and Sunday morning services. Sunday evening the head of the camp, Commodore Clarke—slender, handsome, virile, and moustached—would conduct a campfire religious service. It could not be called Christian. It was mysticism, based on the religion of the local Indians. The loons called from the lake, we all sang psalms. The sun set.

Each section set off on its own series of trips, some to neighboring lakes for a week or ten days, some to shoot the white water rapids of the faraway rivers, and some to take as long as six or eight weeks and go all the way north to Hudson's Bay. We carried all our food in wooden boxes, called by the Indian name "wannigans," or in canvas sacks (flour, cornstarch, and sugar, etc.) called "babies." There were usually three of us to a canoe except in the older-boy sections where there were only two. Rain or shine, wind or calm, almost every day we would cook breakfast, break camp, paddle all morning, cook lunch, paddle all afternoon, set up our tents, cut wood, make the fire, fish, cook the supper, and spend the night.

The food was great. Banack was the Indian name of the bread we baked in reflector ovens. There were pancakes and corn syrup, and we carried lots of fat bacon and ham. Everyone fished, and the guide carried a rifle so that if we should chance on a deer we could live for a few days on venison. Often we would paddle and portage for a week or two from lake to lake without seeing a sign of habitation or meeting anyone. Occasionally a bearded prospector or a trapper would pass, some of them in tiny birchbark canoes. We were totally self-sufficient. Strangely, in the whole history of the camp there has been only one accident—a drowning when a canoe overturned in a rapids and a boy was swept under a logjam.

Although statistically these adventures in the North Woods were safe, there were times when they didn't seem so. One year we lost two of our eight canoes in the fierce rapids of the Des Moines. There were times when we were nearly swamped by the winds and waves of sudden storms. There were times when we were lost, guide and all, but of course the guide had an infallible instinct which led him to follow the waterway to a known river that we could descend to known lakes or trails. There was work all day—at the paddles, at chopping wood and setting up tents and helping with the cooking. There were the silent nights around the camp fire, reflections of the stars glittering on the still water of the lake, stories and sometimes songs. One of these, that I still remember, was about the detested wannigan in which our food was carried:

> W, A, double N I, G A N spells Wannigan, Wannigan
> That is the thing you want to mortgage, mortgage
> Every time you come to a portage, portage
> W, A, double N I, G A N you see
> First you lift it. Then you shift it
> Then you flop it and you drop it.
> So its Wannigan on me.

Sometimes on those silent nights, we heard the yipping of wolves as they chased a deer through the forests. But the main lesson that Canada taught was self-reliance. Anyone who has lived in the woods has learned how to take care of himself, and that person will always have full confidence that despite what happens he will be able to survive. Thank you, Mother, Father, and staff of Keewaydin for that gift.

It was about this time that a conversation took place that I still remember. It was Christmas vacation and my father and mother, my two sisters, my brother, and I were in the upstairs office-library. The children were lying on the floor in front of the fire. My mother, who had been reading *David Copperfield* aloud, came to a phrase that gave her a pause for thought. She put down the book and said, "At this time, I think, our family is at the peak of its happiness. We are all together, all of us are well, and for all of us the future looks bright." It was a prophecy, for it wasn't long before my sisters began to marry and go their own ways.

An example of the interest that my father took in his children and of the way he followed up those interests is provided by his visit to me at Keewaydin in the summer of my first year there, when I was fourteen years old. I had written him about the beauty of this unspoiled northern lake and suggested that he come up for a visit. Sure enough, he did, taking an afternoon and overnight train trip and then a couple of hours on the great *Timagami Belle.*

My father fell in love with the lake and the camp, and wrote home to mother,

This is a wonderful thing for the boys. The best thing I could imagine for them. The entire camp is well conducted, as you would know it would be bound to be. To my mind it will be invaluable to Barney. Wonderful Barney. This morning we talked over everything—the Clinic, real estate [in which my father was deeply involved, both in downtown Cleveland where he had three business properties and around the Knob where he eventually owned more than two thousand acres] and everything. We played chess, pitched quoits and had a wonderful time. He surely is a real promise. There is a slight—a very downy slight— suggestion of a beard, perceptible only to the experienced eye. I don't mean by this that you are going to see a bewhiskered son, but there is a microscopic beginning.

My father, whom my mother now referred to as "the Chief," got so enthusiastic about Timagami that right across the lake from the camp, he leased (the government would not sell) Paradise Island. On this he had a native, who was a Scotsman and a carpenter, build a cabin with a twenty-by-twenty-foot sitting and dining room, a ten-foot porch, a twelve-by-twelve-foot kitchen, and a toilet. For this he paid Mr. McLeod three hundred dollars! "Some of our family's and relatives' boys will be at Keewaydin during the next ten years, and it would give us all a point of contact. Eventually, why not now?" he wrote. This cabin, and a few sleeping shacks scattered in the woods behind it, would still be in use for many years by my sister Peg's children and occasionally by my family too.

The next year, my last year in Waubeno, the middle section of the camp, I won the gold medal in the water sports and was awarded the Harter Cup for being the "all around best camper." Two years later, after two more summers at Keewaydin, I won the same in the senior division. My father's letters from Keewaydin describe the departure of the campers after the midseason base camp recess:

> Barney packed his duffel bag before breakfast and was all set. After breakfast the division rows of white tents came down. "Babies" (bags of provisions), tents, duffel bags, and cooking outfits were as methodically assembled as any squad of soldiers ever assembled their outfit. Each group was at its own dock. Canoes and crews were assigned by Mr. Dow, a bonfire annihilated the debris of the division, and the canoes were methodically loaded and balanced. The divisions finally stacked up as follows: 16 men, six canoes, 1100 pounds of food. Counting canoes, tentage, etc. it stacked up to about a ton of weight for the division. The guide, Frank, is a half-breed Indian. The boys did all the packing and loading. The trip will be 16 days, and they will travel about 200 miles.

The other memorable letter that my father wrote during his visit to Keewaydin was to my mother:

> Here I am sitting in front of my tent—rather Barney's and mine—overlooking the beautiful lake, and on Bob's birthday, which always carries with it the celebration of August of the harvest moon at Winous Point. I am sitting here in the twilight, with a beautiful moon—the same moon—on my left, and the lake and the sunset over toward the right—as a consequence of the August of 22 years ago. What wonderful years, jammed full of every interest life itself can bring. I felt then, as I know now, what a wonderful partner you are. It is only when I get my perspective away from the hurley burley that I can grasp more fully how wonderful you have been. I owe to you all that the children are, or all they will be, and after all, they are all that we shall have that is worth leaving. How impossible all we have built up would be without you, because you have been the builder of what has been worthwhile.
>
> The camp is beautifully situated and splendidly conducted. The air is mighty cool, and I am looking forward to tomorrow

morning's inevitable plunge with unmitigated dread. It is getting too dark to write, but I feel tonight that I ought to tell you that no one could ever have been more to another than you have been to me, from the day we found flowers in the marshes.

The love letter from Keewaydin was typical of my father's attitude and behavior towards my mother. He never seemed to forget an anniversary or a birthday. Usually the token was seven magnificent American Beauty roses which held some secret memory that never was divulged.

In all the years that I lived at home, with a room just across a narrow hall from my father's, I would never hear a quarrel or a fit of temper—not until 1929, when my father would be losing his sight, the stock market in which he had heavily invested would plunge out of sight, and 120 people would die in a Clinic disaster. On a morning shortly after the latter I would hear my father speak sharply to my mother and see her burst into tears, the only friction I ever witnessed. Mother idolized him, and when I was little, spent hours, at my bedtime, tucking me in and telling me how I must live up to the standards set by him. This got very boring, because it did no good at all. I never showed any signs of improving until I got to medical school.

When I reached the dangerous age of fifteen, I showed some signs of being interested in girls. In fact, in a letter to one of my sisters, treacherously passed on to my mother, I had written:

Dear Elo,

We made 6¼ pounds of maple sugar and three quarts of syrup (from the maples in our back yard). The sap ran well for a while but it is too cold now.

I'll show you a thing or two about dancing when you get home. I am a professional now. I like it a lot. My girls are as follows: (1) Shelly Cary, (2) Jean Warner, (3) Fannie Hanna, (4) Elisabeth Chisholm. Shelly is a peach. I like her a lot. She dances awfully well and is the most popular girl at dancing school.

Noting this trend, at the next Christmas vacation when there was a party every night and many opportunities to become involved with girls, my mother banished me to the icebound North. She thought that my failure to become an A + student was due to my mind being on women. So my father contacted his punter (the man who pushed the duck boat through the marsh at the Winous Point Shooting Club) and persuaded him to let me spend Christmas vacation with him. The man lived with a half dozen others in a little shack on Peach Island, across the bay from the shooting club, and spent the winters trapping muskrats. The hides were high, selling for five dollars apiece, the equivalent of at least fifty dollars today, and the trapping was good. The bay was frozen solid and the ice was clear, blue, and windswept clean of snow. Occasionally on cold nights it would crack with a noise like thunder, as a fissure ran the length of the lake. One could wind skate with a sail, take a shotgun down to an open area where the Sandusky River flowed in and shoot ducks, or set and bait the traps or collect the muskrats. In the evenings around the stove, there was good hot food and good salty language and stories, very interesting to a boy of fifteen. In retrospect, I marvel at the morality of that group and of the restraint of its conversation, because I don't remember ever being shocked—well maybe that was my fault, not their credit, because, come to think of it, I never have been shocked. The thing that I marvel at the most is the confidence that my family had in my skill at survival. It was a great experience to be sent off with those trappers, but I'm not sure that I would have dared do the same with my own son.

During the same period in which Mother was so concerned about my budding interest in women, I was writing themes for my English class at University School, one of which must have given my critics some concern. It was entitled "How I Would Spend A Year If I Could Do As I Pleased."

If I could do as I pleased for a year, starting January first, I would go south to the Florida Keys for a fishing trip. I would sail all around fishing for tarpon, spearing sword fish and sharks and making collections of all the interesting things I saw. Next I would come back to Cleveland for the Easter vacation. I would go to plays, dances and movies for about a month, and then I would head for Canada. I would get a guide and take canoeing and fishing trips, and in the fall I would go after big game or salmon fishing. Then I would return to Cleveland for the Christmas vacation, and my year would be over. This would be my idea of a perfect year, but the chances for such a one look pretty small.

My father tried to distract me from my undesirable interests by trying to make a businessman of me. His secretary wrote to me and Jim Milner the following letter regarding our rabbit business:

May 19, 1919

Messrs. Crile and Milner
2620 Derbyshire Road
Cleveland Heights

Will you kindly inform me whether you are in a position to meet the following needs of the research laboratory of Dr. G. W. Crile?

(1) We now have in the coops in the laboratory 21 young Belgian Hares about 12 weeks old. They are not thriving well. Would it be possible for you to raise them for us? If so what would be your terms for their feed and care?

(2) Are you in a position now or do you expect to be in a position at an early date to furnish us with full-grown Belgian Hares for our use in the laboratory?

I shall appreciate a prompt reply and hope we can enter into a business relationship.

> Very truly yours,
> Amy Rowland
> Executive Secretary

Apparently we accepted the offer, because on September 27 I wrote:

Dear Miss Rowland:

Owing to the inconvenience of being paid in advance for the board of rabbits, because it is hard to send a bill for 10 rabbits and have two die, for example, for if so we have to send you a statement telling you that they died and refund you the money for their board. We request you let us send our next bill November first, covering the month of October instead of sending the bill October first paid in advance for the month of October.

> Very truly yours,
> Barney Crile

Again, all my father's efforts failed. I never did become a success in any kind of business. In fact in all my life, I have rarely written a check. Isn't that the sort of thing that mothers and then wives should take care of?

Later on, in 1922, I was still at University School and still writing themes. By that time I had begun thinking, vaguely, about college, and I wrote about it in an essay entitled, "Why I Chose Yale."

I chose Yale for several reasons, the first and most important of which was probably because all my uncles went there and all the family has always wanted me to go to Yale. Next, Yale has always appealed to me more than any other college. I like its spirit and although it has its disadvantages, such as being so big, it also has wonderful advantages and offers many opportunities to those who are willing to take advantage of them. Yale is a wonderful institution as are also Harvard and Princeton, but the Bulldog Spirit of Yale and the loyalty of all its graduates have always appealed to me tremendously. Therefore it is my choice of colleges.

That theme got a mark of B. Obviously the teacher had come from Princeton or Harvard. At about this time my genius in electronics hit its peak. A classmate, Jimmie House, had a radio transmitting set and taught some of us to make little crystal set receivers. I went head over heels into the business, but sadly, in spite of my efforts, I failed to do more than duplicate Marconi's success and did not invent television. A letter written to my parents at the time suggests my obsession with the subject:

Feb. 11, 1922

Dear Mother and Dada,

I am getting wonderful results here with my spider web. This is my hook up. [Here there is a drawing of wires and symbols noting "spider webb, audion, phones, condenser, and ground."] So far I have heard IXJ somewhere in New York talking to KDOW, a boat in the Atlantic about 400 miles out. I heard some radio telephone at the same time, but it was so faint I could not understand it, but the chances are it was the boat. I hear KDKA (Pittsburgh) every night and he comes in loud enough so that I can put a megaphone on the phone and the phones on the table and get music at about three feet.

And so it went—on and on for two pages.

It was during these last two years at University School, before I was sent off to prep school, that I have the most vivid memories of Cleveland's social system. There were my sisters' "coming-out parties"— and later there were weddings. My mother, in a letter to her favorite aunt, described my older sister Peg's debutante ball held in our home:

July 2, 1921

Madame Lipkowska was a great artist, bewitching to look at, with a bird-like voice full of pathos, and she had a wonderful gift of acting out what she was singing—and as simply as a child. The first group of songs were in an old Russian costume, gorgeous in coloring, with a marvelous headdress.

The next group was in an old French costume. They were the adorable little surprising songs, full of the unexpected, and she was bewitching in an old Court costume.

The last were wonderful English ballads, in which she seemed to recall Jenny Lind to every one's mind.

People were mad over her, and we seem to have pulled off a great hit. The house was filled with flowers. I am simply overwhelmed with the interest of our friends and Margaret is swamped, with over 125 notes to write for great baskets of flowers, wonderful corsages, pins, vases, fans, bags, purses. It was like a wedding.

We received in the hall. I wore a tannish, or ecru, lace. George, white trousers and blue coat and Margaret a simple white chiffon with lovely lace applique. Barney and Elo, the latter in a lovely flame-colored chiffon, and Barney in his first white flannel long trousers [age 14], stood in the doorway between the hall and drawing room and gave out programs.

Mother mentioned some of the important people who came and said, "George felt it was a great compliment for them to come as they seldom go to such functions, yet all of them were charmed by my lady and clamored to meet her. The evening was a great success. We took up the drawing room and hall rugs, in the meantime, and danced in those rooms and the ballroom, sitting on the court, and although there were three hundred it was not crowded. At two we played 'Home Sweet Home' and everyone departed."

Margaret's wedding, as recorded under the heading "Society— Crile Garretson Wedding," contained a description of the house:

So beautiful is the home, throughout, that to decorate it in the ordinary meaning of the word, meant to disfigure it, for every part of every room is a decoration in itself. Therefore the simplest scheme was adhered to. In the great hall, living room, drawing room, and ball room, which opens out into the drawing room, tall vases of American Beauty roses were used. The Crile home is one of the most pretentious in the middlewest and one of the most perfect types of Florentine architecture in the country. It is in pure Italian renaissance style with terraces. The hall, ball room, and dining room open upon a red-tiled court built in cloister effect with great stone pillars covered with vines. On this occasion it was closed overhead.

Dancing was a social essential. Once a week, in the school season, I was driven to Miss Flynn's dancing school by our chauffeur, James Kilmurray, a Scotsman who had been a carriage driver and had never really mastered the motor car. Like James, I tried and failed and never did learn to master the waltz and fox trot, but I did meet pretty girls and I remember going so far as to try to kiss one of them. Marjorie was her name, but it was unsuccessful because the impulse hit us when we were standing on opposite sides of a sofa and before we could change that, Marje's mother came in.

I was inexperienced about women. In spite of the fact that in the Euclid Avenue house that we had inhabited until 1914 my bedroom was a converted porch outside my older sister's window and that I had cut a tiny peephole in the curtain over the window that separated the rooms, I had never been able to see things in proper perspective. Before that, when I was about four years old, I had made a brief study of female physiology when a relative of mine who was just my age had been playing with me in a sandbox. We had filled bottles with yellowish body fluid and both of us were contemplating them with interest when my mother came by and asked what was in the bottles.

"Sandy water," I averred, stoutly, a lie that I justified because it spared the reputation of my confederate. Obviously disbelieving, but kind enough not to press the point, my mother broke up the game without sending for a chemist.

A little later my best friend Bernie Towell and I, now aged perhaps twelve, used to sit spellbound in our kitchen while Margaret, the eighteen-year-old kitchen maid whose blouse was always décolleté, would get down on her hands and knees and scrub the floor. I was intensely curious to find out if what I saw contained bones or were soft as they looked. At that time, which was before radios were widely available, I had made a little crystal set which I kept in my bedroom. In fact, I built and sold crystal set radios, and I spent many of my waking hours trying to lure Margaret up to my bedroom to listen to my radio. Luckily I never succeeded, with the result that my curiosity was not satisfied until at least two years later, when I went to a party in the stylish Bratenahl part of Cleveland at the home of a girl whose mother had died. In the absence of an effective chaperone, we played the game "Sardines," in which the boys and girls would pack themselves into a dark closet or basement and hide. There, a brief exploration down another décolleté dress proved to me that beyond reasonable doubt the contours that I so admired were made of flesh and not of bone.

I am embarrassed to admit that, mingled with Bernie's and my sexual interest in women, there was an element of bestiality. My father, returning from World War I, had brought with him Sam, a large, male Alsatian police dog (now called a German shepherd). Although we were still too young to have personal interests in sex, we had great curiosity and noted the dog's occasional erections and his attempts to mount our knees. Soon we found that if we took him to the bathroom and had him lie on his back, we could manipulate him until the ejaculate flew out the open window. This was a pleasant occupation for both dog and boys, but there was an unanticipated complication. Every time Bernie walked into our front door, the dog collapsed on the floor, erect and panting. "Why in the world do you think he acts like that when Bernie comes?" Mother would ask. Although we never answered her questions, we suspected that she suspected.

Those were great days in the Derbyshire mansion. In the basement billiard-and-pool room, next to the workshop, the wall was hung with ancient fencing swords. Bernie and I would take them down and duel over the workbench and saw-boards. This went on, dangerously, until I received a deep laceration of my hand. That's the last duel I ever fought.

I have never known whether my mother's stern prohibition of reading in bed after my light was supposed to be out was made because she wanted me to get enough sleep or because she knew I would be tempted to disobey and get educated. I think it was the latter because in my room was a huge bookcase filled with exciting and educational historical novels—like G. A. Henty's *Treasure of the Incas*. These I would surreptitiously read by flashlight under the covers, or actually by lamplight when I was sure that my parents were in bed.

Then there was croquet. The game was played on the closely mowed side lawn, an area about the size of a football field that lay between the house and the tennis court. One of those games I remember as vividly as any episode of a long and sinful career. I was playing the game with our chauffeur, James, and he was bending over to put his ball through the double wickets. I have no idea why I did it. I've never done anything like it before or since. Suddenly there was this overwhelming temptation. I raised my mallet and brought it down—not very hard, but hard enough to hurt—right in the middle of poor James's innocent and unprotected back. James never said a word. He just groaned, and with his hand on his injured back limped away to his home. He sustained no real injury, but he never spoke to me about it and he didn't tell anyone else about it. Never before or since have I so regretted performing an absurd act.

Not long after we had moved to the Heights and when I was still only about ten years old, the area that formerly had been a golf course was still devoid of houses and I used to walk through it a quarter of a mile up to Coventry Road, on the other side of which was a wooded ravine where in the autumn the ground was strewn with shiny chestnuts. I was gathering them one day when I found myself surrounded by a band of boys about my age who had come up from nearby Little Italy. One of them had a gun—I didn't know whether it was a real gun or a water pistol, and I wasn't particularly interested in finding out. The leader brandished the gun and then commanded me, on penalty of death, to drop my pants and bend over. I complied and can remember no sensation of penetration. Since these boys were no bigger than I it is unlikely that true sodomy could have taken place. The act appeared to be more to prove the dominance of the Italian race than to give sexual satisfaction to its members. After it was over the leader tried to give me a dime but, weeping, I steadfastly refused to take it. Soon they left and I found my way home and told my mother. Miss Hall, my somewhat inexperienced governess, was there and when she heard the story she burst into tears. "Now he never can be married," she sobbed.

How wrong she was! Already I have been married twice and I am only eighty-three!

In Cleveland Heights the great suburban development was in full sway. Houses were going up everywhere on land that used to be pastures, forests, or part of a golf course. The houses, by today's standards, were comfortable, luxurious houses, but to the Criles, accustomed to living in a mansion with a family of six, two or three guests, and a half dozen servants, they seemed puny. We made fun of them. There they still stand, hundreds of them, for they were well-designed and well-built.

The development of housing in Cleveland Heights necessitated building roads, and to make them, piles of crushed limestone were used. I soon discovered that stories were written in this limestone. About one piece in ten had a fossil of some kind or a bit of a shell in it. I collected them and also, in the summer when we vacationed for a couple of weeks at the Winous Point Shooting Club, of which my father was a member, I used to collect shells and fossils and Indian arrowheads. In this western end of Lake Erie, a part of Sandusky Bay, was Squaw Island, a former Indian burying ground. As the water level of the lake rose, the graves washed out bones, teeth, and all sorts of artifacts that had been buried with the dead, onto the beach. Perhaps it was these early experiences in grave-robbing and Henty's book on the treasure of the Incas that would later start me out on my career of diving for treasure.

Our family life was extremely formal. My indefatigable father would return from work about six o'clock and run up the stairs, two at a time, to his second floor library-office, where the secretary, Miss Maloney, had laid out all of his correspondence. After about fifteen minutes he would go back to his room, undress, and slip into the hot tub Mother had drawn for him in the bathroom between his dressing room and their bedroom. There he would luxuriate, as my mother sat nearby and discussed with him the events of the day. At the appropriate moment, my father would leap from the tub, dry himself, and dress in fresh linen and a white summer suit or in winter the tuxedo that had been set out for him by the upstairs maid.

All of the children also used to bathe and dress for dinner. Then we would meet in the sitting room, where in winter there would be a fire in the great fireplace before the sofa. No cocktails were served. This was not because of Prohibition, because if a foreign guest were present cocktails or wine would be served. The rest of the time our family simply did not drink. The dinners were formal. Each of us had an assigned place. The governess, Miss Hall, ate with us. Early, before my sisters matured, there had been a young butler who drove an exciting Harley-Davidson motorcycle, but as the girls grew older Mother thought it was time for Jason (a wonderful name) to depart. I might add that my young friend, the kitchen maid, also left before I turned fourteen.

There was one night of the week when we were not seated at the table and served. That was Sunday. Late in the afternoon we would meet before the fireplace and the one maid who did not have the day off would bring in tea and sandwiches. We didn't need more, because for lunch, in the country, Jack and Mary Bell Kilmurray (Jack's brother was James, the chauffeur) would have served us a full meal of pork loin, applesauce, succotash, Scotch muffins, country butter, homemade ice cream, and fresh peach or strawberry sauce. So far as I know, my mother never in her life cooked anything at all. But she was a superbly competent woman, and I'm sure that if called on to do so, she would have managed, just as my father did. For example, one night we had a guest—the famous Sir Berkley Moynihan—president of England's Royal College of Surgeons. With British confidence, the lord put his shoes outside his room to be shined. When the shoes were discovered, the servants were all in bed. My father, who hadn't cleaned a shoe since he was in the Spanish-American War, contrived to give them a glistening shine.

Before my sisters married and when the family was still together, we took some memorable vacations. The first I remember was when I was three or four years old and we went to Gulfport, Florida—my mother and father, my sisters, Miss Hall, and me. My younger brother had not yet been born. I remember the wonder of the strange palm trees, the green chameleons in the shrubbery, and mainly I remember a cruise to a nearby sand-dune island.

We had rented a motorboat with a captain and a crewman to take us there for a picnic supper. All had gone well until dusk began to fall and we started home. No sooner had we got into the current of the Gulf stream than the motor stopped. The boat drifted steadily seaward. Frantically and with no success the captain tried to repair the motor while the crewman tried in vain to paddle the craft close enough to one of the channel buoys so we could hang onto it and prevent the stream and tide from carrying us far to sea. Finally the crewman fell overboard trying to grab the buoy. Miss Hall became a heroine by pulling him, dripping, from the sea.

By this time it was dark and we were lost. The boat didn't seem to have even a compass, to say nothing of a radio, which had been barely invented. There was a long argument among the men as to which direction was the shore. The night was cloudy and there was neither moon nor star to guide us. It must have been close to dawn, for suddenly, in the distance, far to starboard, came the crow of a rooster. It was then that my father took charge: "Stop arguing and row to where you hear that rooster," he commanded. The crewman got into the little rowboat that we towed, and three or four hours later returned in a new motorboat to tow us home. That was my first vacation expedition in a boat, but by no means my last. Almost all of the subsequent ones also turned out to be adventures or disasters just as exciting as the first one.

It wasn't long after the Gulfport experience that the family went to Asheville, North Carolina, for a week or two. Somehow or other, I got away from them and was wandering through the wooded hills that surrounded the hotel, when I saw approaching me, and baying in hot pursuit, a pack of what looked to me like wolves. Miss Hall had read aloud to me stories about small boys and wolves, so when these dogs chased after me, I knew just what I should do. I lay down, covered my face with my cap, held my breath and played dead. The dogs, whether feral or a pack of hunting dogs, sniffed me all over. One of them raised a leg and moistened me. Then all of them departed. For a long time I thought twice about walking alone in the woods.

Our family's next boating adventure occurred in August of 1914, just before World War I, when all of us went north to the Lake of Bays right in the middle of Ontario. There, with a guide named Tass and a couple of assistants, we camped for a couple of weeks on a pine-clad point which commanded the narrows of the lovely lake. Every day one of the assistants was sent into town fourteen miles away to get news of the brewing war. In our camp I acquired a love of fishing and of canoes that, in spite of a near disaster that occurred to us on the way home, has stayed with me all my life. Miss Hall, who was with us, wrote up the episode in a letter to her mother:

From Bear Lake we went over a small portage to Round Lake, then out through a narrow pass to Hollow Lake, where we met a strong head wind. Since Hollow Lake is very large and deep with many islands and capes it was really a raging sea. However we headed straight into it, three small canoes with three in each canoe. It was no joke, especially as the wind increased very much before we had gone many rods from shore; in fact, so much that we could not have turned around without capsizing, so we had to go ahead. A move would have turned the canoe over, and some of the time we could make no headway. We were over an hour in this sea, and at last landed on the first available bit of land, Squaw Island, I think it was. We were wet to the skin and shipped a great deal of water, our canoe, however, less than any others.

The lumber camps on the lake were closed—because of the high prices of food and hay, we were told—but we found a marvelous family with children around my age—seven to ten—and I played with them for hours in their machine shop making baseball bats on their lathe.

The next vacation we took, but little of which I remember, was in 1916 to the Florida Keys—reached by train or by boat in those days, for the road had not yet been built. I have recollections of palm trees, piles of coconuts, mosquitoes, endless groves of citrus—orange and lime trees. Pictures (filed by my mother) show me holding up two medium-sized mackerels, and a lot of people in boats, none of whom I recognize. For some reason, totally unlike her in her later days, my mother did not fully record that journey. But in a theme that I wrote for my English class at University School and which Mother saved, I recount an adventure in which my father, from the bow of a rowboat, speared a gigantic shark. I was sitting on the stern. The shock of the shark's first tug on the line threw me overboard: "Suddenly I found myself going down, down, down," I wrote. "It seemed forever, but at last I saw daylight. I was on the other side of the boat and still wearing my straw hat."

Captain Dunn, who ran the houseboat that we were on, had invented the Dunn Diving Hood used by sponge fishermen. It was a heavy brass helmet, with a glass window and a rubber hose that supplied it with air from a bicycle pump. One by one, all of us donned this device and descended through the swarms of barracuda and reef fish to enjoy the wonders of the coral reefs of the Florida Keys. My shoulders were so narrow that I had to keep my arms outstretched to keep the helmet from engulfing me. But it was a sensational experience that I never forgot. Nor did I forget the heron rookeries and the diving pelicans and the moray eels and the sea cows that we saw on that memorable trip. All my life I would keep returning to the southern seas for more of it.

In April 1919, the war was over and my father returned to his practice and his professorship of surgery at the Western Reserve University Medical School. Four months later, the whole family set off for a vacation—a month-long pack trip through the Big Horn Mountains of Wyoming. We had horses and pack mules and a big mule-drawn pack wagon that took us up the mountains and across the plains, for my father never got over his love of horses that he had acquired perhaps when he grew up with them on the farm and certainly fortified by his experience with the Cavalry Reserve in Cleveland and in combat in the Spanish-American War. My father kept a journal of the trip. "Through Frank Horton's H.F. Bar Ranch and for $1500 [for the six of us] we arranged for six saddle horses, two pack horses, a supply wagon, cook and guide, two horse wranglers and provisions for 30 days for a horseback and fishing outing in the big Horns." That was less than ten dollars a day for each of us.

I was twelve when we set out on that trip, and my brother Bob was six, but both of us, having ridden at our country place, the Knob, were used to horses. Mine was white-faced "Puff Ball" and Bob's was "Bubbles." We rode up and over the Big Horn Divide and camped at Tensleep where we saw huge herds of sheep—twenty-five thousand or more. My father, an inveterate philosopher, described them:

> These great white herds, black-dotted here and there, spread out slowly over the great rolling mountain benches like slow-

moving white clouds, leaving behind in their oscillations bloated carcasses, fragments of bodies, pelts, bones, horns, manure, earth—earth, rain, grass, cattle or buffalo, elk, deer or wild horse—back through the ages! A given electron has conceivably been moving around, eons immeasurable, from animate to inanimate, now a chipmunk, a fly, a sheep, a mountain lion, a bellowing bull, a leader of a wolf pack, a sheep herder, a wild horse, an Indian Chief, an East Tensleep Trout, and now perhaps the electron is a part of one of our sextet—which one?

On one of the starlit Big Horn nights morals were discussed. The conversation was brought up by my sisters who were seventeen and eighteen, and was recorded by my methodical mother:

1. May we shave under our arms?
2. May we spend the night in other girls' houses?
3. May we go alone to dances with boys?
4. May we ride horseback alone with boys?
5. May we at least powder our noses?
6. Why can't we wear silk stockings all the time?
7. May we wear thin waists, showing our underwear?
8. May we go to movies with other girls or group of girls and boys without a chaperone?
9. May we have our hair waved?
10. Margaret wants a black evening gown.
11. Christmas vacation is to be gay. May we go to all the parties we want, every night?
12. May we travel alone without a chaperone?
13. May we use perfume and cold cream and hand washes that come in prettily shaped bottles?
14. May we use Odorono under our arms?
15. May we go to the Country or Mayfield Club in daytime to play tennis or golf in groups if a boy or girl is running a car?
16. May we ride with Marian when she runs a car?
17. May we ride horseback in groups with boys at the hunt club?
18. May we go off the porch and wander around the grounds or sit in automobiles alone with a boy at the Country Club or other dances?
19. Finally, won't you buy Mother a Buick car, so we can run it?

"The conference lasted two hours," she concluded, "and brought out many surprising and very interesting viewpoints and some agreements and compromises."

These queries and words of wisdom were recorded in longhand by my mother on August 13, 1919, in Island Park, Wyoming, and later were typed by her secretary, Miss Maloney, paginated, illustrated by photographs, and bound into a hardcover book entitled "Personal Memorabilia. Big Horn Outing. August 1919." A copy was made for each of the children, and in similar fashion all of our vacations were recorded. My mother would be the author of two books and the editor of most of my father's twenty-four books. She simply could not keep her pen off the paper. But how did she know how interesting the talk on morals would be sixty-five years later?

My father's notes were rarely devoid of philosophy, even when writing about his daughter.

Scenario
"Peg's Plunge"
one act skit
Charley, the audience
Time of day—Sun down

Heroine with naked knees flashing in the sunset as she sits on the bank. Plump, vigorous, beaming in health and spirits, she transfixes the horse wrangler, Charley. Suddenly this self-confident, vigorous female grows timid, so timid that she screams—screams until Ed the Cook also appears, joining Charley, the frozen man in the gallery! The erstwhile timorous lady now plunges into the cold swift-flowing stream and a full gallery secured, she strikes out boldly swimming like a mermaid to the admiration of the choice audience. It was earlier in the afternoon that the great bull at the head of his herd called his females together with insistent screams. My fair lady on the grassy bank called her gallery in tones equally compelling. Both desired admiration.

My mother at the time of this trip was in her early fifties and my father in his sixties. They were indefatigable. After riding through the valleys and mountains we came to a peak, above the timberline, that towered to 12,500 feet. Up it we went, in spite of nosebleeds from some of the horses. Then came the climax, for a trip with Mother and the Chief was never without a crisis. My father summarized the trip and detailed the episode:

During the 30 days we rode 310 miles on straight trails not including considerable mileage about camp. During this time we caught almost exactly that number of fish. Burned, blistered, cracked, frozen, sore-tired, but wonderfully invigorated is the summary! Peg, Elo, and Bob's horses fell, but no serious injury beyond pride. The physical effect of effort in altitude—the psychic thrill of great heights, beetling cliffs, precipitous canyons, great plains, crystal skies, wild life struggling alongside great domestic herds of cattle and sheep—has been the best I have ever experienced.

At midnight Grace was awakened by excessive light and discovered our cottage was in flames. Waking me, she rushed for the children. Meanwhile I had discovered the coal bucket as our only hope for water. Emptying the coal in the bath tub I poured the bucket of water on the flames, but the fire was on the outside and the wall of the cottage was burning. Grace rushed outside, shouting for help. With our reinforcement we soon formed a fire brigade, Mother handing buckets of water out of the window to me and I over a high barbed wire fence to the lad who poured it onto the burning boards!

In the confusion my father fell into the garbage pit and nearly cut his big toe off on a broken bottle. He never even noticed it until after the fire was out. Blood was seen all over the floor. That was the end of a typical Crile vacation.

2

School Days

M Y MOTHER was convinced that boys should be sent off to boarding schools as soon as or even before they reached sexual maturity. She was certain that thoughts of girls destroyed all of a boy's
ability to learn. So my parents tried to send me to Hotchkiss to repeat
the freshman year of high school. In spite of having had good grades
at University School, I failed the examination for Hotchkiss so miserably that, regardless of my father's prestige, I was rejected and told to
tutor up and try again.

By the time the next year came around I had passed several college
board examinations and had a scholastic standing of seventh in a class
of fifty. The headmaster of Hotchkiss wrote my parents a letter that
must stand out in the archives of Hotchkiss School as the greatest
miscalculation an admissions committee ever made:

> It will not be necessary for Barney to take any school entrance
> examinations. The problem will be to arrange the best possible
> course of study for him so as to use the chance given by his rapid
> progress for a broadening and enriching of his preparatory edu-
> cation. He is far ahead of our lower middle [sophomore] year.
> Whether we can give him enough work to fill up three good
> years is a question. My suggestion is that you let him get all he
> can at Hotchkiss in the next two years, and then, if he has ex-
> hausted our possibilities and you are not ready to have him go to
> college, send him to some special school in America or Europe
> where he can use his time to advantage.
>
> Very sincerely yours,
> H.G. Buehler
> M.A. Litt.D.D.
> Headmaster

So I went to Hotchkiss, entering the lower middle class, and failed to pass two-thirds of my courses. For example:

October 13, 1922
G.H. CRILE
of the Lower Middle Class

Hours	Subject	Grade
4	Latin	52
2	History	48
4	Algebra	60
3	English	50
4	German	70

A pupil whose scholarship during a term falls below 60 in seven or more hours is continued in his class only on probation.

I had failed ten hours! If it had not been that I had gone to Keewaydin Camp where the teacher of this algebra class was a counselor and that he knew my family and was being paid by them for tutoring me on the side, I am sure I would not have attained the 60 in algebra that I got for each term of that year! The whole experience of my disastrous difficulty with the Hotchkiss standards of scholarship was reflected in my interpretation of a letter that Mother wrote me soon after I arrived at school.

September 18, 1922

Barney Dear,

The war, I am sure, is still vivid enough in your memory to recall what the valiant stand of the defenders of Verdun meant to all of us. Their oath—"They shall not pass"—must forever be a clarion note against the might of all evil.

It is because Dada and I believe that you have the capacity for this achievement that on this occasion of your stepping out into a world for yourself—as a tribute of our belief in you—we want you to wear this Verdun fob.

On the fob were the words, "They shall not pass." Unfortunately, this information was passed on to my teachers with the result that almost unanimously they adopted the suggestion and failed to pass me.

In spite of the kind things that, in letters, I said about Hotchkiss, I was deeply unhappy there. I resented the domineering seniors to whom all new boys must bow and scrape along the wall of the corridor, and call sir. I did not like the social organization of cliques, from

35

which I, as a newcomer, was largely excluded, and I was not stimulated by the classwork. Finally, there was an emphasis on religion and religious groups (like the St. Luke's Society) that to me, reared as an atheist, was not only unreal but hypocritical. The boys that I knew used it for social and political advancement. None of this did I put in letters, but all of it I remember. Except for the athletics (that came later), I have few memories of anything worthwhile at Hotchkiss. Let the letters tell the story.

October 8, 1922

Dear Mother and Dada,

The work certainly is hard and I guess I will flunk quite a bit of it the first term, but everyone does that, so it isn't so terrible. I am still playing left end (on the class team). I think I will take lessons on my banjo uke instead of on a banjo because I like it better. [Later I became so expert at this that I played a solo at the glee club concert.]

Fred Jarecky, the boy we met on the train, is awfully nice. I don't think I will start making any intimate friends until the end of the first term, because I don't think it is a good plan to make a friend and then find he is not the kind of fellow you want to associate with, do you?

I've got to stop now and go to chapel.

With love,
Barney

On October 11th, my mother replied to my letter:

I think you are quite wise to settle down to lessons with the banjo uke if you do anything at all in music, for you have it and it will be a good beginner and you can graduate to something else. I should be glad to have you take lessons, but I wouldn't do it this term, at least not until you have struck the gait of the school and feel you can keep an even pace.

I want you always to look up in your friendships. To use the very worn-out old phrase, "Friends are like books," so pick them for what you can learn from them, but always be the richer because of a friend. In other words, see that a friendship adds to your character.

I think you are very wise in having no intimate friends. To me the handicap of a roommate is that it throws you intimately with someone or a group. In other words, be nice to everyone, intimate with no one.

One thing we must always remember—remember as a fact and without any egotism—and that is: We are hitched to a star! Dada has, thru struggle and achievement, sent the name that you and I bear, ringing around the globe. Wherever you go, wherever you are, people will place you. They may seek to know you, they may try to use you. You must try to discriminate, try to separate the gold from the dross, the real and worthy from the unworthy. Bob's and your task in life is to keep that star high in the heavens. Your dream shall be to fling a satellite equally high to accompany it.

> With love and good-night
> Mother

This letter about my father and about my obligations typified Mother's attitude. Often when I was a boy she would come to my bedside to kiss me goodnight, and would sit down and tell me again and again about the miracle of my father and of my obligations and duties to try to live up to the standards he set. Oddly enough, this didn't irritate me at all. I soon got used to it and paid no attention.

A letter from my sister Peg, dated October 12, 1922, is interesting from the point of view of the attitude of its writer towards servants. Peg had just gotten married.

> Well—here I am in the apartment having a wonderful time keeping house. [She had studied for this occasion by attending Miss Garland's homemaking school in Boston.] Our maid, Wilmer, is a wonder. I lost my engagement ring down the drain in the washstand and she, understanding the ways of plumbing, rescued it from some place called a trap, and so she is my friend for life.
>
> I go to market every day, and I have a great time hunting good but cheap food.
>
> > Lots of love,
> > Peg

In those days, in our circles, one could not consider keeping house without at least one maid.

October ?, 1922

Dear Mother & Dada,

I flunked Latin, History and English. Pretty punk isn't it? But everyone does exactly the same and I have some excuse because I have been putting all my time on Algebra. Also I have had one year less Latin than the rest.

It could not have been reassuring to my parents that the rest of the letter was all about football and the banjo uke! The letter ended:

We had a concert on our corridor tonight—two saxophones, a violin and my instrument. Some noise!

With love,
Barney

Then I received a letter from my father which made no impact on me at the time but which I now read with amazement, because as I remember him he never worried, as my mother might have, about the social backgrounds of people.

October 10, 1922

Dear Barney,

I am mighty glad you are in no hurry about making special friends. The boy whom we met is a nice boy I suppose, but I do not think you would find his background specially interesting.

In the laboratory we have some excitement. Fricke worked out a method of measuring the little membranes that surround the brain cells, and found the thickness to be on the order of 1-100,000,000 of a centimeter—just one layer of molecules of oil.

And my father wrote on about the research and how he was starting to build the Cleveland Clinic Hospital.

Mother took a sterner attitude towards my scholastic failures:

October 13, 1922

Dear Barney,

It seems to me that 48 in History is quite inexcusable, for History merely means good concentrated reading. If you can't carry athletics and lessons, remember lessons are what you are there for. If a holiday comes and you haven't arranged time for your work or haven't done your work first, always take work before play. Proper place for play is one of the big lessons to learn. Remember, play should be *earned*.

38

Sadly, no matter how many times Mother was to repeat it, that was a lesson that I never could learn.

The subjects I studied at Hotchkiss—mathematics, Latin, German, English, history, Bible, etc.—were the essentials of what one was required to know in order to get into college. I cannot remember finding any of them interesting except certain episodes in history and in the Bible, which I thought were very amusing because some of the people seemed to take it so seriously. In retrospect I find it astonishing that Latin, for example, was taught as an end in itself instead of as a way of getting to know the derivation of our own language. In the vocabulary, when an English equivalent of a Latin word was used, it was always the Anglo-Saxon translation rather than the Latin equivalent that was given. It is such a boon to memory and to spelling to understand the derivation of words, and later when I studied medicine, it was so helpful to be able to understand the meaning of the Latin terms that I still don't understand why Latin cannot be taught as a means of understanding English instead of as an explanation of why all Gaul was divided in three parts.

The German class was wild. The professor, Mr. Buell, nicknamed "The Bull" because he was so violent, was prone to fits of temper or exhibitionism in which he roared and hurled chalk and erasers or whatever was handy at the heads of the students. Purposely, I presume, he never hit them.

After the first disastrous year I began to pass my courses. I also was on the varsity football team, playing right end. I was great on defense but could never catch a pass. I tried to play hockey in the winter, but never made the team. In the spring I trudged away from all the budding track athletes who were sprinting or jumping, pole-vaulting, or hurdling. Dragging the twelve-pound lead ball of the long-handled hammer behind me, I joined the javelin and hammer throwers on a remote part of the grounds where we could throw our missiles without too much danger of killing anyone. About once a week a coach would come by and give us advice or criticism, but it seemed to us that we knew more than he did because he wasn't a thrower and could give us nothing but opinions. In spite of this I did pretty well. I won most of the varsity meets and, in my senior year, won the Yale interscholastics in which most of the eastern prep schools competed. The winning throw was 152 feet—about six feet farther than I'd ever thrown before.

But athletics was not my only preoccupation while I was at Hotchkiss. Even at that early age I was beginning to have those distracting thoughts that my mother had for so long feared would be my ruination. I had "fallen in love." The girl's name was Marjorie Adams—one of the best dancers in Miss Flynn's dancing school and also very pretty. Back and forth went our letters. By today's standards, they were utterly boring. But, if one looked closely, the love in the signature "with love," was occasionally underlined!

Looking back at it I find it extraordinary that my family went to so much trouble for me. There was a senior prom at Hotchkiss, and I had asked Marjorie Adams to come. Of course she couldn't come unchaperoned. So my mother took her all the way from Cleveland to New York by overnight train, and then from New York to Lakeville by train. Mother stayed there for the festivities and then brought Marjorie safely home. She was such a good chaperone that I didn't find a way to kiss Marjorie even once, even if she would have let me.

In the 1920s, in Lake County, north and east of the Knob, my father had more than two thousand acres of land. A deep, wooded ravine ran through the center of it with a creek filled with frogs and minnows. There was a trail beside the stream, and beside the ravine were acres and acres of fields, where once the farmers had raised wheat and corn. Now the fields lay fallow, for the hundred-acre family farms, plowed by horses and operated by the owners, were no longer profitable. The machinery that was used on the huge farms of the West was too expensive for use on small farms, and the land close to the city was too expensive and taxes too high to make it profitable to enlarge them. So the farms and orchards and vineyards were abandoned and, through them, every Sunday morning, our family and friends and the groom Barnicoat, and occasionally some of our neighbors, would ride.

My father, trained in the cavalry for the Spanish-American War, was a superb and fearless rider. He had jumps put up in some of the fields, and over them all of us would hurdle, all but Mother who rode sidesaddle and discreetly skirted around the obstructions. She was wise because we had several accidents. My father fell and broke a couple of ribs, but never missed a day of operating. Twice we had visitors fall, to say nothing of the several falls that each of us in the family had when we raced our horses through the woods and over slippery wooden bridges where the hoofs slid and the horses fell.

There was much drama to the riding. Not only did one of our neighbors, Elton Hoyt, have a pack of hounds with which he hunted the foxes, but another neighbor, Livingston Mather, had a large stable of horses on which he mounted a dozen or more friends and was wont to take excursions of four or five hours into the mysterious wildernesses of Carver's Pond and the ravines to the south of Little

Mountain. And at night, of course, there was coon hunting with the trained dogs that the King family brought.

One day my cousin and I were galloping home from a ride when my horse, Juanita, suddenly slowed to a canter, then staggered to a trot, then fell on her side stone dead—heart worm, the veterinarian later said. I was able to leap off and, realizing what had happened, put my foot on the mare's shoulder and raised my arm, before dissolving in tears at the loss of my favorite horse.

In retrospect, perhaps this was a blessing because I have yet to see a young man who was deeply attached to a horse who ever amounted to anything!

3

The College Years

AFTER the first year at Hotchkiss I passed most of my courses, and in my senior year, in spite of the fact that I can't remember working hard, I got better than average marks. I even got a highest mark in the college-entry algebra examination—a true miracle. This success let me coast through the College Board Examinations and into Yale, where I found the freshman year dead easy and got honor marks. The same thing happened in the next year in spite of the fact that I spent every night of that sophomore year playing poker with six other amateurs who lived next door to me above the YMCA in the fourth-floor remnant of an ancient dormitory. Presiding over the poker game and raking in a steady profit was a professional named Walt. He came from Texas, was four or five years older than the rest of us, and was wise in the ways of the world. In the sophomore year it was Walt who contributed most to my education.

Although I had played football at Hotchkiss and was used to trotting out on the field in front of the cheering crowds, it was different doing that in the Yale Bowl. I had played all year as end on the freshman team. So in sophomore year, when I became eligible for the varsity, there I was on the first squad. I wasn't a regular, but I played a lot. I was excellent on the defense, but still couldn't catch a pass. That was in 1927, before they allowed a change of teams for offense and defense. As a result of this I never was a regular, but I started some games, including the biggest of the year, against Army.

In the 1920s the Yale-Army game was one of the major sports events of the nation, and the Yale Bowl was packed with more than seventy-four thousand people. Ivy League football was tops. It attracted its audience from all over the country and commanded top billings on the radio and sports pages, if not on page one of the *New York Times.* I took it all fairly seriously, but not as much so as my father and mother, who, with my mother's brother Malcolm McBride (who had been captain of Yale's 1900 football team), used to come on for almost every big game. Their loyalty or curiosity was astonishing to me then, and is incredible to me to this very day. It meant taking an overnight train to New York, a change of trains and a ride of two-and-a-half hours on the New York–New Haven and Hartford, every car jammed with fans. Then they had to hang onto the open streetcars that went from the station to the bowl. All this they did and then fought their way back through the same obstacles to Cleveland.

Track was a different thing. I was a fairly good hammer thrower for my 170-pound weight. I had won the Yale interscholastics, and in college the twelve-pound high school hammer had grown to weigh sixteen pounds so that at Yale I was getting only about 140 feet. But that was good enough to win most dual meets.

With me in the hammer throw was my friend, Bebe Spiel, one of those with whom I'd played poker all through my sophomore year. Bebe was five feet two, weighed about 240 pounds, and was unmovable, an asset for a football guard but a liability for a hammer thrower. To throw the hammer, one has to be agile and able to twist and turn.

I always seemed to throw farther if Spiel were around, so pretty soon the coach began sending Spiel along on all track trips, in spite of the fact that he could hardly throw the tool out of the circle. Spiel's greatest triumph was against Harvard, which had only two men entered in the hammer throw. For Yale there were Spiel and myself. One of the Harvard men was also a hurdler and was trying to decide whether to hurdle or throw. I was warming up, Spiel was sitting on the bench in his track suit watching. I took an easy windup, twirled twice, as smooth as glass, and the hammer sailed out for about 145 feet, farther than I'd ever thrown it. Spiel leaped to his feet. "Crile, how many times do I have to tell you to keep your head down?" he shouted. "If that's their second man," I heard the Harvard hurdler whisper, "I'd better get on over to the track." He departed. Spiel threw the hammer barely out of the circle, automatically got third place, and in so doing won his Y. Bebe Spiel remained to his dying day one of the country's great talkers.

A turning point came in my third year at Yale when I happened to take a course called "The Science of Society." It was based on the original research and scholarship of Professor William Graham Sumner, one of the world's first great anthropologists. The course was taught by Albert G. Keller, a hard-headed, no-nonsense, no-religion, all-science German of the old school. He was just as demanding as he was tough. His science of society was a sort of Social Darwinism that included the entire world, all the queer customs of people everywhere. Our own customs, too, were discussed critically, appreciatively, and rationally, and always from an evolutionary perspective emphasizing survival of the fittest. This was a point of view that my father had given me with his weasel stories and problems, but which I had never heard of in school. For the first time I was excited with learning, an excitement that has persisted. It was the inspiration of Keller and the transition to courses like biology and physics which I liked. It was this experience that changed me into an interested student and made me graduate with second honors from Yale and later magna cum laude from the Harvard Medical School.

In addition to studies and athletics there was social life. During freshman year at Yale I roomed with two old friends from Cleveland—Boots Britton and Ted Williams. We lived in the freshman quadrangle which was right in the middle of the city of New Haven. We had two small bedrooms and a living room on the fourth floor of the ancient brick building. Some of the Yale dormitories were almost as old as the college, but they had dignity and from our room we could see the town square with its cannons and walks beneath the stately elms. Just across the street was P. Ring's Drug Store where a bite of breakfast could be procured, and a block away was the Commons, where we ate lunch and supper. But most of the time I was eating at the training table—good fat, rare beef to build you up and make a man of you! No consideration then of heart disease, cancer, or stroke.

The year passed peacefully until the first warm day of spring when, as had happened so frequently in the history of Yale, a freshman riot broke out. In the past, Yale had been famous for the town-gown riots between city boys and Yale students. Rifles and cannons had been used and injuries had occurred, but I guess we had become sissified because we didn't fight anyone, we just broke windows and overturned cars and pulled the streetcar pulleys off the wires and ran around yelling and setting fire to piles of paper. There was no reason or plan for the riot. It just occurred. It was spring and time for breeding and no women were available to absorb the energy. My roommate, Ted Williams, lit pieces of toilet paper and dropped them out of his window, a crime that was easily traced by the campus cops. He was suspended for a month.

The next year we lived with the poker players on top of Durfee Hall, which was next door to the chapel and above the YMCA. Our only prayers were for a pair of aces. The Williams family held Ted strictly accountable for his allowance. They were religious and were gratified when Ted's accounts indicated that he gave so much to charity.

I have never been a politician and have never been elected to official positions because I have never been good at associating names with faces and have never been much of a conformist. But the miracle happened, and for the first and last time in my life I was elected to office. I became a member of the student council. That was because I had come from Hotchkiss, where a lot of my classmates had known me and because my name was known as a member of the football and track teams. Never since then have I been elected to any office whatsoever.

In sophomore year one becomes eligible for election to fraternities. A new one, named Chi Psi, had been started at Yale just two years before, and it had permission to "pack" for three years, i.e., make advance offers to the men they wanted to elect. A group of us from the football and track squads signed up. Some of them I had known at Hotchkiss, but most of them came from Exeter along with representatives of the *Yale News* and other extracurricular activities.

We ate our suppers at the Chi Psi House, and attended weekly meetings there, but we did not live in it. We remained at large in the social life of the University. It was in the Chi Psi House that I was introduced to beer, and after a couple of bottles I found myself dizzily bumping down the stairs and trying to sing. On the whole, however, fraternity life was innocuous and innocent.

When I was at Yale, the Sheffield Scientific School was socially and residentially as well as scholastically separate from the academic school. We knew the Sheff students through participation in sports and extracurricular activities, but they lived in their fraternities and were socially separated from us. One of the tragedies of Yale was that some years later its excellent scientific school was merged with the rest of the college with the result that Yale became the Home of the Humanities. Her science did not die, but it has never regained its pristine vigor. Whit Griswold, my friend and classmate at both Hotchkiss and Yale, was in large part responsible for this trend at Yale, for he became president of the university.

Since there were no female students at Yale and since it was an unwritten rule that one did not date the town girls, there was a lot of yearning going on. I remember long conversations with a beautiful townie who was a secretary in the Yale-in-China office, but it would have ruined my reputation if anyone thought that I was dating her.

In the 1920s students were not permitted to have automobiles until their senior year—a good rule because the roads of New England were dangerously narrow and winding. In 1927 Dr. Harvey Cushing's son had been killed in an auto accident, a victim of those treacherous roads. Thus our best bet to find a cooperative female was to hop on one of the excellent trains that would take us to New York or to Connecticut College for Women in New London, or to Smith in Northampton, or even to faraway Wellesley or Vassar. On weekends, when I was not tied up in athletics, I often took the New York–New Haven and Hartford Railway to New York where, or near which, several girls I knew were in school.

Prohibition was in force and although there were bootleg joints, like Moriarty's Bar, I can't remember using them. We used to go to the Roosevelt Grill and dance to the soft pulse of Guy Lombardo's music. One night at the Roosevelt Grill my partner was Jane Halle, a couple of years behind me at Smith College and whom I was to marry about seven years later. We were dancing cheek-to-cheek—in those days a breach of etiquette. The maître d' threw us off the floor. I still blush when I think of it.

There was no place in New York where one could go to make love. I usually stayed at the Belmont Hotel right next to the Grand Central Station and the Oyster Bar, but hotels threw you out if they suspected you of having a woman in your room. Life on those trips was mainly cultural—the movies, the theater, once even the opera. And there were museums, tours, Broadway, visits to the Statue of Liberty—and dancing in Harlem. We weren't afraid, at that time, to walk the streets at night.

More productive than New York was visiting the girls at their colleges because there, the sophisticated ones could lead you in the evenings to wooded retreats where one could recline in shade and solitude. In retrospect it was all so innocent that it seems incredible. We were in our late teens and early twenties, and yet we had no dangerous habits. I never heard of anyone who got pregnant or contracted a venereal disease, and I didn't know anyone who took a drug except an old lady, a friend of my father's, who often in public would sniff cocaine. It had been prescribed for her by a doctor (not my father) so why not?

We didn't smoke, at least I didn't because most of the year I was in training. Except for beer parties and an occasional bottle of bootleg liquor there wasn't much drinking—almost none when in the company of the girls. But lest anyone think that there was something odd about our behavior, I hasten to confess that our sexuality was not suppressed or perverted, it was only shielded. Instead of penetrating, and running the risk of pregnancy, for which at that time the penalty was a shotgun marriage, and also instead of taking a chance of contracting a venereal disease, for which in those pre-antibiotic days there was no cure, we employed the safe and satisfactory procedure of "Dry Fucking." Everything was carried out in the way it was designed to be, but we kept our clothes on. The employment of this technique, which I had learned late in my high school years, was greatly reinforced by subsequent experience.

In my first year of medical school I worked in the clinics where the poverty-stricken came for free treatment, and I saw their huge penises dripping with pus and helped to perform the painful irrigations of those organs with a stinging antiseptic solution. That gave me more morality than later on was instilled even by the orations of the evangelists.

No one, male or female, of the age of my children or of my grandchildren will believe what I am now going to confess. I, and most of my male friends, I would say 80 percent of them, were virgins when we graduated from college. During medical school, because of the above-mentioned introduction to the reason for morality, very few deviated from the course. Even in that day there were Fish Skins and condoms, but we were afraid of them. We had developed a safe way, and it seemed to us to be satisfactory. Few of the girls complained. The laundry bill for the underwear was costly, but not much compared with the price of pregnancy, syphilis, or gonorrhea.

I have no way of proving exactly what proportion of my friends in medical school who were twenty-two or more years old were still virgins by the technical definition of not having penetrated. But I know that I and several of my intimate friends were. My recollections of that era were not those of frustration. I loved it, and went home feeling safe, sated, and happy.

In my sophomore year at Yale, for no reason at all, a very frightening thing happened. I came down with lobar pneumonia. I was perfectly healthy; I did not smoke; but then it struck. I was admitted to the infirmary. The next day my father and mother and Dr. Phillips, the head of the Cleveland Clinic's Medical Division, were there. I had Type 3—the worst type. There was no known treatment. All that could be done was to wait for the "crisis," the time when the fever was highest, the pulse and respirations the fastest and the patient the sickest. The crisis was the dividing point at which some of the patients died and others made a quick and dramatic recovery. After a period of delirium, from which I remember horrible and gory dreams, the crisis passed and I made a good recovery. Except for one thing. There was some damage to the airways of the affected lower lobe resulting in bronchiectasis that for all my life has made me susceptible to a productive cough.

After my recovery from pneumonia, Mother took me to Atlantic City where the fresh sea breeze was supposed to restore my lungs. Instead I began to run a fever. I felt miserable. Mother phoned my father and promptly he came on. He brought with him a renowned medical consultant. They examined me and thumped my chest and had it X-rayed, looking for abscesses and empyemas. I got sicker and sicker and felt more and more miserable. I told Mother about my mouth being sore. She looked at it. When my father came back, she said, "George, I think Barney is coming down with measles." She had recognized the oral manifestations of the disease.

"Absurd," said my father, impolitely, but the consultant looked. By then the rash had started.

"She's right," the consultant said, and everyone was happy. It's the only time I ever knew my father to admit that he'd made a mistake.

At home, life was more conventionally social. Our family belonged to the Country Club, the Mayfield Club, and the Kirtland Club, all of which offered golf, tennis, and swimming. Downtown there was the Tavern Club (men only), the University Club, and the Union Club (for men but with a ladies' annex). My father was also a member of the Winous Point Shooting Club and the Castalia Trout Fishing Club. Besides this we had a tennis court at home, a swimming pool in the country, and a stable of eight or ten riding horses, groom and all. Also in our house on Derbyshire Road there was a huge ballroom. Why did we belong to clubs? I never could figure it out because none of us played golf and we almost never used them, except Saturday nights in the summer, when I used to go to the dances at the Kirtland Club. Before college much of our social life was spent in Bratenahl, the then-stylish lakeside residence of many of Cleveland's millionaires.

It must be remembered that in the 1920s and 1930s Cleveland was the country's fifth largest city and it was famous for its wealth and culture. By 1980, Cleveland would fall to eighteenth in size, and its population from over 900,000 to only a little more than 500,000. It would be at this time that Cleveland would become the subject of defamatory jokes.

There were seasonal balls and coming-out parties in those baronial mansions where, to the tunes of nationally famous imported orchestras, we danced till dawn. All of this was duly recorded in Cleveland's society magazine, *Town Topics*, and, of course, on the society pages of the papers. At that time we knew the names of almost everyone mentioned in those columns.

Since there were pools and tennis courts in all of the girls' houses, we never went to the clubs. All of us had met one another at Miss Flynn's exclusive dancing school and had grown up together, under the vigilant eye of Miss Flynn and the small, furry monkey that crouched on her left forearm. In her right hand she had clicked the castanets.

Among my friends of this period were two homosexual men. Both were popular and well accepted by society. One became a famous photographer, the other a society reporter. Both were good friends of one of Cleveland's older philanthropists, whose sexual preferences and social acceptability were the same. "Fairies" we called them in those days, and they elicited curiosity and wonder, but as I remember it, no criticism.

Those were strange days because we, or at least I, really took the girls and the social events fairly seriously. They seemed to me to be an important part of life. Sometimes I got so serious about sex and society that before calling up a girl to make a date or tell a story I would write down a series of notes to remind me to say all the things that I wanted to.

I remember one day soon after I had become old enough to get a driver's license, I was on my way to see my friends in Bratenahl when three or four children dashed out from a house and hand-in-hand started to run across the street. The older ones saw me coming and stopped, but a little three-year-old kept right on running, straight into the rear fender of my car. She was so small that it was her collar bone that hit the fender. I felt the bump, and it was then that I had my first inkling of the kind of impulse that causes crimes. "I hit her," I thought to myself, although really it was she who had hit me. "No one saw it. Shall I stop?" I did, but I am ashamed to admit that it was about one hundred feet from the spot of the accident that I put on the brakes. I then took the little girl to the Clinic, where her fractured clavicle was treated. Ever since I have felt a chord of sympathy with those who have been arrested for hit-skip driving. The instinct of survival dictates the necessity for escape.

By the time my senior year at Yale came round I was thoroughly enjoying the courses in physics and biology, but I never liked chemistry. Physics and the sciences of life always seemed reasonable and explicable, but chemistry I could never make any sense of, and hence never could remember why the various elements reacted with one another as they did.

On an appointed day in the spring of every year all of the members of the junior class assembled on the old campus and stood about waiting to find out what would happen to them. It was "tap day." The members of the four "secret" senior societies would, one at a time, stride out and seek the man they wanted to elect. When they found that man they would raise an arm and strike him (tap him) hard on the shoulder. The elected one would then either shake his head in refusal of the offer or accept by following his tapper to the secret domains of the society. This was a tradition almost as old as Yale and a very harsh and cruel one, for it made a public spectacle of social success or failure. I, along with most of my closest friends, was tapped for Skull and Bones, the most secret of all the secret societies, and so I was imprisoned in the Skull and Bones Tomb each Thursday and Saturday night for the entire senior year, without benefit of either booze or blondes. I led a life devoted to philosophy and the secret rites that on penalty of *(censored)* I dare not describe.

In the summer before senior year, all fifteen members of the newly elected Bones Club of '27 met at Deer Island, one of the Thousand Islands between Canada and New York, and spent a week together in a luxurious camp owned and monitored by a venerable and delightful senior member of the Bones.

During this time there were summer vacations, of course, and many of these I spent as a counselor at the same Keewaydin Camp where I had gone earlier as a camper. One of my best friends, Dave Lowry, who also was in training for athletics, usually went with me. We used to drive up together in his flashy yellow Cadillac touring car. He was a handsome young man and we had no problems in finding young ladies to spend the evenings with when we would stop in Toronto on our way up. But we were innocent and I had memories of Canadian girls that still frightened me.

A few years before, my cousin and I and a friend who was even more innocent than I had gone on a moose-hunting trip to Mattawa, Ontario. There we had outfitted ourselves with provisions and rented canoes from an amiable operator of a general store. At the time we had been about seventeen years old. "Would you like to spend the evening with some women?" the operator had asked. We had assented, not eagerly, but with considerable curiosity as to what was in store. So the operator drove up in his large seven-seater touring car, in which were his sixteen-year-old daughter and two of her friends. We piled in together, and as we whispered and snuggled, one of the daughter's friends almost mounted my friend while the father drove us on through the night.

By now Dave Lowry and I were considerably older but still quite innocent and not seeking involvement with women. Prohibition was in full force, and on our return the customs agent at the border saw handsome Dave at the wheel of the flashy car and motioned us out of line. Then the search started. I have never seen anything like it. They simply took that car apart. After about an hour of it, they finally gave up.

"You win," the agent said, "we can't find it. But if you will tell us where you hid it, we'll let you keep it and give you a reward." They simply could not believe that we were not bootlegging a bottle.

There were other moose hunts too, when a group of us from college would hire a guide we knew and go up for a week to paddle the lakes and streams. We would portage the canoes and call the moose, and sometimes shoot one and clean it and eat its liver and its ribs and carry the haunches back out with us. Those were glorious nights of adventure beneath the northern lights. Max Eddy, Dutch Wells, Count Costikyan, and I were the four that went—all of us members of Skull and Bones.

There were trips abroad also—with the family—usually on a medical tour with a group of my father's friends and their families. On the boat I fell in love with a New York girl who was about my age, but she rejected me completely in favor of older and more mature companions. Mother took our family through the museums while my father visited the clinics, and in France we revisited the battlefields where my father had been stationed in World War I. One of my most vivid memories is of the so-called bayonette-trench where a squad of soldiers, standing upright, were buried in a trench by the blast of a shell and the ends of their rifles, bayonettes attached, protruded from the ground. They remain there still, just as they were, as a memorial.

I remember my arrogance about the United States and the way we continually compared our culture with that of the Europeans, always belittling everything they did. "They don't even know how to make a milkshake. They don't understand ice cream. Look at their shabby cars." But in Venice my cousin and I loved the gondolas. Our gondolier introduced us to Italian beer. "Bona biera," we would shout as we passed beneath the beautiful bridges. "Bona biera!"

In 1929, my senior year at Yale, I became eligible to drive a car, and so in the prosperity of that time, just before the Great Depression, I bought one. It was a fourth-hand Chevrolet touring car, about ten years old, for which I paid thirty-five dollars. It had only one defect. At night when I put the brakes on, the lights went out. That made it exciting on those dangerous curves of the narrow New England roads.

Senior year was much like the other years at Yale—varsity football, class hockey, and varsity track, but by now I had become fairly monogamous with Jane Halle, a sophomore at Smith. I had known Jane in Cleveland for at least ten years in dancing school, the country clubs, and as not too distant neighbors both in town and at our country place at the Knob. Jane was an excellent athlete—swimmer, diver, tennis player, and field hockey too, as I remember. She was the third of four daughters of Sam Halle, owner and operator of Cleveland's largest department store.

Sam Halle had been born of an orthodox Jewish father who ran a fur business, but when Sam started Halle Brothers store and fell in love with Blanche Murphy, the beautiful young Irish Catholic girl who ran the corset department, he renounced the family faith. From that time on neither of them attended religious services. Mr. Halle was an intellectual, a patron of the arts, a lover of classical music, a horseback rider, and a country gentleman. His wife was a lady who devoted her life to the love and support of her family and the store.

Mr. Samuel Halle was a dominant figure in Cleveland's business and philanthropic communities, but in the 1920s Jews, even if they had renounced their religion, were not elected to clubs and rarely were their children admitted to private schools. There was only one Jewish boy in our class at University School, and he was noted for that fact. Kay, the oldest of the Halle daughters, was a pioneer, for she was admitted to the exclusive Laurel girls' school and to dancing schools. She was popular and was invited to all social events. All of the Halle children followed the same path, none of them practiced any religion, none of them married Jews. No one thought of them as Jews, and they weren't. They were as much Catholic as Jew. But Walter Halle, the second child, who went to Princeton and who later became president of Halle Brothers, was never elected to the Union Club, whose building stood across the street from the Halle store.

Although my mother never said anything to me about the Halles, I always suspected that in the early days she was not too happy about my consorting with a girl who was not of the Christian faith. My father, of course, couldn't care less. He was an atheist.

In the summers I worked at the Clinic in the Research Department, where my father assigned me problems to solve. I watched him operate, occasionally assisted, and then transferred my newly acquired techniques to the laboratory, where we operated on dogs, rabbits, guinea pigs, and white rats. I don't think I learned much about science in those summers, but I did learn how to use instruments, sew, and tie surgical knots. In the summer of my first year of medical school my father set me and my classmate, Max Eddy, to work in the dog laboratory. Operations had to be done on dogs and pouches made to collect and measure the stomach acid we were studying. The supervisor of the dog lab and dog surgery on the seventh floor of the old research building was Ralph Edmonds, who had come to the Clinic as "diener" of its first animal laboratory. He remained in that position until his retirement. Ralph not only took care of the animals but anesthetized them, prepared and draped them for surgery, and sometimes assisted at operations. He had seen everything done so often that I am sure he could have operated on the dogs just as well as many of the surgeons. Ralph was an unperturbable, pipe-smoking, slow-moving philosopher. He was always accompanied by a black dog that lived with him at night and all day lay on a rug in the corner of the operating room. We never knew what the dog thought of the unending procession of his kinsmen who were being brought downstairs, injected, put on the operating table, and then removed never to be seen again.

In the summer of 1930 Max and I first observed a fundamental and effective principle of fee-for-service, medicolegal medical psychology: i.e., when anything goes wrong, try to make the family of the patient feel responsible for the tragedy. Ralph asked Max and me if we would be interested in practicing surgery by spaying cats and dogs. "Of course," we shouted. We were delighted, so Ralph let it be known that for a small service fee he could arrange to have cats or dogs neutered by the Clinic surgeons. All went well for several weeks. Max's and my skills were increasing and Ralph was prospering. Then tragedy struck. Cats are notoriously prone to die while being anesthetized. The large black cat that the owner of East Ninety-third Street's largest boarding house had sent over typified this trait. After a brief struggle during induction of ether anesthesia the cat simply died. Cardiac arrest, but that was before we had learned about resuscitation. Max and I stood beside the animal aghast. Ralph was at the head of the table, calmly smoking his pipe. We offered to call the owner and explain. "No, no," said Ralph, "just leave it to me. I'll tell her tonight." The next day we asked Ralph how the owner had taken the news. "Oh, I didn't tell her," Ralph said. "I just said the cat hadn't taken the anesthetic very well so we decided to keep her overnight."

"Now what will you tell her?" we asked. "Wait and see," Ralph said and went to the phone. "Tabby isn't doing at all well," Ralph told his friend. "She seems to have a stoppage of the bowel. She is all blown up and nothing has gone through." There was a reply that we couldn't hear and then we heard Ralph say, "You didn't feed her the night before she came over here, did you?" There was a brief reply and then Ralph went into a tirade, "Look, you live right across from the hospital, and guests at your boarding house are patients there and go over there every day for operations. Did you ever hear of one of them eating a big meal of fried fish just before having an operation?" There was a pause and then, "Look at all the trouble you've put the doctors to, operating and all that when the poor cat hasn't a chance of making it. Oh well, we'll keep working on her, but I don't think we'll be able to pull her through." Ralph put down the receiver, drew on his pipe, walked across the room to pat his dog and turned to Max and me, "We'll let that cat die tomorrow."

Every weekend our whole family would head for the Knob and every Saturday evening I would leave them and take Jane to the dance at the not-too-far-away Kirtland Country Club. Sometimes, due to post-dance delays at the Halle house, I wouldn't get home until three or four o'clock A.M. Then I had to be up for breakfast at eight-thirty so we could saddle up and go off on our twenty-mile ride on the trails that wound through the twenty-five hundred acres of forest field and valleys that my father owned. In season, there were delicious concord grapes, apples, and succulent pears in the vineyards and orchards. My brother Bob and I raced through the fields and over jumps, and my father always was just ahead or just behind. By this time my sister Peg had married Hiram Garretson and they too would accompany us, for he was the son of General George A. Garretson, a horseman of note and president of the Society for Savings Bank. Peg and Hi lived in a house that they built on the west end of the Crile's in-town lot. Soon they would have two children who would be mounted on ponies and join us in our rides.

After the rides, we would all go down to swim in the pond made a few years before by damming up a stream that ran out of the caves of Little Mountain. It was filled with frogs and tadpoles and newts, but not a fish could live in it. They went belly up in twenty-four hours as the result of the acidity of the water from the sandstone caves.

After lunch there was the meal of the day—roast loin of pork with homemade applesauce, roast new potatoes, thick brown pan gravy, corn, lima beans, peas—whatever was in season, followed by dessert of home-turned ice cream made from the cream from the dairy of our neighbors, the Kings. This cream was so thick that it would hardly pour. Needless to say, the senior Kings would die of heart disease and the two King boys who were my sisters' ages did the same before they were fifty.

We used to beat the cream, turning the handle of the old-fashioned freezer. Then we added freshly sliced peaches drenched in maple syrup, and usually there was a frosted cake that had been baked by Mary Bell. All of us children were urged to drink as much as we could of the rich, whole milk. Eating lots of fat meat and milk was what made a man out of you, we thought, and our parents seemed to believe.

Although Jane and I were mostly monogamous when we were together in the Cleveland area, we never talked about and I never even thought about marriage. In the 1920s, if you were married it was impossible to get a good internship. "How could he have his mind on his patients and his work if he were married?" the professor would ask. Since internship was five years away, this was no time to make commitments. So Jane and I would ride together at the Knob, or on the horses at the Halle farm where her family spent their summers, and we would play tennis on their courts and swim in the clear cool Halle Pond, and then, after a supper somewhere and a dance we would make love in our sanitary fashion and say good-night. There was no alcohol and neither of us smoked. Except for all the milk and meat and cream it was a healthy life.

What Jane did when she went away to Europe with friends or family I never did find out. Or on her trips to Thomasville, Georgia, the famous quail-hunting area where Cleveland's sportsmen covened in their winter hunting homes. Jane often was invited to Thomasville by a young man who I thought was more attractive than was good for me; and when she was in college other young men came frequently to visit her, but Jane was a wise woman and never would talk about this. All I knew was that I believed in the Roman law which said that when the soldiers of the legion had crossed the second river, all marriage vows were suspended until their return.

My mother was the world's most orderly woman, with an almost obsessional interest in collecting and filing memorabilia. As a result, I have inherited a series of volumes of letters, clippings and cards all bound, dated, and gold-inscribed with year, subject, and all. These were put together by our secretary, Miss Maloney, under the direction of my mother who did the same thing for my father and for my three siblings.

The largest of my twenty-two volumes is from my senior year at Yale, memorable not only because I graduated but also for the May fifteen Cleveland Clinic disaster that killed 123 people, 43 of them staff or employees of the Clinic. Then, in October, came the stock market crash and the Great Depression. Because life in our family, and indeed in the United States, would never again be the same, I will quote at some length from the material that Mother collected. Oddly enough there is little mention of the stock market. It would be years before we would feel the full effects of the depression. The first of the two senior-year volumes is inscribed:

Dear Barney,

You've been very generous in letting us share so completely in your years at Yale and these diary files have been as good sport for me to put together as they were for you—in the acting.

The first poetic inclusion in the memorabilia of my senior year was copied under the heading "Odds and Ends of Verse Found Among Barney's Papers." It was entitled "Wall Street" and it was modelled after Robert Service's "Shooting of Dan McGrew." It was appropriate for the times because before the crash the stock market had climbed to $380 (about $3,800 in today's dollars). All of my friends were putting every odd dollar that they had in the stock market, and many of them were planning to move to New York to make their fortunes on Wall Street. The poem started like this:

> Oh Wall Street's world is a dissolute world
> That mothers a bloody brood
> And its golden arms hold hidden charms
> For the sinful, the greedy and lewd.
>
> And Strong men rust from the gold and the lust
> That sears the Wall Street soul.
> For their minds are bent and their labor spent
> To add a bill to their roll.
>
> But of all the men who inhabit this den
> I often have heard it told
> Wall Street Jake was the most on the make
> To gather a pile of gold.

Included also in Mother's collection were some weird products of my imagination that were written for a course called "Daily Themes" and a letter dated February 11, 1929:

Dear Mother,

Why am I always so far behind? Today was the first day I looked at my calendar, and I find that your anniversary was Thursday. This time I am really ashamed, for I had made a strong mental resolution to observe the occasion befittingly. We arrived back here after an uneventful journey, and I got the rest of my marks. I got 85 in organic evolution and science of society, 89 in history, 90 in English, 70 in art and 80 in Daily Themes—an average of about 83. That cursed art irritates me, for an 81 would

have put me on the Dean's list. I may drop it and take Seymore's
Contemporary European history instead, as I feel I can learn art
from you. Enclosed is the term bill, which I do not feel able to
meet at this juncture.

My father had turned over the income from the Kensington Hotel
and a few shops that he owned on Euclid near Sixty-third Street to
his four children, and I was supposed to put myself through school
on my share of the income. Apparently I had not yet learned to
economize.

My father, the one-time calvary officer, was a dedicated and sometimes dangerous horseman. Witness this letter from my sister Peg to
my mother who was in Memphis with my sister Elizabeth who was
having a baby.

September 16, 1928

Mother dear

Dada, Bob and Hiram went riding this morning and had only
been gone about forty-five minutes when with great clattering of
hoofs and blowing of horns Barnicoat [the groom] arrived, saying that Dada had had a spill. Don't worry now, for he's all
right—badly bruised around the shoulders and neck and pain-
fully stiff, with perhaps a cracked clavicle (not displaced at all, if
it is broken) and a beautiful black eye and skinned face. Apparently they were jumping over in those fields just off the new
stone road [Auburn Road] and had gone down the jumps and
then were riding back up them. Dada went first, the others
watching him, and when he came to the last and lowest jump,
no one knows how and what happened, but the horse was on its
back with its feet in the air and Dada, of course, thrown on his
head. He was knocked unconscious for about five minutes; his
face was cut by his glasses and badly skinned by sliding on the
ground and quite swollen from the fall—no deep cuts, just abra-
sions, so the doctors say. We had a terrible time getting him into
my car, for his back and neck hurt terribly and we just crawled
all the way home.

My love to Elo and yourself,
Peg

At this time my father was sixty-four years old. He continued to
ride and had several more such accidents.

September 21, 1928

Dear Dad,

I had heard nothing of your accident until Mother wired me last night. It is certainly a tough break, especially at this time when Mother is away and the remainder of your family spread about in education of body and mind. Anyway you have my best wishes for a speedy recovery. Why not come East and convalesce and visit your sons?

The car [that 1924 Chevrolet "touring car," for which I had paid $35] is still running finely and has given me hundreds of dollars of fun. I drive it to the field (for football practice), loaded with humanity until it creaks all over, but it seems to stand up all right. Today I got my Connecticut license. You have to pass a driving test, and I began by stalling the dern thing. It then gave a great leap and nearly jerked the poor man's head off.

Football is going along the same as ever—no scrimmage as yet. McEwen is right end on the first team, Lenehan on the second and I on the third today [etc., etc. about football].

Love,
Barney

Mother wrote me about the accident:

Barney Dear—

I telegraphed you today about Dad's accident. It certainly was a miraculous escape. Your letters mean so much to him and he is so eager for all your little football gossip [which, of course, was all my letter contained]. I felt sure that if you only knew you wouldn't let anything interfere with sending him a few lines each day. We just scan the papers for football news. I never see him that he doesn't ask if there is any mail from the boys. So just take a minute off and send a line each day. [Mother had given me a pile of stamped and addressed envelopes.] Dad slept last night with the help of morphia [morphine] and today looked and acted 100% better. —I'm just holding my breath lest you or Bob get hurt—and I'll be called upon to make rounds in triangles or squares. Imagine—Cleveland to Memphis, Memphis to New Haven, New Haven to Lakeville! [And indicative of the opulence and elegance of those times in 1928, Mother went on to speak of Mr. Palmer, the interior decorator who had an almost full-time job decorating and redecorating the Crile Mansion.] Mr. Palmer is dashing down to New Haven to decorate a freshman's room. I'm mad with curiosity to know *whose:* But he has guessed my

58

criticism and won't tell me. You didn't take any of your oil paintings or pictures for your room. Don't you want them or are you
waiting until you are more settled in order to see which ones you
want? If so I'll ship them when I return. [Under the influence of
my Aunt Lucia McBride, who had given me some now almost invaluable Orosco etchings, I had picked up in pawn shops a few
decorations that I thought were great art.] Your letters have been
a godsend. He lives by them and the football page of the Times.

Mother

And from my father, a letter:

September 24, 1928

Dear old Barney,

I appreciate your many letters keeping me up to date. I can
well imagine the fun you have had out of driving your own car.

I am following day by day the moulding of the team. You are
sure to have a lot of fun in your lively competition and in a few
years from now it will not so much matter, as you have already
won your letter. The fellows in assured positions will not have
the same kick and discipline. Happily, you have bigger games
this year, whatever the outcome as to the team.

However, here's the best of luck to you.

Dad

September 24, 1928

Dear Dad,

Sunday Hoot [Ellis] and I rode down to New London [Connecti-
cut College for Women] in the Chevrolet and had a horseback
ride and picnic lunch and came back that afternoon in time for
supper. All went well on the way down, but then trouble began.
First something gave way in the clutch and the old buggy
refused to move forward or backward or any way. We towed it
into a garage where a man said we had "lost the rear end" and
that it would cost about $35 to fix it. I said to go ahead and tear it
down to see if he could do it cheaper than that as I refused to pay
that much. He did so and found it to be only a loose coupling
and the parts cost only 18c.

Wednesday the coaches are playing the varsity. I hope I get in
for a while. They have a good team too but they will lack training.

Love
Barney

Telegram from Memphis   September 26, 1928

Hold a place for a broad-shouldered fullback from Memphis.
Weight seven pounds 15 ounces, with a mop of brown hair. Punts
well and certainly good at tackling—all well.

Mother

September 26, 1928

Dear Dad,

I heard the good word about Elo [my sister Elizabeth] and am
rejoicing in being an uncle once more in a different direction. . . .

The car suffered another breakdown today in which the carbu-
retor became loose and I put it in the shop to get it and the brakes
fixed. This cost me one dollar. The car is now a $36.18 car. Tonight
we ran out of gas on the way back from the hospital where a
bunch of us were out seeing Bobby Hall who has a torn knee. Max
Eddy, Hoot and Butch Laud and I pushed the thing about two
blocks and got it going so fast that we nearly ran over the keeper
of the gas station and then nearly carried away a pump.

I spoke to Toots Farr about making Phi Beta Kappa. My average is 83$\frac{1}{3}$. I have only half a year to pull the average up to 85
which is a prerequisite. This means I would have to get an average of exactly 95, which is impossible. However, I will try to get
as near to it as possible just for the fun of seeing how close I can
miss it.

Love
Barney

September 27, 1928

Dear Dad,

Last night the President addressed the University in Woolsey
preparatory to the speech, and in order to get the people over
there, there was to be a parade for which the University band
played and which was led by the "Y" men, in sweaters, carrying
lanterns. [I go on to say how the "Y" men, I and a group of
friends, waited for the crowd to assemble, but it didn't.] A vision
of what Woolsey would look like with the band and "Y" men sitting in the first row and the tiers and tiers of empty seats yawn-
ing in the President's face. So we decided we would have to get
more people, and back we marched through the Freshman Oval
and managed to terrify great quantities of freshman into joining
the throng. Max and I found an old bum out on the street and
invited him in with us in order to help fill the place. But the man

turned out to be drunk and horrified us by waving his cap and shouting "Hold 'em Yale" after the first song. Thereupon we had him removed.

Football goes on about as ever. I don't know what team I rate on now. I am glad to hear you are coming along better.

Love
Barney

September 28, 1928

Dear Dad,

Yesterday I had an unfortunate experience.

Coming down Chapel Street in my open job I slowed down for a street car and put her in second. I then raced the motor, in order to get a fast start to pass the car and let out the clutch. There was a high-pitched musical shriek. The car bounded forward like a wounded antelope and came to rest with a series of sonorous thuds. At first these thuds were deep and vibrant like a bass drum, but as the car slowed down, they became thinly metallic and degenerated into a quick succession of tiny clicks. As I listened I heard the musical tinkle of the small parts gently dropping from the rear end while the deep thuds of the inner noises accompanied the melody like a drum to a piano.

All of this music was much more expensive than sweet, for the garage man says it is a broken pinion in the differential and it will cost $12 to fix. . . .

Love
Barney

And from Mother, after the Georgia game that she and my father attended:

October 15, 1928

Barney Dear,

Yesterday was indeed gratifying. Dad, Hank and I all felt that you outplayed your rivals and that you have increased a lot in speed. . . .

Mother

In the Army game—except for Harvard the most important of the season—the bowl capacity was always overflowing. Tickets were at a premium. Apparently I had been improving, for I was chosen to start that game at right end. Uncle Mac wired:

October 26, 1928

Delighted to see that you have first call for tomorrow's game. Good luck to you and the team.

Sadly, my uncle's hopes and mine were crushed by the Army, for we lost, eighteen to six, and I tore a ligament and was out of action for most of the rest of the season. However, my day of glory was recorded by the press:

But there had been a shift in the ends. Barney Crile was guarding the right wing now, McEwen had gone to left end and Hickock had just come out. Crile was in like a bullet as Cagle started his sweep. With all the power of a runaway buck Crile threw himself at Allan, the interfering back who was leading Cagle.

He hit Allan low, and so hard that he spilled both Allan and Cagle, who was running close to his interfering back. The ball bounced away from Cagle. "Firpo" Green, the Yale guard, gathered it in and ran 15 yards for a Yale touchdown.

My father, apparently unaware of the extent of my injury, wrote me from Cleveland:

Sunday

Saturday you gave me a great thrill. I do not know what the authorities will do, but I put you on the first string for there you belong. I was proud of you. I hope the coaches will see as I do. At all events it was a great day for me.

Dad

But not everyone was so enthusiastic about my performance. A New Haven newspaper wrote, "The game Saturday proved that Yale's ends are a miserable failure. McEwen, Crile, Walker, Hickock—there is little to choose between them. They were not only boxed on every play but they were wrapped in burlap and crated for shipment."

Although I did play in the Harvard game, my injury had put me pretty well out of the running. So that was the end of my football career. What's more, I was getting old—twenty-one on November 3.

November 1, 1928

Dear Barney,

I am not sure I shall see you this Saturday [until I was hurt he had come on for almost every game], as there is something here I cannot manage otherwise.

By the time this reaches you, you will be twenty-one. I hope the watch which Mother and I are sending you will arrive properly marked in time for the day.

Did you ever think much about the biologic and social aspect of the 21st birthday?

Apparently it is the average age based on millions of observations at which youth has experimented with the meaning of life and found out by means of trial and error about how much of all the advice he has had is valid, has found out many of the mysteries of life; has had some illusions shattered; many hopes realized; has gone through the most acute period of rebellion; has tested all the codes; and has learned something about almost every phase of life—and in consequence has reached a more certain and stable position. In consequence, he is invested with the responsibility of citizenship including the right to title and use of money—in other words has acquired legal rights.

For you, Barney, I hope you have found the meaning of life. It seems to me you have been ready for several years for your twenty-first privileges. Surely if your next period finds you as commanding as the one you are leaving has, you will have a happy and successful life. I am proud of you—your fine restraint in the midst of intensive experimentation. [I have no idea what he was referring to because as yet I had not experimented that much.] Your fine achievements along so many lines have meant to Mother and me, something which you cannot understand, for this experiment [paternity, I presume] you have not yet made and this experience is yet to come.

I could not wish for more from you than that you may be as fortunate as I when you find yourself in my happy state. So here's the best of luck for the second half.

Dad

At the same time there was a similar letter from Mother:

November 3, 1928

Barney dear,

Your twenty-first birthday, yet it seems only a span of years when on a Sunday morning you came to us. And surely no one ever was more longed for or more anticipated than you.

There was more along this line, but the letter ended on a different tone, describing the arrival of one of my father's patients—Begum Saheba.

She is a queen regent for the young heir apparent Gulam Moinddin Khan and reigns over Mananeder and Nangrol which occupy the Peninsula of Zingaret and are in Kathiewar just north of Bombay. She has an exophthalmic goiter and travelled all the way from India to be operated, if operation is indicated. She came with a suite of 16, her brother and four children being among the number. The young prince is 16. The ladies all wear the East Indian costumes—silken robes, sandals, shawls and silver scarfs over their heads. They are small and mild with sweet intellectual faces. In her own language she is a poetess and scholar. They were met officially, and having been handed along by the British Ambassador to this country, request having been made that they be accorded all the prerogatives of royalty.

Mother wrote on for a page or two about the Begum, who by the way had a successful thyroidectomy by my father, and then she went on to rave a little against Smith who was running for president against Herbert Hoover. "I simply can't follow the arguments for Smith," my staunch Republican mother wrote, "and I can't endure the mudslinging in his speeches, the capital I and his poor English—city slang—and poor oratory and rasping voice." Mother, when she had an opinion, did not hesitate to express it.

The football season went on, even though I was largely out of it. Excerpts from letters from the family, first Uncle Mac:

November 12, 1928

Yale should have won! That is all there is to it. It does no good to make excuses but you can't make me believe that the Yale team felt themselves to be Yale men last Saturday or they would have smothered Maryland. Princeton will be ready to pounce [Princeton Tigers] on such carelessness if it appears for a minute. I hope you are all right again [I wasn't] and will be from now on. Remember the past is over with and spend no time in vain regrets.

This continued for four pages. Uncle Mac and all of us were a little up-set because the year before, Yale had won all but one game and was declared the nation's champion, and in 1928, with almost the same team, they lost all but one game.

From Mother:

Wednesday, November 14, 1928

Dear Barney,

No matter how it goes this week, don't mind. You have made your fight. You won it and it was just a bit of hard luck that knocked you out at a significant part of the season. However the benefit of the fight is forever yours while a bit of limelight ages and grows dim.

Mother seemed to fear I would be deeply depressed by not being able to play on the first team. I can't remember feeling any regrets. Mother went on, mentioning a Yale professor she knew:

D. Thompson Reid has asked me and Dad and your girl, if you have one, to his house before the Yale-Harvard game.

Today I was counting your profits on the ten oils I purchased for you—only five shares each—and it amounts to $895.87 [that would be $8,958.70 in today's dollars].

We are cutting down the dead and dying chestnuts about the shack and tents at the Knob [a great blight in the 1920s killed all the chestnuts, which were the dominant trees of our woods] and today we found some flying squirrels, a mother and two young ones, that are at present nesting in the cookie tin.

Elo's cook went after her nurse maid the other day with a butcher knife [in 1928 everyone had cooks and maids] and Gus [Elo's husband] with a pistol in his hand, discharged her. It all sounds exciting for America.

My Indians [the children of the Begum] are crazy over University School.

Anticipating seeing you, and with every bit of energy I have, rooting for you and old Yale.

Yours with love,
Mother

And from my father:

Pennsy Train
November 17, 1928

I am just proud of you. Jim Greenway says of your playing

that you are the best defensive player on the squad. You were able to fight your way up to first place on the Army game. Your injury took you out for two critical weeks—almost three—and here you are again playing Princeton, and judging from your performance today, you are on your way back to your position on the Army game.

But, old man, it is not so much this that makes me proud of you, rather it is that I recognize in you the quality that the English call "playing cricket," namely playing a sportsman, as in an uphill game playing your best, and as well whether you win or lose, for after all, it is the playing rather than the winning that reveals the quality of the player. You are playing fine cricket. The score, in the longer view, is a detail.

I am all for your way of playing football, for this tells me how you will play greater games.

Dad

Rereading this, I find it small wonder that many young athletes are so spoiled by their adulation that they never accomplish much else.

November 19, 1928

Dear Mother and Dad,

I wish I could have seen you longer Saturday. There will be more opportunities this week.

I called up Toto tonight [Flora Mather, whose family owned a huge country estate next to ours and whom I dated alternately with Jane Halle] and found out her plans. [I had invited her to the Yale-Harvard game.] She expects to meet her family [also Yale people] in New York Sunday. She arrives in New Haven at 9:45 Saturday and is going to the game with Mory Everett. Our responsibility does not start until after that. Then we are going to dinner at 8:00 at the Chi Psi house. Then to the Sheff [Sheffield School of Applied Sciences] parties. Home about 1:00.

I have two tickets for theatre Saturday night and three for game. Let me know what time you plan to arrive Saturday. *Please don't forget to bring me my derby!*

Love
Barney

My father closed the football season with this letter which sums up the pleasures and the risks:

New York
November 21, 1928

Dear Barney,

In the ten years your sports have given me a great interest, I wonder if you really got much more kick out of it than I did. I can tell you, now that it is over, I shall miss the spectacle (and the Yale Bowl crowded with cheering people in coonskin coats and bright dresses was indeed a spectacle) and shall miss your interest. I am greatly, more than I thought, relieved that you have come through safely, without serious physical or moral injury. I am sure the moral injuries in football are more serious than physical injuries. Taken as a whole Football Stars have a most unhappy showing in after life, and I am sure that the moral casualties are greater than the physical. The whole sport must have seemed to you to be a sort of miniature life itself. It has the lights and shadows and certainly the discipline that comes with the play of the game of life.

I am glad you played in the Harvard game just to complete the record, but I know how far from fit you were at the Princeton game. You put up a fine show of being well recovered from your muscle injury. I know better, of course, but I respected too much your good sportsmanship to discuss it with you.

I am much more glad than sorry tonight closes the season and the period for you.

Lots of love
Dad

On December 2, 1928, there was a letter from me to Dr. A. T. Bunts, son of Dr. Frank Bunts, who was my father's lifelong friend and colleague and cofounder of the Cleveland Clinic and who had just died.

Dear Brud,

It is needless for me to tell you how much I sympathize with you in your loss. Nevertheless I want you to know how keenly I feel it.

We are of a different generation. Your father and mine have built up an unequalled idealism in medicine, and I keenly regret the opportunity that I have lost in never having been in the profession in his time. You who have had the opportunity of working with him and imbibing his spirit are to be greatly envied, but at the same time more greatly pitied in the more poignant realization of the loss.

In future days my ambition is to work with you and Dad and to absorb from you two as much as I can of the spirit of your father. My hope is that you and I can carry on the Clinic in the spirit in which it was founded—the splendid idealism of your father. Again my deepest regrets.

Barney

An example of my parents' support and of the depth of their interest in me is in a letter from Mother dated December 18, 1928, written shortly after the death of Dr. Bunts.

By the way Brud showed Dad your note to him. He was enormously pleased, and Dad was so gratified to read it that he asked if he might bring it home to show me. It certainly was perfect, Barney. I just wept over it. You will never know until you stand in the same place what it means to have a child of your own come out 100% in what he undertakes. That note showed real comprehension. You caught the psychology and if you go through life with such a deft touch, success will have to come.

Since that day I often have wondered where that touch went.

In my next letter I describe the wedding of the sister of a classmate, Ed Manville. In our class at Yale were the sons of many rich and prominent families including Manvilles, Mellons, Duponts (Wack), Ashforths, Baldwins, Binghams, Dodges, and Seiberlings. On the front page of the *New York Times* the headlines read:

Miss Manville Wed in Military Pomp

Marries Count Bernadotte in Brilliant
Church Setting at Pleasantville
First Royal Bride Here
250 Guests in the Church—1000 at Reception
Couple to go to White House Luncheon

Dear Mother and Dad—

Count [my roommate, Granger Costikyan] and I had a good drive out to Pleasantville where the wedding was, and after some argument with the doorman, who insisted on seeing our cards which we had forgotten to bring, we finally got in. There were as many cars parked there as at a Yale-Harvard football game, it seemed. I've never seen so many people. Three thousand were invited and it seems to me they all came.

68

The men wore the blue uniforms of the Swedish Army with their decorations, swords, plumed helmets etc., and the girls had lovely red evening gowns that blended perfectly. . . .

I only made two breaches of etiquette during the whole affair. One was the addressing of a New York State trooper in blue uniform as a Swedish duke, and the other was to steal a pair of the heir apparent's socks. One of these Dutch [Wells] has and the other I have. In later years when I meet him as king, I shall return mine to him. It was a very ordinary-looking black silk sock with a clock on it and a plain name-tape marked "S. B.", his initials.

Since that time nothing of note has happened.

Love
Barney

The sons of the rich and famous in our class were affable and some of them were able people who participated in extracurricular activities and usually did better than the average in their studies. It seemed to me that they received no special acclaim as a result of their socioeconomic status. The ladies did not flock to them any more avidly than they did to the athletes, and from the standpoint of election to offices or societies it did not seem to me that they had any advantage. Perhaps Yale in the 1920s was a true democracy, or even a little communistic.

In 1929, high society existed not only on Long Island but also in Cleveland—witness this November 30 letter from Jane:

Barney,

Mary Harriet asked you to her dinner—she isn't having it now—Patty is having it instead—but is only asking girls. They are to ask any boy they would care to take. If you haven't been asked I would just as soon carry a cross that night. Will you go to her dinner with me and the Princeton Triangle after? From there on you may do as your principles demand—Walter [Halle, Jane's brother] can take me to my dance [coming-out party?] as I have to get there early.

If I seem to be a precious child to be asking one Barney Crile— then think over the conditions and you will find a reason—but if you think I am a bit of concentrated adorableness to ask you, then think that I want you to go with me.

Address is 13 Belmont
Smith College
Northampton, Mass.

I accepted and five years later she would accept my hand in marriage.

In those days, the Christmas vacations were a round of formal dinners, theatrical events, and dances. As I remember it, there wasn't a night free. Everyone knew everyone at those parties because we were a tight-knit group, whose parents had known one another and had sent us to the same private schools, clubs, and dancing schools. (Gone are those days. Now the majority of one's children move away to some strange city, and the whole process starts all over again.)

Suddenly, in the middle of this unreal world of athletics, dances, and dinner parties, came my first shattering experience with reality. My cousin and best friend, Henry Sherman, who was a year younger than I and a junior at Yale, was kicked in the head by a horse.

Henry was taken to the Clinic to have the wound sutured, but he didn't seem quite right. My father and I went in to see him. A neurosurgeon was called. Soon Henry was unconscious and the surgeon operated to remove a clot that had formed between the skull and the brain. Apparently there had been internal hemorrhage too, because he never regained consciousness. I had memories of the funeral of a great-aunt, whom I had loved, but at eighty or so death seemed appropriate. Henry's was not. I watched it, heard his stentorian breathing, felt his slow, full pulse, noted his failure to respond. Although I did not witness his last breath, I was a part of it. Then a strange thing happened.

There was a funeral, of course, and our car was filled with young men about my age. I remember how we laughed and joked and told stories. The reality was just too real for us to face. It wasn't until after it was all over that I cried.

On December 15, I sent a telegram to my father congratulating him on the opening of the Clinic's new Research Building. I then went to Cleveland for Christmas vacation, carrying with me a copy of my application for admission to Harvard, the medical school that I and my friends who were going into medicine thought was the best. Regarding my decision to go to medical school, I was just brought up to believe that that was the only thing that I would do. In response to the question of "What reading or what actual information about the science or practice of medicine have aroused your interest in the study of medicine?" I answered, "My father being a surgeon, I have been brought up in a medical atmosphere and have always been in and out of his hospital. My interest in medicine originated in problems regarding cases that my father explained to me. Research work carried on in the summer under his direction has added to my interest as have certain scientific courses, especially biology, psychology and physics.

Books such as 'The Microbe Hunters' have also stimulated me, but my chief interest has always been in the cases that I have seen in the hospital and in the animal surgery I have done in summer research."

In response to the question of what were my college activities and distinctions, I listed "Two years varsity football. Two years varsity track [a third would be coming]. Third honor roll for three years, Chi Psi fraternity, Skull and Bones Society, two years Student Council."

The Crile children's governess, Miss Hall, was in her late sixties and was suffering from some debilitating illness that was soon to be terminated by pneumonia. Since my parents always were loyal to their employees, Miss Hall stayed at home, in her room, and was nursed there instead of being sent off to a nursing home. The following is from a Christmas Eve, 1928, notation that Mother dictated to her secretary, Miss Maloney:

All had been bustle for weeks before. Miss Hall had been invalided in her chair all year, and in order to have her participate in the fun of Christmas we arranged to do a little wrapping each day, she helping with the packages stretched out on the sofa in the study. Sam [the German shepherd dog that my father had brought home with him at the end of World War I] at her feet, a table piled with colored paper, cards and Christmas ribbon, she worked, I doing the carrying, she the wrapping. Long before Christmas the drawers were filled with alluring red packages tied with silver ribbon, and the great basket of gifts to go under the tree was full to overflowing.

Instead of having a spider-web party with a gift at the end of every string, we decided to play handkerchief games and to have the last game "Find your place at the table"—where monogrammed handkerchiefs served as place cards as well as Christmas gifts to all assembled. The individual tables were decorated with red candles and fruit.

Tall silver candelabras and Santa Claus with his reindeer—on a field of snow, red ribbon ending in a fluffy white popcorn ball—graced the dining-room table, while a big cake, three tiers high, each piece bearing a China figure, had the place of honor on the tea table.

While playing games [it must have been a party for the friends of the children]—the bell rang and behold, The Begum Saheba of Manawadari. She was wrapped in red tissue striped with gold. Her two daughters. Choga and Kulsum, were in rose and light green. She had been a patient of George's for several months but she had never seen a Christmas tree. Slowly she walked in, her gorgeous eyes almost melting in wonder. She was like a little child. She was spell-bound over its glittering beauty. She could not seem to get enough and pulled up a chair—almost sitting under its branches. The children took part in the games, tumbling about in musical chairs, the handkerchief game and blind man's bluff, but the Begum sat silent, gazing. After the party the boys brought Miss Hall down in their arms and the little group remained—Henry, Mary Helen and her boys, Aunt Ella, Mrs. Lyman—and we opened our gifts.

Mother's reminiscence goes on for five more pages and summarizes the events of the year including the details of the accident in which my cousin, Henry Sherman, was killed. One of the next entries in her collection of my works is a little light verse I wrote for Jane, inspired by the popular song, "I'd Be Lost Without You," and written during the flu epidemic of that year.

> You're the germ in my nostril
> You're the cold in my head
> You will always be
> The necessity
> For my staying in bed.
>
> You're the bug in my sinus
> As I've already said
> You will always be
> The necessity
> For my staying in bed.
>
> Some girls have mild ways
> Some girls have wild ways
> Your ways are bold ways
> Always—cold ways.
>
> You're the bac (k) to my teria
> You're the B (ee) in my bed
> You will always be
> The necessity
> For the cold in my head.

In Mother's wishfully thinking footnote she writes "Barney had sat next to Jane at dinner." (If I remember correctly that was not the way the disease was transmitted.)

After the Christmas holidays in Cleveland, I wrote to my mother and father:

January 13, 1929

Dear Mother and Dad,

We had an uneventful trip back, made delightfully peaceful by the departure of all the girls on a different section of the train. Our train was 30 minutes late and we made connections with two minutes to spare by getting off at East 125 Street. . . .

By the way, my last exam is on the first of February—Friday. Helen Chisholm's wedding [to Jane Halle's brother, Walter] is Saturday. Classes don't start again until next Thursday. This is the time of the Prom. Shall I come home? Will you be there? I would rather come home as I don't feel the urge to attend the Prom.

This letter told no lies but omitted the fact that I was beginning to be in love with Jane, and that she would be at the wedding and not at the prom.

The first volume of Mother's memorabilia of my senior year ends with a very characteristic paragraph in a letter dated January 28, 1929:

I sent Jane Halle flowers for her coming-out party and received from her one of the best notes I ever have received from a youngster. It had charm and finish, and said thank you without saying it, which you know is an art. I don't know whether it was the Irish blarney or the Jewish diplomacy which gave the result. . . .

Love
Mother

A few days later my reply is recorded, ending with my own form of diplomacy:

Enclosed is a Bursar's bill which I find I am not able to meet. A letter follows tomorrow.

After having forgotten the anniversary and being sick and not sending you a birthday present, I decided to make up by a splendid Valentine message. But I got the date wrong. You didn't mark it on the calendar.

This is in haste, as I leave for a class—

Barney

My first literary work of the year 1929 that Mother collected was a story entitled "The Occult Power." It must have been inspired by a course in zoology! Soon after writing it, I sent it and others to a literary agent. I wrote my mother, telling her that my agent said that "she thought she could sell them for me and would not have taken them if she hadn't thought so. She said I wrote with some clarity and aptness for phrasing, so I think I'll keep on with it."

But the stock market crash was around the corner. Nothing would be sold!

On February 22 Mother, in reply to an apologetic letter of mine, wrote:

Dear Barney,

You talk like a "second generation." It's always "darn hard to accomplish things because there are so many distractions" [it was distractions by women that Mother was worrying about] and what is true now in that regard, will be far more true as life goes on. I'm quite serious. Your problem is to get yourself organized—to get really hitched up to your ideals. There is no trouble when you have something pushing you—a man looming up ready to pop you into your place gives you a real urge; but what I want you to do is to get the mental urge for knowledge that will make you search out problems.

Then, second, I still am Victorian enough to be skeptical of girls who drag other men in on the pretense of seeing their brothers and sisters. Bob might call it "wet." I call it "thin." Family parties I'm suspicious of! With these words of wisdom I'll pass on to the apple—Eve's famous artifice.

It breathes, it can be suffocated, it suffers a loss of potential when one bites it. The potato is negative but the sprouts are positive. The onion seems to be the apple's perfect mate, for when you bottle them up together, each takes what the other doesn't want, and they live along happily together. A positive and a negative, in fact a potential can be established between them.

Mother here is talking about my father's bipolar electrical research into the nature of life which culminated in his book *A Bipolar Theory of Living Processes.* She continued:

Today Dad had pages upon pages of telegrams from New York asking for comment on Laville's new theory of treatment for cancer. It is based on the Chief's [my father's] work. Laville feels the cancerous cell and its growth and multiplication is nothing but a short circuit in the electrical mechanism of an animal and his treatment consists of applying to the affected area certain strengths and rhythms of discharge of negative quantities of electricity with the idea that it will aid the cellular nucleus to reestablish its electrostatic equilibrium—Laville speaks of it as merely carrying the Crile theory a step further and making a practical application. Dad, of course, can't venture to comment, but he is awfully excited about it and we are going to start measurements at once on our own cancer rats, which strange to say, are in order.

So, my dear, don't you see how important it is to set your mental prod—within yourself—and to get such a sharp one that no one—no thing—no distinction—no argument—can dull it—or lessen it?—You have ambition in your soul, I know; you have ability; you have been given every opportunity. Don't, don't, don't, ever for one minute take the course of least resistance, Barney. It is a deadly subtle thing that, before one knows it, gets under one's skin.

Mother closed her letter by saying that I probably would by now have regretted writing her that letter about my needing too much prodding:

That is what startled me, for it is just that which has made many an honor man slowly toboggan downhill in the accomplishment of life. I want—oh! I just couldn't bear any tobogganing for you. I know the climb that is ahead of you, and thank God, it is not a climb unless one has to make effort. One star has been flung high in the heavens. You and Bob must make of it a constellation.

Mother

February 24, 1929

Dear Mother and Dad,
The trip to Boston was lots of fun. We called the Cushings and found them out. The next day we had an appointment at eleven with the Dean. We got up early and called Dr. Cushing, who said he was going to operate and we could watch him, and to meet him at nine. We went to his office in the hospital and his secretary told us he wasn't there yet, but we could watch his assistant work. He was draining spinal fluid and pumping air in the ventricles of the brain preparatory to taking an X-ray.

When this was over we wandered around watching all sorts of operations and spent the whole morning in this way. It was interesting to me to see the differences of technique between

Cleveland and Boston. Here it is all so unorganized and slow, while your operations are so fast and perfectly organized in every detail.

After a while Dr. Cushing came but he didn't operate that day. We had lunch with Mary [Cushing, who was about our age] and Mrs. Cushing. You can't avoid the Cushing hospitality, no matter how hard you try. We invited Mary to lunch and ended up having lunch on Mrs. Cushing, try as we might not to, for I begin to feel embarrassed at accepting so much. [The Cushings were originally from Cleveland and were lifelong friends, as well as rivals, of my mother and father.]

The Dean was quite encouraging to all of us, and told me that there was no need of my applying to any other school. He said Max's chances rested on what kind of a breakfast the committee ate the morning they passed on him. Bud will be in all right, I guess—

Love
Barney

Max Eddy was not famous for his scholarship, but he was captain of the football team and an acknowledged leader in student affairs. Dr. Cushing, who had a strong influence over the dean's office, had played on the Yale baseball team. He would be a staunch supporter of Eddy, not only getting him admitted, but when Max fell in love at the end of sophomore year and flunked out, it was Dr. Cushing who had him reinstated to repeat the year. Interestingly, Max became one of the most successful and nationally recognized surgeons of our class.

On March 1, 1929, my father sent me an eleven-page handwritten letter telling of and fully explaining the causes of the death of Miss Hall. In the closing paragraph he said:

I was glad to hear that you are entered in the Harvard Medical School. I was perfectly sure it would be so wherever you applied. Now your way is open for your final goal—your role in life in what I think is the finest from any view that one could take. It will be great fun when you finally get under way. You will soon be here again and will see the new building has grown taller [the hospital building].

Lots of love
Dad

And Miss Hall left a letter for me, whom she had reared as her own:

February 1929

Dear Barney,

I have tried to think of something that I have which you might like as a bit of a remembrance.

I do not seem to have anything except these four Greek coins which I had planned to have made into cuff links. They are supposed to be real coins, and I did buy them in Athens. They were probably made in Waterbury, Connecticut or in Germany.

Please accept them as a farewell gift with much love from

Your own,

Marguerite L. Hall

Miss Hall was a classicist until her dying day—and also a warm and loving woman.

Nineteen twenty-nine was a great year for the rich and for the lovers of the arts as shown in a letter to my parents dated March 3:

I saw "Caprice" Friday night and certainly enjoyed it. I think it about as well done and delightful as anything I've seen. [Apparently I thought nothing of shuttling back and forth from New Haven to New York to go to the theater.]

Mr. Santvold of Lucas & Company arrived in town yesterday and fitted me for all the African clothes. The hunting suit is a very sporting job, and caused a great deal of comment among those of the boys who saw it. Picture me in my 185 dollar hunting suit, trying to stalk a lion and still not spot the trouser or rip a sleeve.

The $185 would surely be more than a thousand today, and to this was added the cost of sun helmets and special footwear. The safari suits were specially made of beautiful tan fabric with a layer of red woven into it so as to "block the infra red rays of the sun and avoid sunstroke."

I concluded my letter:

I studied for my history essay, read some Poe, and then began and finally understood about 50 pages of the best book I've ever read, "The Nature of the Physical Universe" by Eddington. It is a layman's edition of advanced physics—relativity—quantum theory, etc.

I shall be very learned when I see you next. Will you please send me the story I wrote at Christmastime?

With love

Barney

On March 4, the *Yale News* carried the headline "College Seniors Vote Phi Beta Kappa Most Desired Honor in Annual Poll. Major 'Y' wins in Sheff." My friend, Fred Simmons, who roomed with Max Eddy next door to Costikyan and myself, was voted the most popular. Max was voted second most popular. Joe Lowes, another of the group we lived with, was voted as having done the most for Yale, with Paul Mellon a poor eighth. Simmons, who was editor of the *News*, was also the most admired. Joe Lowes, the business manager, was most likely to succeed, and G. H. Crile made twelfth place with three votes, one of them probably his own. It is interesting that most of those who were voted "most popular" did well in later life, whereas few of those voted most likely to succeed ever amounted to anything.

On March 15, I had a letter from Dean Hale of Harvard:

Dear Mr. Crile,

On account of your very excellent recommendation and scholastic work, my committee on admission has voted to accept you as a member of next year's First Class [the first fifteen or twenty men accepted]. The announcement about the dormitory will be sent later.

My roommate, Bud Yandell, received a similar letter, but my two other friends who were applying were not accepted until later.

By now my father was sixty-five years old and Mother was beginning to show concern:

Barney dear,

Dad has been very tired. Sometimes I wish I could squeeze money out of the skies so that we would never have to feel the urge to make it. The drive to make The Clinic a well-rounded accomplishment has been stupendous, but sometimes I wish we could take more of what he earns himself—just to give him ease—but he says when that time comes—your work is finished.

Yet I think, in the last five years, Dada has given back into The Clinic one million dollars [equivalent now to ten]—i.e., in the last five years he has given up one million that he has earned and hasn't taken. He's the biggest thing I've ever known.

Mother wrote on about her preparations for our projected trip to Africa and to say that she thought that Hoover was going to be one of our outstanding presidents. She told also of a German surgeon who was visiting:

He had been at Ypres setting up one of those observing balloons that Dad so hated. In fact he directed fire against our station. Isn't it futile—enemies ten years ago—trying to kill each other and today chatting lazily together in front of a fire—Dada telling him the latest doings in his own private laboratory and he asking if he may translate the Bipolar book into German?

On March 27 a delightful two-page letter from Harvey Cushing invited me and my three Yale friends who were by now admitted to the Harvard Medical School to have breakfast with the Cushing family, two of us to stay with the Cushings, the other two at the Harvard Club. Dr. Cushing and my father had been in medicine together in Cleveland and they were together in the war. Dr. Cushing's name is mentioned twenty-one times in my father's biography, and he described him as "a fascinating and stimulating personality, intense, meticulous and brilliant."

Easter vacation was coming up. I wrote home to say that Jane was going to join me for a dance in New Haven on Tuesday and after classes on Wednesday we would go to New York, and that I would put her on the train to Northampton, and I would take the midnight to Buffalo, getting home at two o'clock P.M. on Thursday. Then in the files there is a formal invitation from Mr. Brigham Britton and Mrs. George Crile for a reception on Saturday, April 6, at eight o'clock to meet Miss Ingalls and Mr. Warburton. Anne Ingalls was one of Boots Britton's and my favorite girls, and she was the first of our group to marry. Her fiancé was a distinguished English gentleman, and their marriage would be a long and happy one.

A letter from Mother, April 19, 1929, told of the Begum's recovery from surgery and of "arranging to get guns off to Africa this month. Bob, Dad and I shot at the armory one night, and Bob peppered the bull's eye—I hope you'll make this term count for a lot in earnest work—long sleeps—and little foolishness. I do feel now that you are beginning to near the long road toward medicine there are just a few things I would be glad to have you forget—such as smoking, drinking." She continues:

> Not that I feel any criticism for I know you do neither to excess, but because I know that you'll take that long pull better physically, intellectually and that in the end—in itself it will reflect back and help you, if you are classed among those who don't do it.
>
> Of course as far as drinking is concerned I feel strongly about it [a close relative of my mother's had been an alcoholic]—as I'm

so afraid of it these days [Prohibition]. I found an empty bottle of Bourbon in my room [in the Roosevelt Hotel, New York] when I arrived and felt about the same in regard to it as if it had been Prussic Acid.

It is six—I must fly as Dad is waiting downstairs.

> Lots of love
> Mother

The next letter from me told of Anne Ingalls's wedding, the bridal table, the toasts, the dancing, the pranks, and of the trip back to New York in the private car of Mr. Howard Ingalls, a member of the railroad-rich Ingalls family. The letter ended:

Would you please send me "Nature and Origin of the Emotions" which I left in the library and also "Man—An Adaptive Mechanism" [two of my father's recent books]. I'll also need my cutaway this June for the weddings, so you'd better send that. Also my good butterfly tux tie.

I'm sorry I didn't see more of you both this vacation. It was most hectic.

> Love
> Barney

Next is a letter to Jane that starts:

After an extensive research into great volumes of psychology and after a most meticulous study of your letter I have decided that you are in reality perfectly madly in love with me. Don't fool yourself, young woman. Don't try to evade the facts of life. Admit them both to yourself and to the world. I have completely psychoanalyzed you and will now tell you the findings of the investigation.

The first sentence in your letter confessed to missing me poignantly at the moment of stepping on a worm.

Freud, you know, interprets all association pertaining to elongated objects as being phallic in nature. Hence my association with the worm is distinct proof of a repressed passion towards me.

I continued in this vein for several pages, which indicated that I was taking a course in psychiatry. In it I apparently did not learn anything about being faithful to women because next in the collection is a love poem—written to a different lady—Toto Mather. Mother was the detective who found it.

*Verses Scribbled by Barney in His
Science of Society Text Book*

In days of yore
There roamed galore
O'er plains of vast dimensions
A bird more rare
But passing fair
Whose fame I now will mention.

Her body was
with downy fuzz
Covered quite completely
While both her legs
Were bare as pegs.
(She dressed most indiscreetly.)

Her neck was thin
From breast to chin
And wound in undulations
Whose frequent knots
Were cause of lots
Of eating complications.

The bird would lay
An egg a day
Of vastly large dimensions
And howl in glee
Whenever she
Exceeded her intentions.

This bird of fame
Was called by name
The Dodo Predignesson
Now Toto, dear,
I warn you here,
To learn from her a lesson.

To live and thrive
And keep alive
Be sure to dress discreetly
Don't let your knees
Get cold and freeze
And always answer sweetly.

From the same period, when Mother was worrying about my relationship with Jane and the Clinic disaster was two weeks away, Mother wrote:

April 21, 1929

I didn't mean to get into a dissertation [about Jane], but I'm not keen to be included in such a family party, if you want my honest opinion, yet I would like to be present at your graduating exercises.

I know Dad feels the same, for when he told me, I said, "What did you say?" He said, "I had nothing to say. Barney knows it could not meet my approval."

College is a terrible crucible, Barney, and it is right that it is so, as it is an acid-test for the start of one's real life. Tradition, however, is a pretty safe thing to cling to, and if it can become such a part of one's self that it is unconscious—in other words, that good traditions become instincts—then one is safe. That, to me, is one of the fine things of the Englishman. His tradition has made him stable.

Were you surprised at Betsy Cushing's engagement? And do you know James Roosevelt? She'll have to be a democrat now.

I just can't understand these engagements before one is out of college. Harvey Cushing and Kate were engaged seven years without announcing it, for he wasn't willing to be engaged until he could offer support. There's something about that kind of a code of honor that rings success. The other "let father do it" would never satisfy me in my King or Chief.

Dad is having a dinner of sixteen tonight—members of The Cleveland Museum of Natural History. They are considering taking on quite a famous ornithologist in the Museum and he is here tonight.

There are some few things—such little things—that still trouble me, although I'm deeply grateful and appreciative of the many fine qualities that you possess. Perhaps if I didn't hold so high an ideal for you, I wouldn't mind, but Dad and I so longed for you, my dear child, and you always have seemed so perfect in our eyes, that I can't bear even a tiny disappointment, unfair as it may sometimes seem to you, to demand so much.

Anyway, I love you dearly, and always believe in you—and am not only very proud of you, but ambitious for you.

Mother

And again from Mother, on the same day:

April 21, 1929

Dear Barney,

I'm glad I had the teeth out as I was harboring strepto-coccus virulens, for which I have no sentiment. It certainly let loose an avalanche to absorb however, and I've had the worst sinus and antrum blockade I have ever experienced; and it came simultaneously with the extracting of the teeth—almost with the injection of novocaine. I've been laid up ever since, but today worked up enough misery and temperature to try out my resistance, and as it is going down this afternoon, I've ceased feeling frozen and depressed and miserable generally. I think now I've really beaten the germ, altho I still have lame shoulders, lame knees, lame toes, lame neck. I'm certainly in no kind of "repair" for either a dance or a safari now, but give me time!

Really, I think your plan of no girl at the Commencement Dance the best. You are going to be awfully rushed to get off for our midnight sailing and to get all packed up; and I want an organized son, not a disorganized one. That's first.

Second, Lucia [my aunt] sails one day after we do—or one day before, I forget which. Anyway, we will be in New York together. Not inviting Lucia before has been simplified as she wasn't available, but I don't think I could explain your racial proclivities.

Third, Commencement at Yale—your PhB—is a goal for which we all have struggled. It means something but "entre nous" I've heard twice since you left, from grown women and Mr. Sherman of how much you liked Jane Halle. Someone is doing some talking; and I know it doesn't pay—for you!!!

Love
Mother

I replied as follows:

I was greatly interested in the point of view you took in your long letter. I think I agree with you in every detail of it. But there is one fundamental difference in attitude between you and me that makes us differ on this point. You seem to feel that I am about to fall in love with Jane and offer her my hand in marriage, whereas I know that I not only entertain no such feeling and idea, but never could.

Perhaps we also differ on the matter of having Jane as a friend. Whether Jane were white or black, I'd like her if she had the qualities that she has, and I don't see any reason for getting snobbish about races. She is a very fine girl in most respects, although I don't consider her the kind that could inspire love—in me, at least. Again, there is something lacking. But what difference does it make if my friends are half or wholly Jewish, if they are smart and attractive? I believe in weighing heavily race and family connections when marriage is involved, but not when it is a college friendship.

As for the Commencement dance, I don't care a bit whether I have a girl or not. I observed that a number of my friends were having them and thought it would be nice. But on second consideration I am convinced that it is impracticable.

I really enjoyed your letter, as it was very interesting from the serious point of view. I merely think it is inapplicable to my situation and feelings which are of a lighter nature. So get your joints in shape and be my Commencement Prom girl.

Love
Barney

About this time I called Jane and asked to see her Saturday. She said she had a theme due and didn't have time. I was confident in my ability as a writer and sure that the standards of Smith would be very low compared with those of Yale, so I said I'd write the theme for her—a review of a book on psychology. I skimmed through the book, dashed off a four-page typed summary of it that I thought was deserving of an A +, and got it back to Jane on time. To my infinite chagrin the theme was graded C. But I had the satisfaction of a letter from Jane, saying "If you knew how much it means to my peace of mind to have that psychology report gloom removed you would think it worth the effort. I appreciate it. It was rather a dirty trick—mercenary or something on my part—Love and handshakes—Jane."

May 9, 1929

Dear Barney,

I hope all goes as you wish in these last days in New Haven. One thing, Barney, you must not fail to do. Get your typhoid inoculation in New Haven. And by association, if you can find time and opportunity do rifle shooting. It is settled now that we hunt on the Serengeti Plain, where the Martin Johnsons and others found so many lions—in troops, as many as 15. There have been reported so many surprises there that we must all be prepared.

Mother and I shall be in New York on Friday, perhaps on Saturday as well.

> Lots of love,
> Dad

May 11, 1929

Dear Mother and Dad,

I'm naturally rather troubled about Bob [who was failing some of his courses at Hotchkiss], not so much because of the things he does, but rather due to the fact that he seems oblivious of the danger he is running in doing them. . . .

I'm beginning to get genuinely steamed up over the idea of Africa. It seems to be getting very close now. Will you keep your eyes open for interesting books that are really worth while? For I'd like to accomplish some reading this summer. I'll also have to begin to decide exactly what I am going to take along with me in the way of clothes. The more I think of it the more wonderful I realize it is going to be. Have we gotten another hunter yet?

> Love
> Barney

That was the last reference to the African trip. Four days later, dated May 15, 1929, came the telegram:

> Explosion at Clinic. Dad all right.
> Mother

Forty-three members of the staff and employees died in that explosion and eighty patients and visitors—a total of 123 people.

The cause of the disaster was the ignition—by a light bulb or a cigarette—of inflammable X-ray films stored in a room that had a ventilator that connected with the four-story Clinic's main ventilating system. Instantly, the building was filled with deadly poison gases, carbon monoxide, and nitrogen dioxide. The latter, when in contact with the moisture of the lungs, is converted to nitric acid and destroys the tissues. At the time of the explosion, my father was in the hospital building, although unhurt; but the cofounder, Dr. John Phillips, and several other physicians who were my close friends, did not survive.

My father's leadership and genius were used to their best advantage in the days following the disaster. He had the offices moved across the street into an empty school building and he rushed the completion of the new Clinic building, so that in a matter of weeks the Clinic was functioning normally, although handicapped, of course, by the loss of some key personnel and by the prolonged convalescence of others.

The public contributed generously to sustain the Clinic in this emergency, but all that money was returned to the donors. The Clinic was able to go right on, and eventually it was able to settle the several million dollars' worth of lawsuits that the explosion generated. The tragedy has been described briefly as follows:

> During the confusion of that tragic morning persons trapped within the building were entirely ignorant of the nature of the gas that filled the halls, corridors and examining rooms. They knew only that it caused severe irritation of the throat and lungs, with coughing and difficult respiration. Those who reached the examining rooms at the sides of the building and closed the doors behind them had a chance of survival. They opened the windows widely and leaned out into the fresh air. When ladders reached them many made their way safely to the ground. A few jumped.

For days the lung-damaged survivors kept dying, but those who survived made complete recoveries. In the entire episode there was only one absurd thing that happened to me. The newspaper had a headline, "Dr. Crile Goes Through Holocaust Unscathed." Although I was a senior at Yale and had majored in English, I had never heard of a holocaust. Until I looked it up in the dictionary, I had thought it must be something like a skylight.

After a visit to Cleveland, I returned to college and finished the term. Actually, I finished it in the headlines of the *New York Herald Tribune*'s sports page which featured an article on the Yale-Harvard track meet:

YALE DEFEATS HARVARD
Conner, Crile Score Necessary
Points for Blue in Field Event

> Trailing by 15 points near the end of the day Yale athletes came through with an all-conquering rush to reestablish track and field supremacy over the Harvard foe. Four successive victories in the discus throw, pole vault, 220 yard sprint and hammer throw climaxed a great battle between the Blue and Crimson and sent the Elis out in front 71 to 64.

Of course, the drama of it was that the hammer throw, which always for safety's sake is held in some remote area far from spectators, was the last event to be finished and led to an extraordinary concentration of the audience on this usually secretly conducted sport. I had missed the Princeton meet because of the Clinic disaster, but third place against Harvard gave me my third letter in track.

Although it was only a little over a month since the disaster, my parents decided still to attend my graduation. And there was some correspondence:

June 5, 1929

Dear Mother,

Graduation expenses contributions, $50 fee for registration at Harvard and bills in general have me just about broke. Could you deposit my July allowance at once, so that I'll be able to clear these matters up? You see it is going to cost me a lot to stay around the East from now over the races, and I can't get through on what I have.

I've taken my history exam and passed it, I think, although not very creditably. I had a beautiful idea in writing about the "development of towns in the thirteenth century", but my dates were two centuries off. I intended to explain the matter by showing the non-existence of time except as an illusion created by the fourth dimension.

I broke the back of one of my studs and can't get it fixed here; so will you send me the other one that I have in the little black case in the back of my drawer?

(Imagine my plaguing my parents with trivia at this time, two and a half weeks after the disaster.)

June 1929

Barney dear,

These days are awfully hard—oh so drab! Do write often. Dad is pretty well, but I know his heart is broken. So many of the boys are still ill. Sherrer is again in the hospital and Swafford and McCullagh are awfully ill.

The ray of hope—it's a big one—is the way the patients pour in—300, 325, 350. That is the rainbow. But of course no one knows where destiny will head for the legal problems are manifold. — But it's over. The task is ahead of us. It must be rebuilt again, and we must all square our shoulders and keep our eyes on the sun.

Write whenever you can no matter how short.

Mother

June 8, 1929

Barney dear,

Just a line. Be careful about expenditures won't you—for there are so many problems.

Half of our staff, eleven out of twenty-four are dead or ill. Those salaries have to be maintained for a year including Bunts and Phillips [the two dead founders]. We have sent for more oxygen tents. Nothing is being spared for their recovery, but it is a terrible business and one's heart aches for their families.

Are you sure that this galavanting all over the country is a safe preamble to exams—and a desire to make high marks? It is easy to make resolutions and to build ideals. The acid test is to put them through. . . . I want this summer [in which I was scheduled to work in the Clinic's Research Department] to count as nothing in your life has counted before. I want you to feel that this is the first step over the threshold of medicine and that you are going to face it with shoulders squared for that task alone and that you may keep your eyes on the sun.

Did you see the Literary Digest of yesterday? The picture of Dad, to me—terribly in the depth of sorrow—yet beautiful in its humanity—is the essence of human emotion—controlled emotion. It reminds me in quality of that veiled face in Sim's picture [my father's favorite painting]. That face seems to be weeping for mankind yet it is dauntless, courageous, enduring—

Goodbye dear and loads of love—

Mother

On June 11, in the midst of all the confusion, my father found time to dictate a two-page letter:

Dear Barney—

On entering your medical career you will find your work quite different and your life more simple. In Yale and at home you have had more freedom for social life and I imagine by now its novelty has worn off. In starting your career you will have more joy in the pure achievement and progress.

For this summer I am proposing, subject to your approval, your joining Dr. Farrell and our group in a research into the gastrointestinal tract. . . . Farrell's work is a continuation, with use of measurements of potential, along the lines I mentioned and involves difficult operative technique.

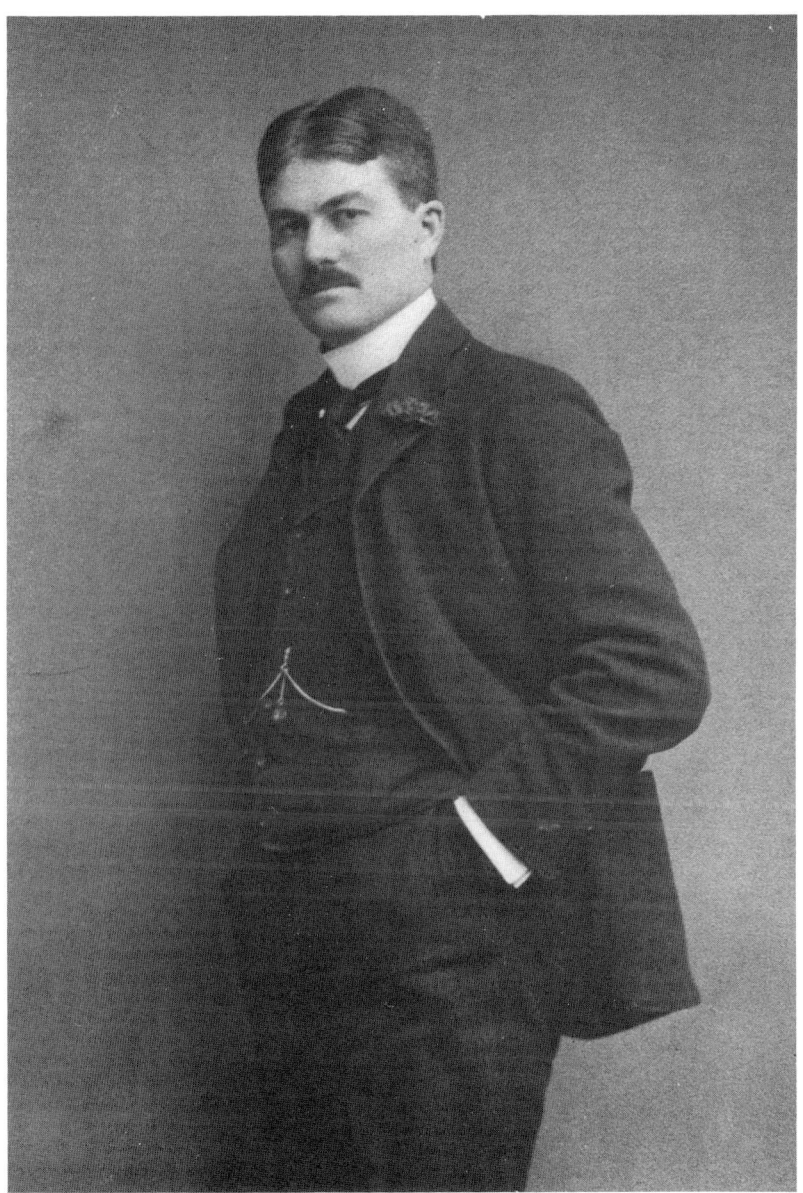

Dr. George Washington Crile in 1899. He later used the name George Crile, Sr., to avoid confusion with his son.

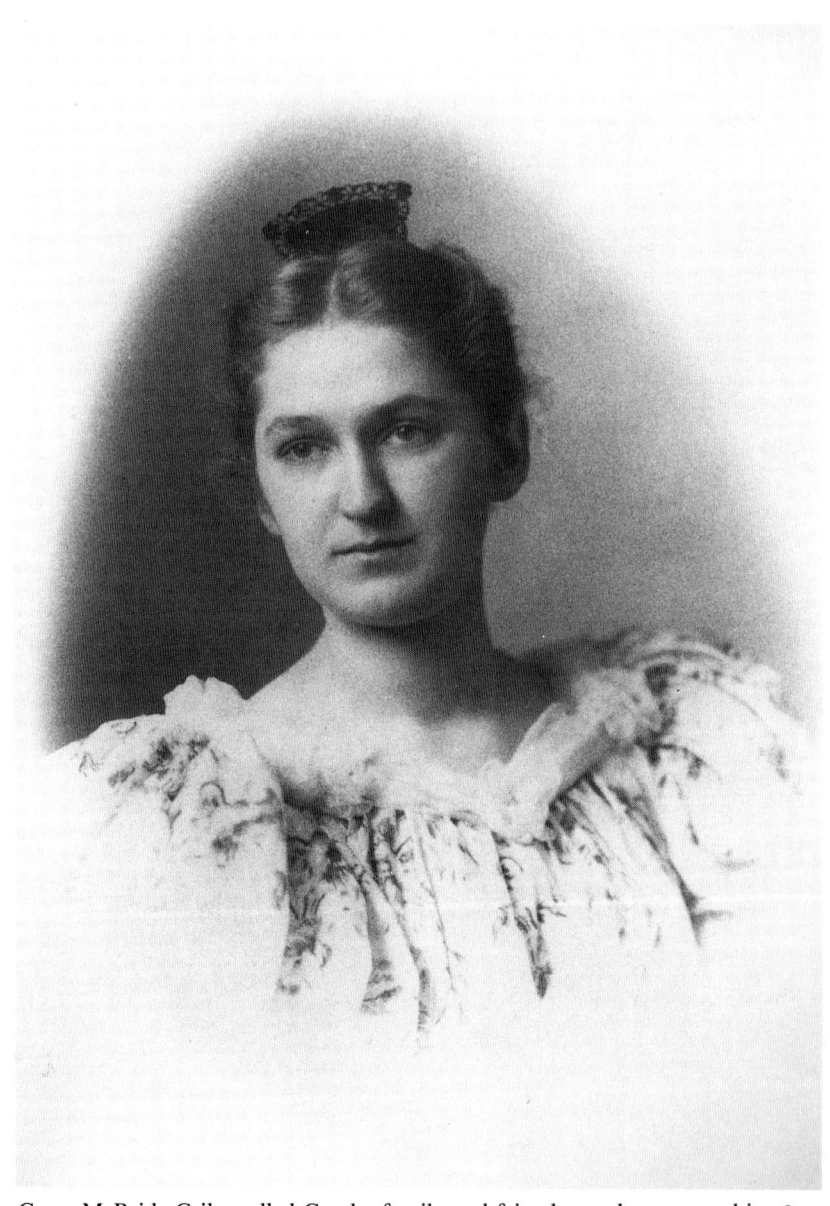

Grace McBride Crile, called Gay by family and friends, as she appeared in 1899.

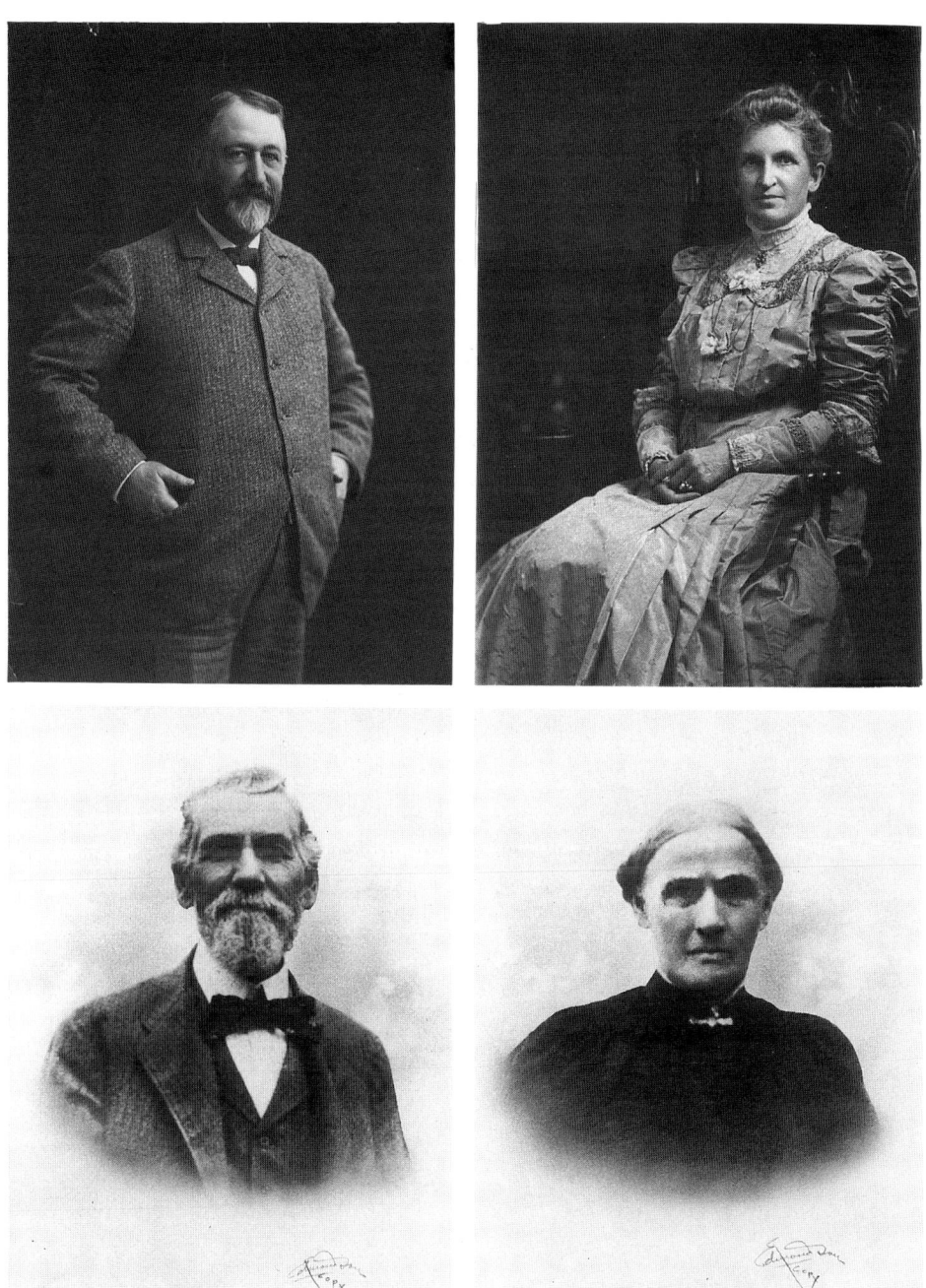

Barney Crile's grandparents. Above, his maternal grandparents John Harris McBride and Elizabeth Ama Wright McBride. Below, paternal grandparents Michael and Margaret Dietz Crile.

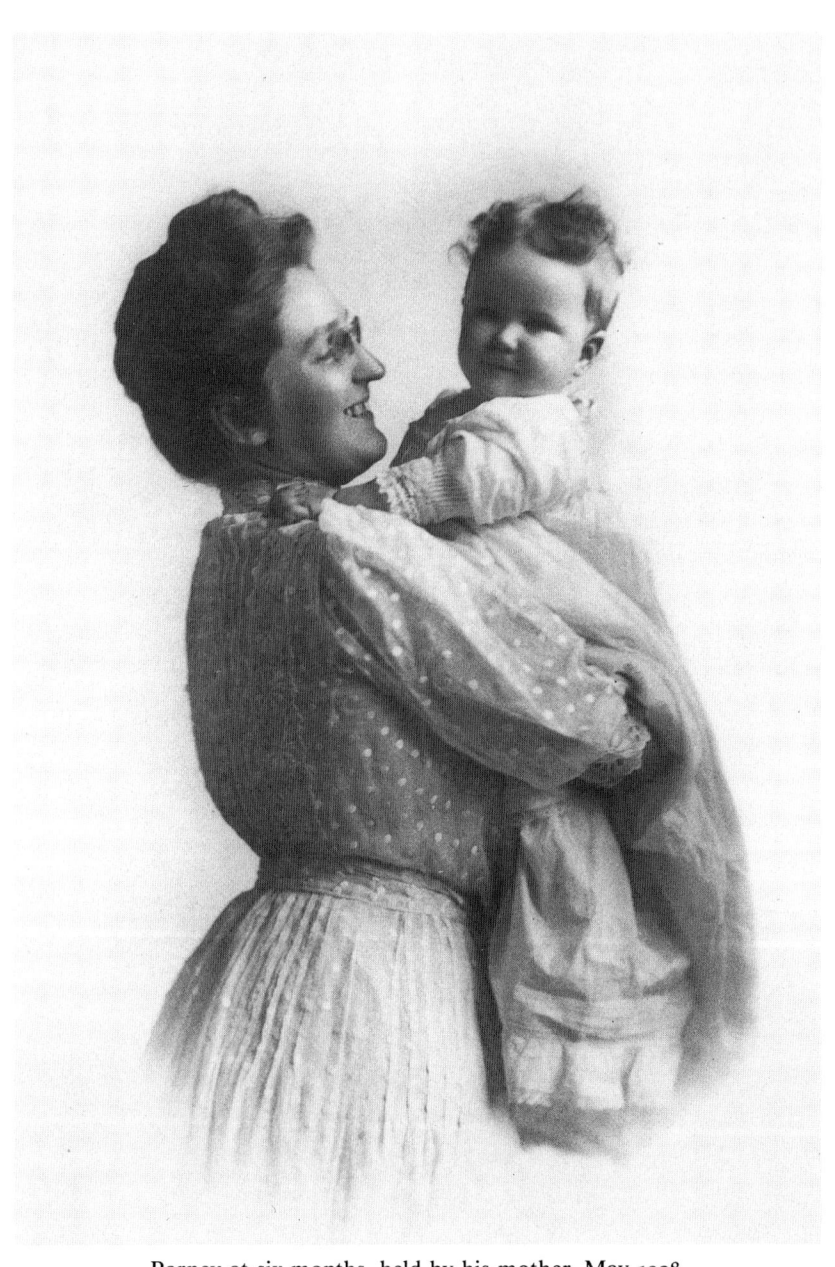

Barney at six months, held by his mother. May 1908.

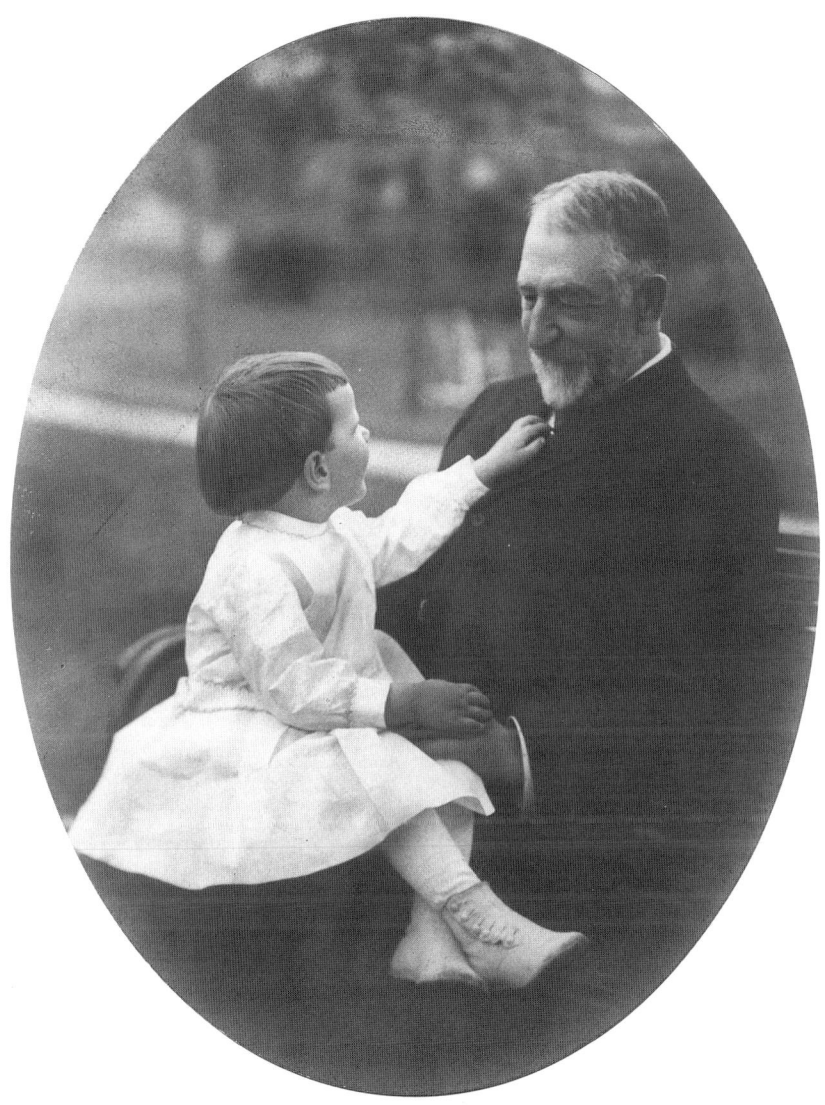

Grandfather McBride and Barney, who is not yet two years old, summer of 1909.
John McBride died later that year.

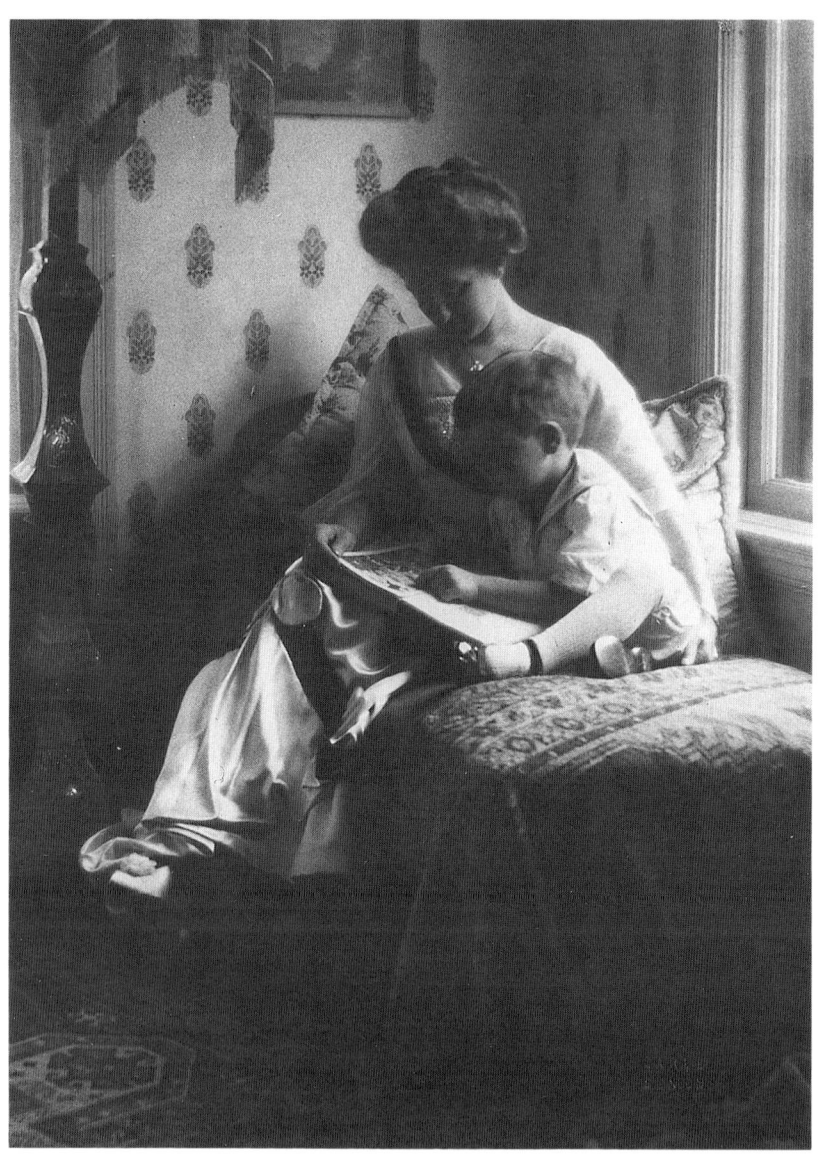

Portrait of mother and son: Grace Crile and Barney, ca. 1910.

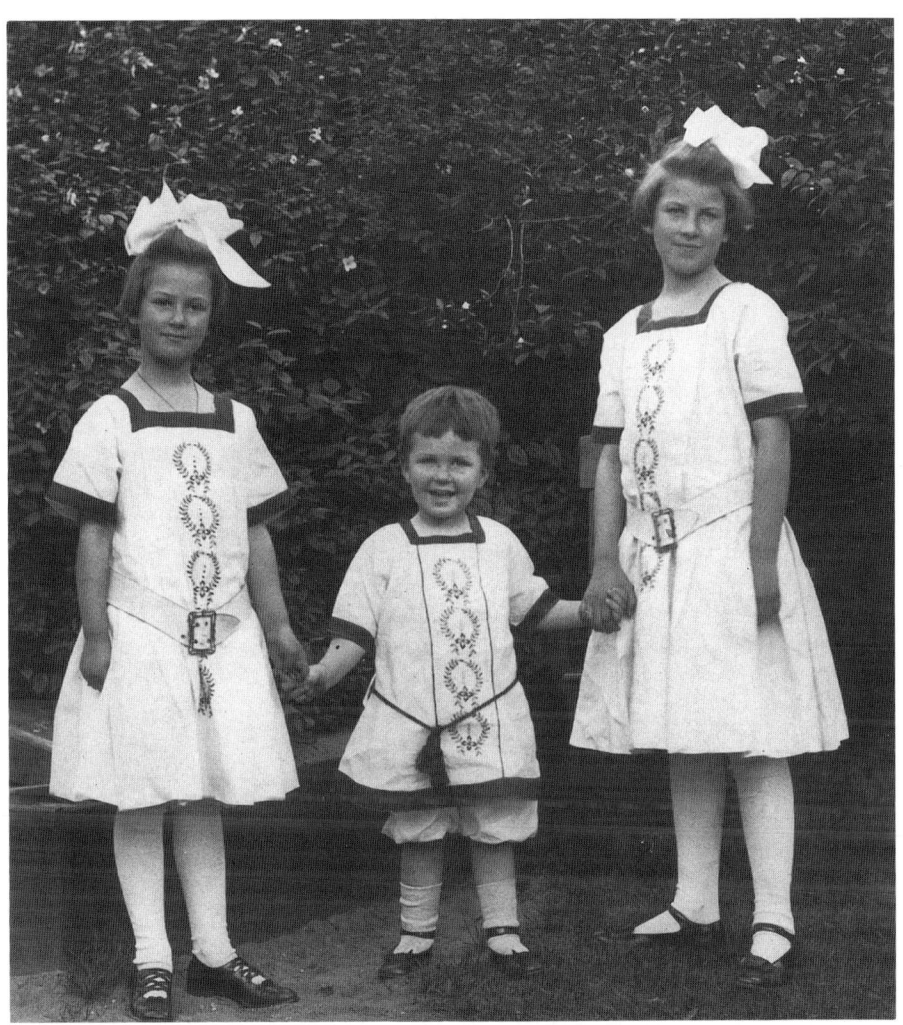

The Crile children in 1910. Elizabeth (Elo) at left, Barney, and Margaret (Peg).

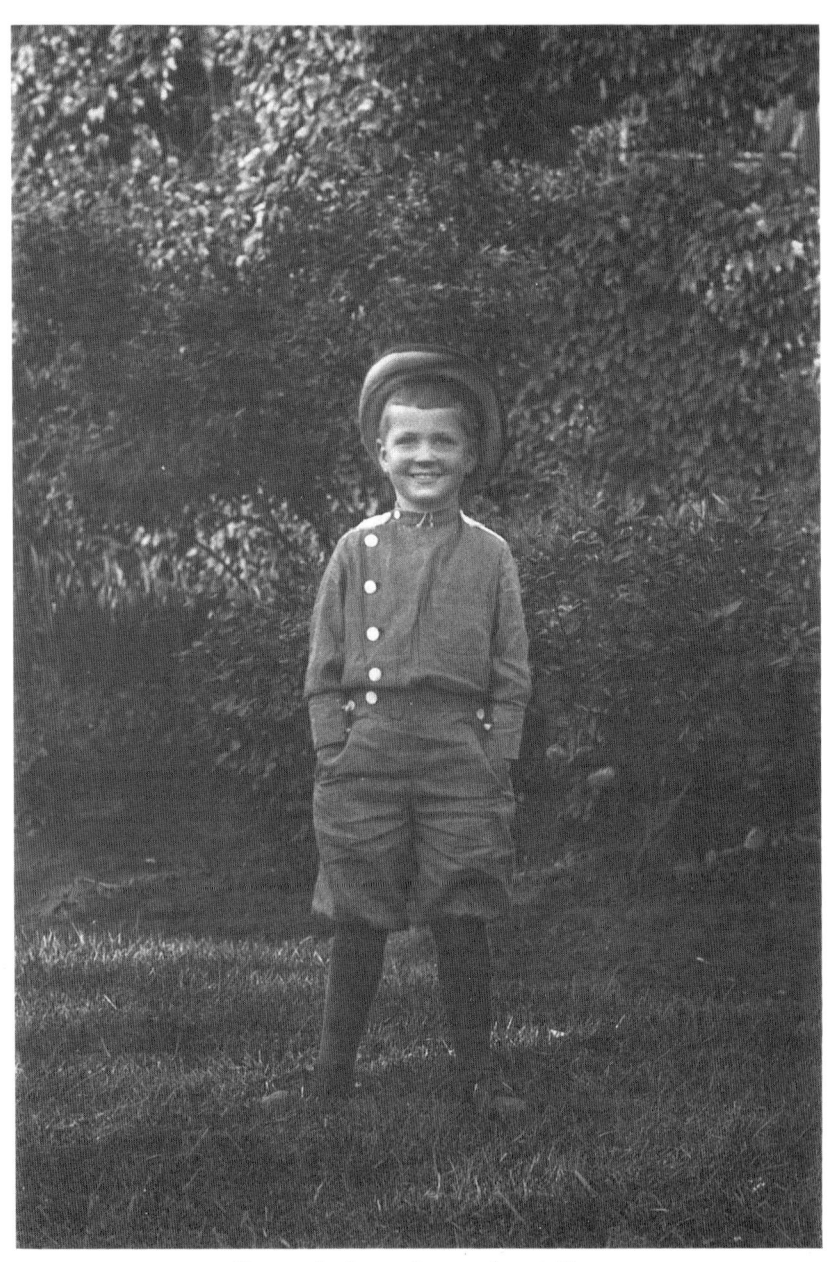

Barney in June of 1912, almost five.

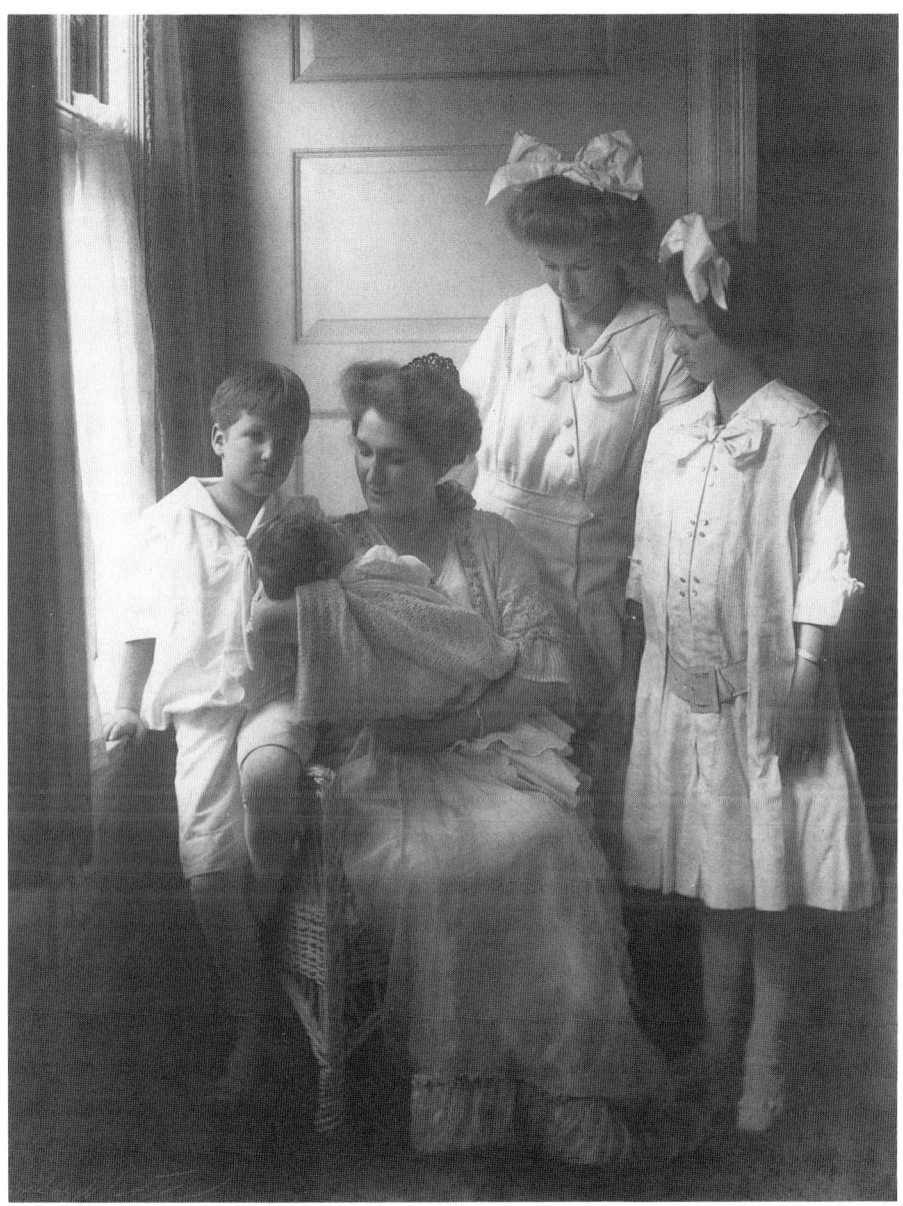

Grace Crile with her children in September 1913. Barney is at left, Robert (Bob) in his mother's arms, Peg, and Elo at right.

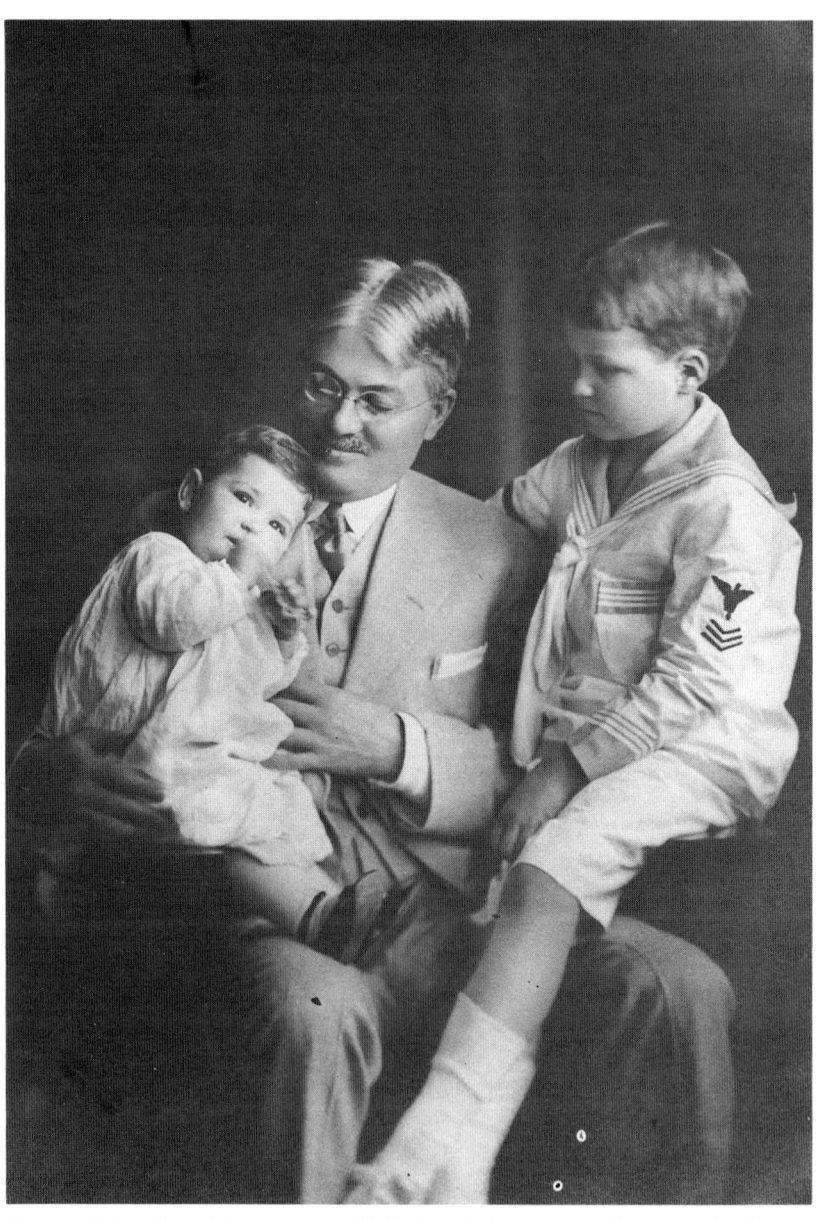

George Crile, Sr., with one-year-old Bob and Barney, nearly seven, in August 1914.

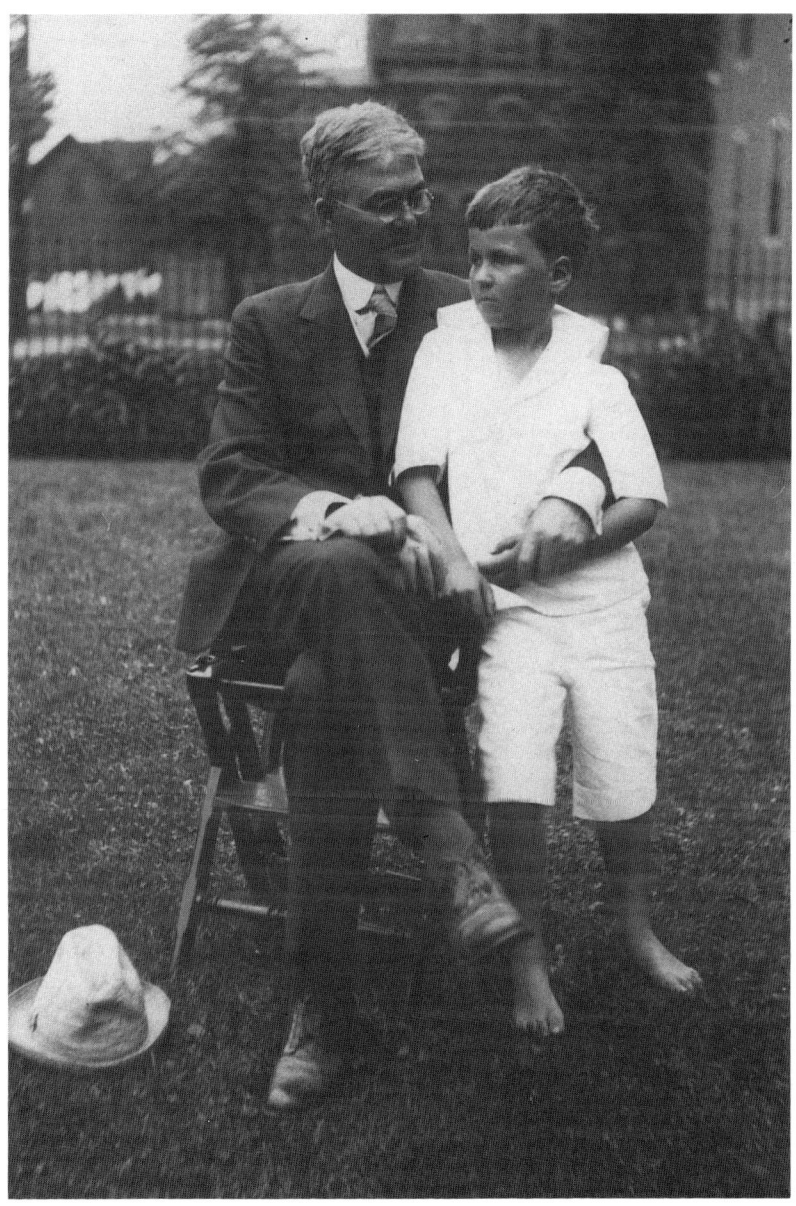

Barefoot Barney with his father, summer of 1914. Still at the Euclid Avenue house.

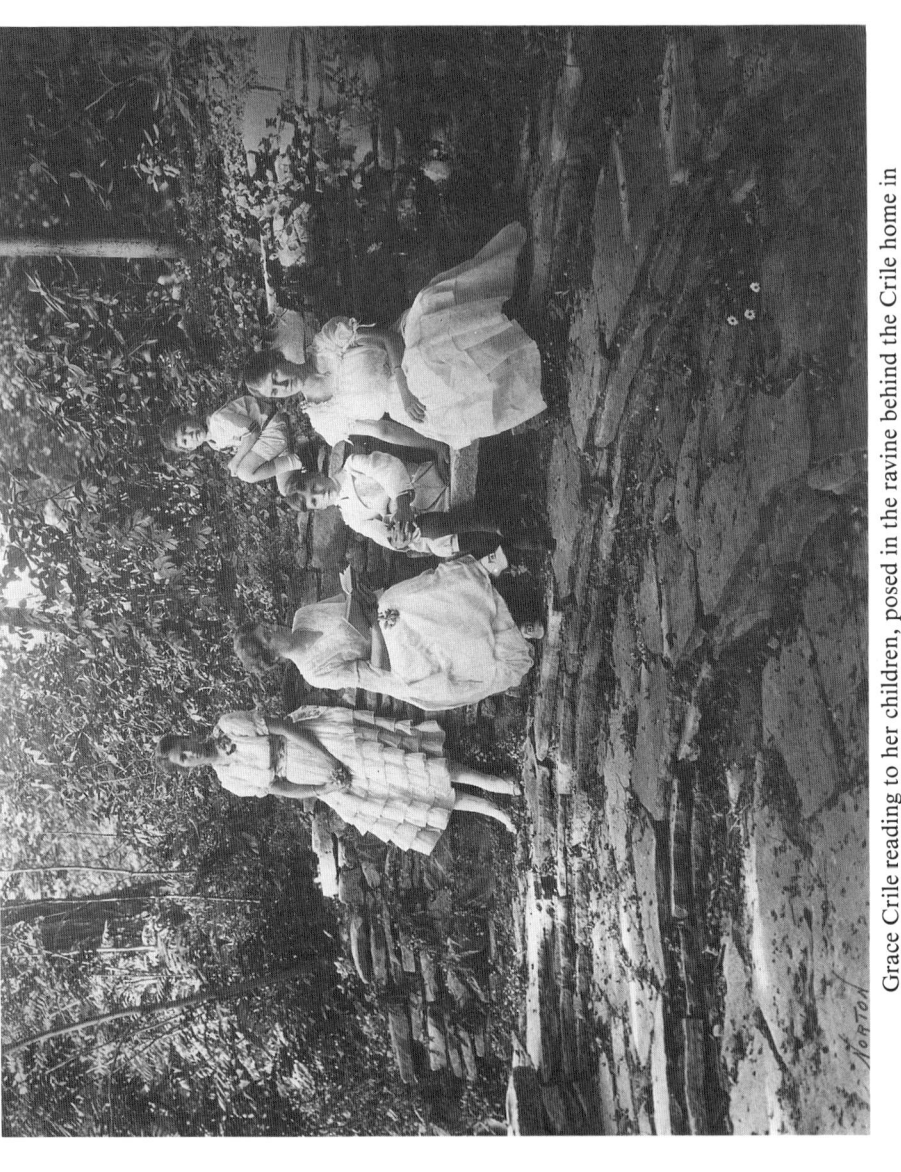

Grace Crile reading to her children, posed in the ravine behind the Crile home in Cleveland Heights, 1917. Left to right: Elo, Grace, Barney, Bob, Peg.

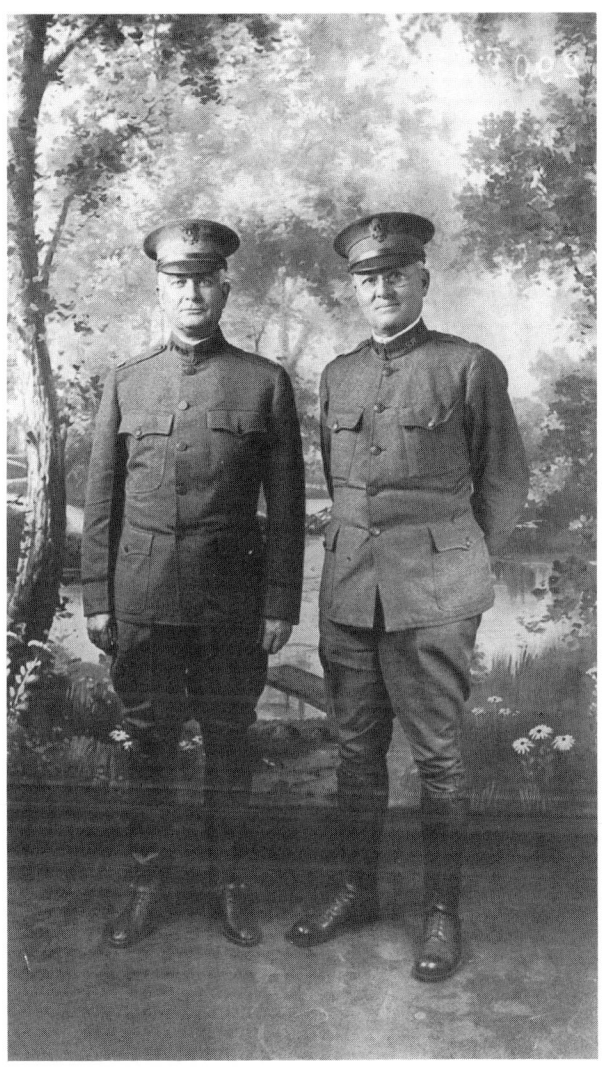

Major Will Mayo of the Mayo Clinic, at left, and Major
George Crile, October 1917. They were with separate units
but met while "over there."

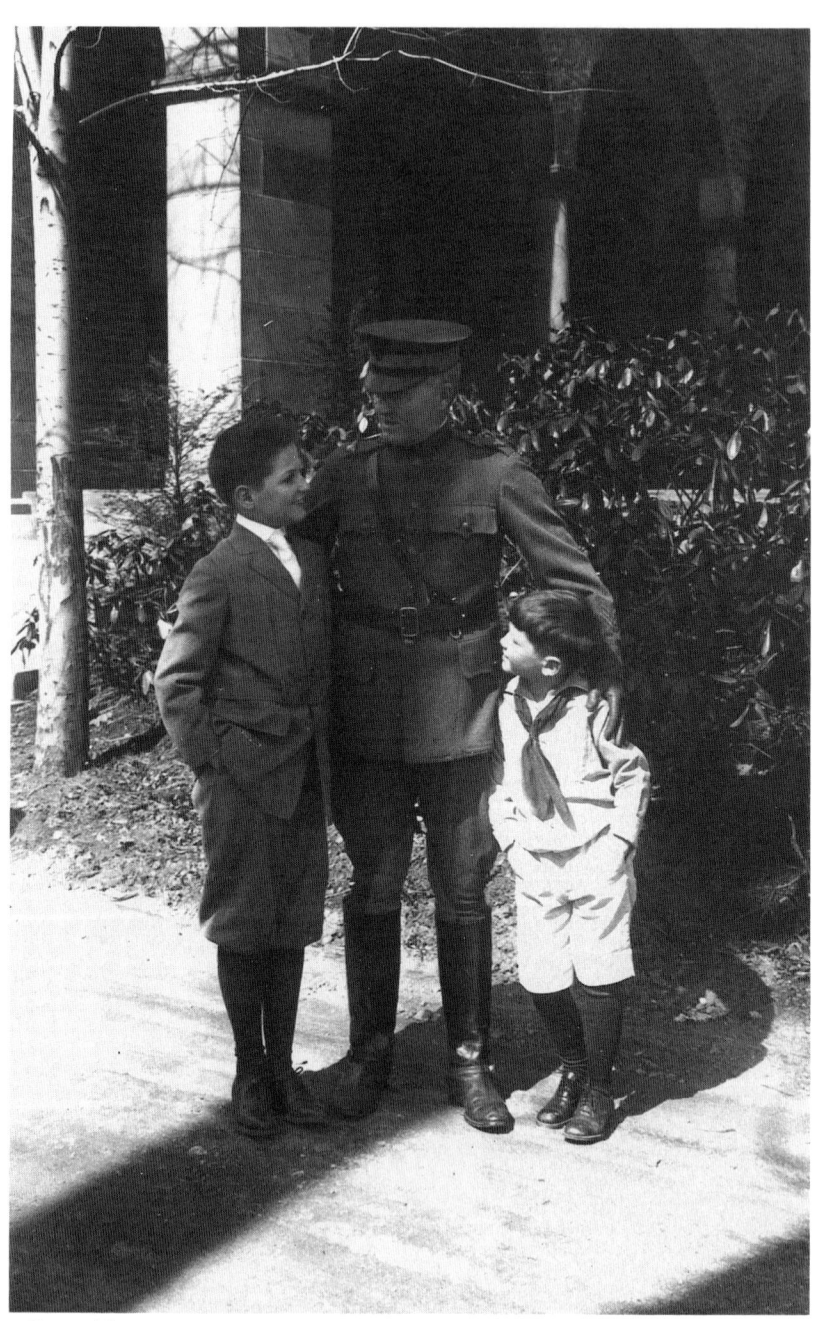

Greeted by sons Barney, left, and Bob, George Crile returned home in 1919.

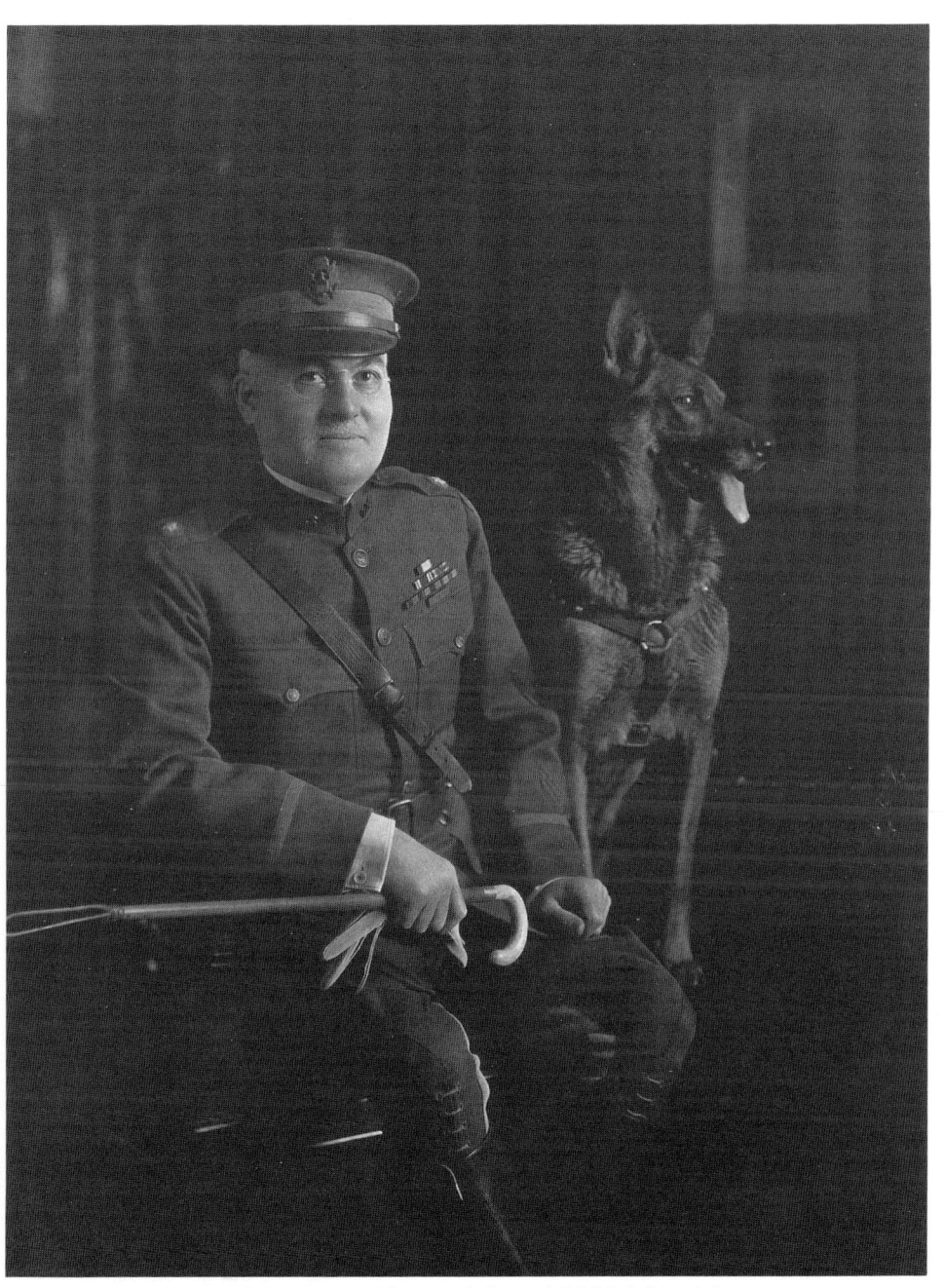

General George Washington Crile and faithful friend Sam.

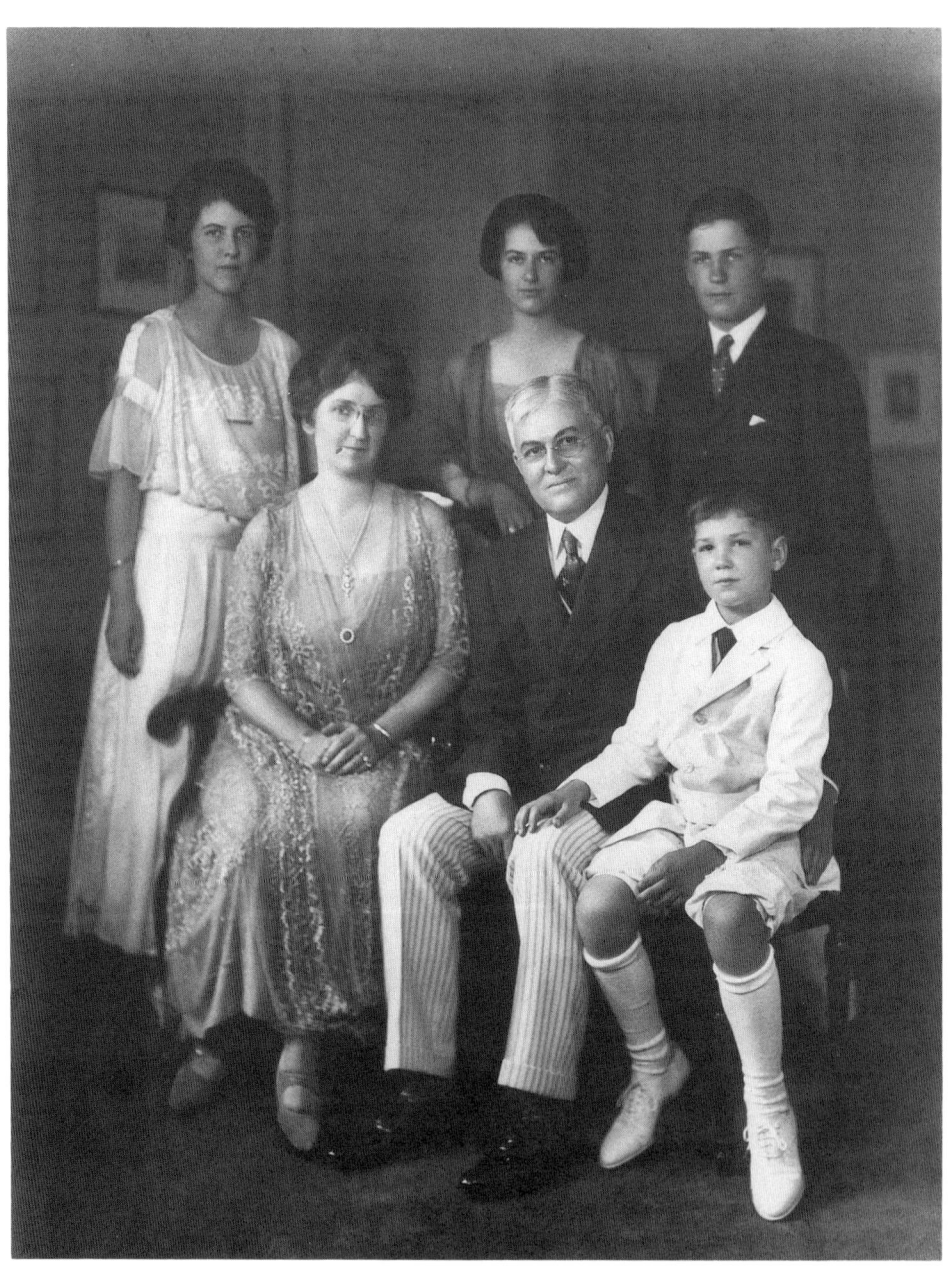

The Crile family poses on the occasion of Peg's coming out party in 1921.

If there is any other problem you would rather attack, it will
be open to you.

—Lots of love and appreciation.

Dad

In the middle of all the tragedy of the disaster and the confusion
of the reorganization of the Clinic, my parents came on to my graduation, and Mother, on her return, dictated a two-page memo describing it:

Sunday came the Baccalaureate Address in fine old Woolsey
Hall, and Dad and I felt a real thrill when Barney, capped and
gowned, walked down the aisle. [And she went on to talk about
the son of one of my father's best friends who had] just flunked
out of Medical School and has announced his engagement to Dr.
Wood's daughter. He probably sees no connection between the
two, but those of us who are older and wiser regarding Sher-
rington's story of "The Final Common Path," and surely Dick did
not keep to the single path in medicine. It is thus that the second
generations decline to mediocrity and never will understand
Why.

In view of these opinions of my mother, my hopes for a love life in
medical school were rapidly fading. And so ended my senior year at
Yale. After school, we spent a few days with my club mates at the
Skull and Bones Deer Island Camp, in the Thousand Islands.

Then it was back to Cleveland for the summer—in the research lab.
and weekends at the Knob—riding, and dancing Saturday nights at
the nearby Kirtland Club, and becoming progressively more monoga-
mously involved with Jane, whose love of riding and whose country
summer place near ours made our companionship both pleasant and
convenient. Still I lived up to my ideals and there was no talk of love
or marriage.

I submitted a six-page typewritten report on our summer studies of
gastric ulcer. In our laboratory dogs we had made "Pavlov pouches"—
little pouches off the stomach, which allowed us to study the acidity
and other characteristics of the secretions of the stomach. We observed that, contrary to my father's anticipation, injection of adrenaline into the dogs increased the amount of mucus and decreased the
amount of acid. I concluded the report with a comment that must
have horrified my father, who was accustomed to have his laboratory
technicians find what he had predicted they would: "It is difficult in
light of our adrenaline effects to see how the adrenal medulla [which

was what my father was denervating in patients with gastric ulcer in hopes of causing the ulcer to heal] could create ulcer. As yet the work is not clear in any indications except that the secret to ulcer lies in the kinetic system."

This was the first time that an idea gleaned from my experiments conflicted with my father's theories. It would not be the last, but in spite of our differences, there was no open conflict.

The senior year volume at Yale ends with two telegrams, sent on a moose-hunting trip to Canada, where I'd gone with friends from Cleveland, the Manuel twins. The first telegram was from Hailebury, Ontario:

> Fine trip. Address is Angliers, Quebec. Going in north of Lake Expanse. Arrive home sixteenth. Please call up Kate Hanna and accept invitation for dinner dance which I regretted. Barney.

And on September 14 from Angliers, Quebec:

> Shot at three bulls and a bear. Lucky we didn't go to Africa. Having motor trouble but hope to be home late the night of the fifteenth or sometime on the sixteenth. Will wire later. Barney.

In the files there also was a letter from me to Jane:

> Hotel Hailebury
> The Most Modern Hotel North of Toronto
> Hailebury, Ontario
> The Tourist's Paradise

Jane my dear,

This life of a hunter is something very fine. Bill Manuel is sitting across the way in this palatial motor boat which is the last link between us and civilization, singing alternately "I think we ought to have a drink" and "Drunk last night, drunk the night before." Tomorrow we get in position for hunting. It's really the greatest sport in the world to be up in this country again where there is no care or trouble, and no shaving or tight-fitting collars. You can say what and act as you please. The only other time I've felt this way this summer is when I've been with you. If you were only here it would be perfect.

We are on the Lac des Quinze. Why the Quinze? Fifteen—an abstraction. A meaningless digit whose very vagueness enhances its charm. Why Quinze? What were the fifteen? Why were they here in this remote and Godforsaken puddle of loneliness? Does the mystic symbol signify the tragic fate of fifteen men drowned deep in the cold, green waters? —Whether sincere or in jest and mimicry the Lac des Quinze has for me all the mystic lure of the Great Unknown. Fifteen lives—fifteen loves—fifteen drinks—fifteen fish—fifteen attacks of acute indigestion. What does it signify? And the rest of our trip I am going to devote to the solution of this mystery.

Jane, my dear, I return the 16th and leave for Harvard the 20th. Can you save me the 17th? The 18th I must be home, but I want to see you on the 17th.

> All my love
> Barney

It was after my last year at Yale, when I was working in my father's laboratory, that as a result of a shameful episode I was forced to change my name. My old hammer-throwing colleague, Bebe Spiel, wrote me at the Clinic and correctly addressed the letter George H. Crile. The "H" stood for "Harris" which was my middle name. My father's full name was George Washington Crile. When written fast an *H* and a *W* look much the same.

Since my father's eyesight had failed, Miss Rowland read him his mail. When she came to the letter from Spiel she slammed it on the table and stalked out of the room, saying "And this, Dr. Crile, I know nothing about."

My father brought the letter home and when Mother read it to him, both of them collapsed in laughter. The letter started, "Dear Dr. Foreskin, Do you remember those two babes that we were with in New York last month?"

It was then and there that my middle name was dropped and I became George Crile, Jr., and my father George Crile, Sr.

4

Medical School

THE "DIARY" (September 1929–September 1930) that Mother kept for me and much of which was typed and filed by her secretary, Miss Maloney, was prefaced by an inscription:

> Barney dear,
>   At last the dream has come true and you are in Medical School.
>   As the years roll on—These Diary leaves will tell you what it has meant to us—as well as to you—
>
> Mother

On September 22, 1929, I wrote my first letter to Mother from medical school. My roommate, Bud Yandell, and I were furnishing our two rooms in the dormitory. To read my letter you'd think my room was a small house. I asked Mother to send me a few colored pictures and etchings, and "the hunting print that Aunt Lucia gave me, the old German coach scene, the etchings, 'Family' by Orozco (three pyramids), the Kent named 'Revisitation' with the woman silhouetted grimly against a dismal sky, the Moose and the Bear; the Horse and anything amusing or good that you happen to think of, also Orozco's 'Requiem' of the nuns and candle." Also "curtains if you have them" and so forth, including requests for "a china cat and horseman, a bureau cover, and a cover for a round table. If you look carefully in the bottom of the envelope you'll see a tiny piece of the green plaster, giving you the dark green shade that it is."

Apparently I thought that life in medical school was going to be as relaxed and social as that in college had been. A letter mailed the next day, however, began to reveal the realities:

Boston, Mass.
September 23, 1929

Dear Mother,

I have a box of bones and am learning the vertebrae. Dissection starts tomorrow.

I need any cushions you have for the room—preferably the Yale ones. Also a medical dictionary. No time at present. Will write later.

Love
Barney

On the same day, I wrote my father about the first days at school and remarked that "at present I am confronted with a huge Gray's Anatomy, whose aspect is not mellowed by the parting thought you gave me that its 1417 pages contain no repetition and not a single unnecessary word."

I went on to comment that I was impressed by the appearance of my classmates. "They are an extraordinary keen-looking group—and I can see it is going to be real competition." I asked his advice about joining the R.O.T.C. (Reserve Officers Training Corps) and asked if he thought it was worth sacrificing one hour a week and six weeks of summer training.

My father replied, "As to R.O.T.C., it is not worth any time—I do not want to publish this idea as I am in the guild myself. I certainly would let it alone for want of time."

I had also asked him about joining a medical fraternity, Alpha Kappa Kappa, of which he was an honorary member, and had told him that I'd had enough of fraternities at Yale and saw no need to join a medical one. He agreed, saying, "but I would miss saluting you as my brother—which is about the case anyway. I could never see much place for frats. in medical school unless it provided houses to live in—eating places etc., but you have all that now."

And again, a handwritten letter about a day that he had spent duck shooting at Winous Point in "the quiet of the marsh—only four absent-minded ducks all day," but plenty of time to work out and write a medical paper and to tell me more about the challenges ahead of me in medical school. There were four pages of this, yet he was at the height of his surgical career and off the next day to speak at several meetings.

And from Mother—in the middle of an equally long letter: "This morning I dashed over to your interior decorator. I didn't feel quite satisfied with the bedroom scheme, so changed to a pictorial curtain. It represents a book—a novel. Sim [my friend Fred Simmons], the literary light, will have to guess, but I'll tell you. It is 'The Bridge of San Luis Rey' and the design was drawn by your beloved Rockwell Kent and the fabric stamped, so you see it is really modern." I wondered if Mother knew that a dormitory bedroom was supposed to be used for sleeping.

Boston
October 2, 1929

Dear Dad,

The first few days with our friend, whom we have named Lord Plushbottom, were rather amazing. We were turned loose in the lab with a set of instruments and the idea that we should skin the back and separate it into layer of skin, superficial fascia, and deep fascia. We were shown a dissection and were told what each layer looked like. With that instruction destruction began.

After about an hour of attempts at skinning, Bud [Yandell] condensed the ideas of the four of us by remarking "If there is one thing this guy is not like, it is a banana."

Then we were lost amidst the lumbodorsal fascia and mazes of trapezius, spleniuses, rhomboids etc. and not until Sunday, when we spent all day studying and catching up, did we feel that we could master anatomy.

I spoke to Professor Cannon the other night and introduced myself. [Walter Cannon, the Father of American Physiology who was professor of that science at Harvard.] He asked to be remembered to you. He has a son in our class—a darn nice boy—sort of a hereditary competition. [My father's and Cannon's theories had been competitive and Cannon's son and I became best friends and went through medical school and internship together.]

Love
Barney

P.S. I took your advice about R.O.T.C. and kept out. The first look at the stiff [cadaver] is a real thrill. Especially the first sniff when you have as soggy a one as ours.

The letters of that autumn went on to describe the inexorable advance of our dissection through the ramparts of the body and spoke of histology and embryology which also we were studying. "Instead of trying to learn first and dissect after," I wrote, "I take Gray along with me after just reading it over to get the idea, and read it in the dissecting room, looking up and dissecting as I go." I added, "We all finally decided to join the Lancet Club"—a social club with occasional meetings—"instead of a time-taking fraternity, and we enjoy it very much, as we have had no meeting and don't know anyone in it."

And then amazingly, in the middle of all this, "We went to New Haven Saturday and saw the game. The team looked pretty good although Vermont was a pushover and you couldn't really tell." I didn't say it in my letter to my parents, but I think it is likely that Jane met me at the game and we spent an evening together! I don't think that football alone would still have had me so interested.

October 12, 1929

Dear Mother and Dad,

We are now dissecting the axilla and having a terrific time with the intricacies of the brachial plexus. I would never have dreamed after watching breast cancer operations that there were so many things there. I don't think I would ever again have nerve enough to cut a dog anywhere. The whole darn body seems to be full of structures of whose existence I was totally unaware but have now become of grave importance. . . .

Don't forget to tell me about the Harvard tickets as I must get going if I have to dig them up in New Haven.

Love
Barney

As an example of my father's speaking schedule (this was before air travel):

October 14, 1929

Dear Barney,

Since I wrote you I have addressed meetings in Detroit, Hamilton Canada, Buffalo, Omaha, and Kansas City and have presented a practical application of our general theory everywhere. For the first time it seems to be well understood by the average man and received with greater enthusiasm than I have ever seen before. I trust there will be some practical results later seen at the Clinic here. . . . Patients with ulcers treated by adrenal denervation were "coming along finely so far."

This was a matter of opinion. Later on my objective review of the records failed to reveal any long-lasting improvement; subjective or objective.

On October 22, I wrote my parents that "I decided that I'd take a break Saturday afternoon and took the train to Northampton and back again Sunday noon. It's a darn good break and gives a chance for study on the train too." It must have been Jane whom I was seeing because I didn't mention the dread name to my mother. Bert Dunphy—my friend and classmate and later one of America's most distinguished professors and president of most of the important surgical societies—would accompany me, for he too had interests in that remote town. Nancy, whom Bert would later marry, was a classmate of Jane's. At the end of the letter I speak of surgery at Boston's Brigham Hospital: "I saw Cheever's clinic Saturday, in which he did a breast cancer and removed the pectoral muscles and dissected the axilla. A beautiful piece of dissection, but more practical for a stiff than a living being as it took nearly two hours. It makes you realize the importance of your anatomy to see the clinical side."

If Cheever really did a radical mastectomy in two hours, it was some sort of a record because the ones I saw later used to take half a day. One time Dr. John Homans, associate professor at Harvard and author of *Homans Surgery*, is said to have passed through Cheever's operating room at 8:30 as Cheever was starting a mastectomy. At noon, as Homans passed by again on his way to lunch, he told Cheever, "Hurry up, David, or it will metastasize."

Some sad and some funny things happened that fall, and Mother wrote about all of them including how she went to Dodd's to buy a stereoscope for me to help study anatomy slides. When she called, Mr. Dodd told her to bring along a slide to see if it fitted. She did, pulling the first one she came on. When she arrived "Mr. Dodd recognized me," she wrote, "and asked 'Did you bring the card?' I handed it to him. He looked up rather queerly. I said, 'Does it fit?' He said, 'Yes—Do you want to see it?' I said 'Yes,' took it—and heavens it was the lower section of a man's abdomen. I was just horrified to have been so stupid. I suppose he felt I was merely modern. Well, no more. Love. Mother."

She wrote of Dad's brilliant presentation at the Chicago meeting of the College of Surgeons when he spoke of and interviewed patients with goiters and ulcers: "I was thrilled over Dad's paper. The room was jammed, even the aisles were filled. He walked away from the microphone yet his voice filled the entire hall. Dozens of people spoke to Dad afterwards. This week we've had a lot of interesting people here, a Dr. Morris from Melbourne, Australia and a Dr. Doppler from Vienna, Dr. and Mrs. Terry from San Francisco." That is the way our house was in those days—a true hostel for overseas visitors.

Mother went on to mention for the first time the stock market crash which had started in September 1929. "Did you ever know of such a fall? I suggested selling before I went East and then when I returned the slide down had begun. Oh! well they are sound investments and we can forget them and someday be surprised!" Surprised Mother must have been, because the value of the average share would fall from 380 in September 1929 to 41 in July 1932. That would be followed by the bank holiday. Suddenly there would be no money. But all that would come later, about the time I would graduate from medical school.

Although my mother seemed a bit perturbed by the behavior of the market, my father made no mention of it in an eleven-page handwritten letter touching on a myriad of topics. There was (1) my medical education, in which he said, "Everything you are now learning is as permanent as the multiplication table." (2) "The fact that every cell in the anatomy is there by evolution gives a good chance for reasoning through the laws of struggle and survival. You no doubt are setting up a mechanistic theory as to the muscle-nerve mechanisms. Certain movements must be made and the limb returned again. Theoretically one should be able to construct an animal completely." (3) "The experiments are coming along as you left them. The drastic fall in potential, acidity, and total volume of juice on injecting adrenaline"—which was the opposite of what my father's theory had led him to expect—"may well find an interpretation along the line of the precarious state of cells when the temperature is lowered near to or to zero." (4) "Several days ago I did another adrenalectomy for ulcer and again the symptoms were abruptly cut off." Which was natural, I later discovered, for who would complain of ulcer discomfort when there was the dominant pain of the newly made and still-unhealed surgical wound? "There seems to be a relationship that concerns the nerve—adrenal as well as the thyroid influence. We shall find out more about it." (5) "The concentration cell—collodion film—glucose—apple ash solution on one side, distilled water on the other side showed respiration." (6) "The operation that you saw me do so ruthlessly on the shoulder on which I put a rubber tourniquet through the anterior and the posterior folds of the axilla and around the shoulder came out well. He was in town to see me today." (7) "One thing you must remember—that is our ancestors fought face to face with their enemies and also went against environment obstacles the same way, making the contact parts rich with resistance elements—the internal parts correspondingly poor so that in operating we take that into account. Then too we take into account that the whole man is worth more than a part." (8) "I hope that all went well with you in your tests. One more thing I will tell you about when I see you, and that is molecular pathology. But I must let you off for your Gray. Dad."

This condensation is of a letter five times as long. Such a letter, handwritten as it was by a man with so many responsibilities, remains beyond my belief or comprehension.

An example of the description of medical school life that I was sending home is this section of a letter describing an anatomy examination:

Then we were sent down to be quizzed by another man on the thorax. He asked me which lung was which of a pair lying with the root up so you couldn't see the lobes, and I cracked that one cold by examining the relation of the bronchus and artery. Then he asked Bud to show him the internal mammary artery. The thing was gone and only a stump remained, which Bud found all right. He asked him to show him more of it. Then he asked me, and I said it was all gone. He shook his head gravely and pointed to it, cut off completely and adherent to the sternum which was completely reflected back and lying on the neck. That was a dirty question because he might just as well have hid it under his chair and told us to find it.

We certainly put in a terrible two weeks of study for these things. I was fed up on the exam because I had the brachial plexus down pat and he never asked me a thing about it.

One thing that helped me through the anatomy was my father's sage advice to remember that every anatomic part has a function, and if you think of its purpose it's easier to remember where it is and what it looks like.

November 6, 1929

Barney dear,

I really think it is best to leave the Harvard game situation as it is—Dad is so keen to see you and your group and I know you will get a different kind of visit with him if you have him all to yourselves. He wants to see your cadaver and chat over a lot of things with you—your letter just thrilled him. He is so excited over the daily unfolding of the old trail.

Mother was right. My father came on and it was a good visit in the dissecting room and in the dormitory with all of the old group who had come down from Yale, whom Dad knew and who were working together and living with me or next door. Incidentally, I got a B in the anatomy exam and was ashamed of it because three of my classmates got A minuses. My father, after his visit to the dissection room, wrote to say how much he enjoyed the visit with us. "This is just like being a grandfather—no responsibility, just a fine unadulterated enjoyment."

In spite of the Great Depression, we still seemed to be living comfortably at Harvard. On December 7, after receiving a few ducks that my father had shot, I wrote, "We knocked off for an extra hour Tuesday night, and invited Dutch Wells who is now in town and had a duck dinner in the private dining room here (in Vanderbilt Hall). It was a great dinner and lots of fun."

And things kept moving along at home too. Mother wrote that "Mrs. Carl Akeley, wife of the great explorer, blew in for overnight." She had colored moving pictures of Africa featuring gorillas, and Mother promptly arranged for a dinner party in her honor and for a hundred people to come to our ballroom and see her films which were "simply entrancing. She is quite a fascinating person—pretty and young. Dickson brought along a book by Mrs. Carl Akeley to be autographed—But it was the *first* Mrs. Akeley's book. Poor Dickson!" Mother continued:

> We left Sunday night. That afternoon we had the Clinic staff and Fellows and their wives for tea. We stopped at Nashville (all of this by train, of course, as Dad gave a paper there). Nat Shofner (a former resident) met us, and they gave a lovely dinner. He is doing awfully well and everyone speaks of his ability and hard work and that he is bound to be successful. Nothing short of the success of you and Bob so delights Dad as the success of his "Old Boys." And why not? He has given them of his knowledge, his skill, even his patients—and they, in a way, are his immortality. They are the hope of carrying the torch.

After that visit, my mother and father went on down to the Circle M Ranch in Macon, Mississippi, as the guests of Dr. J. A. Crisler, whose son Gus had married my sister Elizabeth (Elo). The rest of the family, including me, as well as Mother's sister's family (the Shermans) and my father's cousin's family (the Lowers), joined them there for two weeks of sport: quail hunting, duck hunting, horseback riding, fox hunting, and rabbit chasing. We lived in the guest houses of the huge plantation, and were fed, waited on, and catered to by a horde of what then were called "darkies" who worked on the plantation.

From New York, a club mate of mine from the days of Skull and Bones, who was now working for *Time* magazine, typed a three-page letter to Max Eddy and me, telling of the horrors of his life in New York. "Some call it Apartment 2C, 455 East 51st Street. Some say it is

Hangover House; others Villa Vicious; some cynics say it is Villa
Vomit. Yet who indeed would call it home? It is a strange prison where
Tristam, Borneo, and Faustus and even the Barbarous Blish have lost
something—something unnamable. Lost it perhaps in great kegs of
peach brandy, long rows of scotch bottles, glittering gin bottles. Lost it
in an everlasting flow of alcohol in which for one moment we try to
strike out for shore and then float languorously down broad rivers of
sunshine and warmth and tropic trees and great winged birds only to
awake amidst storm and hail and darkness and bewildered, to plain-
tively cry, 'Who got drunk? Why?' " And so on for two more pages.

The problem of alcohol, which seemed so acute to my friend in
New York, did not exist to any such extent in Boston. Prohibition was
still in force, but there were many ways around it. We in medical
school were too busy to find those ways, but we did brew our own
beer in crocks and in the bathtub, and under the competent direction
of Rex Ross, later to become a distinguished West Coast vascular surgeon, we bottled the beer in big quart bottles that we'd carry with us
when we went out to parties. All went well until once when Rex
wasn't around to supervise at bottling time and we apparently put the
corks on too early. On a hot day when no one was around and when
the bottles were lined up side by side in the huge bookcases that lined
the wall, one of the bottles exploded and it set off a chain reaction in
which all exploded. You can imagine the mess to which we returned,
as well as the tragic loss of our passports to the hearts of our favorite
women.

Boston
January 12, 1930

Dear Mother and Dad,

This has been the most terrific week I've ever gone through.
We have covered the entire morphology of the brain and its nuclei, the tracts of the spinal cord, and the nuclei tracts etc. of the
medulla. Besides we've dissected and are supposed to have
learned the pelvis, perineum, external genitalia, thigh, anterior
and posterior gluteal region and posterior aspect of leg and plan-
tar foot. I figured that my average work for the week is 14 hours a
day.

I did pretty well in the exams, receiving "Excellent" in anatomy and
histology. Mother wrote that she was "perfectly delighted" and that
"Dad is treading air and wears a smile that won't iron out." "You have
won a victory over your greatest obstacle," my father wrote.

On January 28, 1930, I wrote them:

Physiology started today, and we conducted a wild experiment on metabolism. As usual things started "in media res" and none of us had any idea of what went on. We were turned loose in a room that looked like the boiler room of a steamship all full of pipes and tubes and weird tanks, and were told to measure metabolism.

To do this, one of each group of five offered himself as a subject and breathed into a machine as we added oxygen to it and observed the rate of its use. Max was the subject and turned out to be terrible because, contrary to all principles of physiology, he used up more oxygen before lunch than after, and more when he rested than when he worked. As a fitting climax, he had to run around the block and come in nearly fainting of exhaustion and breathe through that foul tube until he was blue in the face. To cheer him I read him the next experiment as he was recuperating. "With the same subject as in the preceding day again reporting at the laboratory without breakfast, conduct three periods while he is on the stationary bicycle instead of reclining." At this he made it clear that he was resigning his position! This is going to be a great course!

I was still persuaded that my father's "Bipolar Theory of Living Processes" was able to explain most of the phenomena of life, and on February 2 I wrote him saying, "The Physiology is great. We spent the afternoon doing electric stimulation of frog's muscle and recording the results on a smoked drum. I'm crazy about that course. The more I read the more convinced I become that the entire bipolar theory is absolutely sound and is the only conceivable explanation of it all." As time went by, I was to learn that there are many electrical phenomena in the processes of life, but that my father's theory was a vast oversimplification of the world's most complex problem. He had some notion of that, because in response he wrote, "When you come to your Physiology exam you must be careful as to what you write down—for if you write an exposition of your pagan ideas you will be expelled and the place fumigated."

Then on February 7, 1930, less than a year after the Clinic disaster and only a few months after the 1929 crash of the stock market, there was a letter from my father that said, "Today at a board meeting—and John Sherwin, Jr. is now a member—we voted to prepare plans for a new building." Certainly that decision celebrated an extraordinary rise of a phoenix from its ashes. And the man that made it possible was my father.

At about the same time, my Great-aunt Ella died at the age of eighty-one and my father wrote to remind me that Aunt Ella had taken my mother abroad for "almost two years of travel and education. This I believe was not a little responsible for Mother's keen interest and understanding of the history and culture of Europe which she has put before you all your life in so many ways." Whether or not my father was right in attributing the genius of my mother to her travels in Europe, there is no question that somewhere she received the educational equivalent of at least one Ph.D. Mother's reaction to Aunt Ella's death was philosophical. "Aunt Ella was 81," she wrote, "and most people should die when they're 80 and so everything was just right." At the time I didn't question the truth of Mother's remarks, but now I begin to wonder if she was always right.

While I was deeply engaged in physiology and biochemistry, the latter of which I was having a hard time with, my father was busy working on a paper on memory that he was scheduled to give at the Philosophical Society. He had a concept of "vast numbers of dialectric films of the fibrillae, and he presupposes a particulate structure of the jelly-like white matter, for if the microscopic pathways have insulation, they of course would hold an electric charge." In one spot his paper read, "If an educated atom could wander about the brain in an aeroplane and examine the molecular structures of the action patterns, he would identify everything that could be recalled to memory by that brain." I never cease to be amazed at the infinite variety of my father's interests and of the drive that enabled him at the age of sixty-five to see thousands of patients, perform hundreds of operations, manage the operation of the Clinic and Hospital, plan the construction of a new Clinic, shoot ducks in season, ride horseback the year round, and write me longhand letters a couple of times a week!

In retrospect I have often wondered whether my father's obsession with the bipolar, electrical explanation of everything he saw was not a portent of impending senility. More and more as the years went on, his conversation, his letters, and his papers spoke of nothing except these theories. For him, it was a fascinating project, because he interpreted everything he read, from quantum theories up and down in terms of molecular biology, electrical energy, and life. Before long, this began to separate him from the scientific community and finally even I began to realize that sometimes the results reported from his laboratories were given to him by workers there who did not care to displease him. At about this time, I began to think not that my father was senile, but that he had become aware of the inevitable end of his career, and was just trying to explain everything in life while he still had enough life to do so.

At Harvard Medical School, in the spring of 1930, I wrote my parents about our initiation into the Lancet Club which was composed of students, some members of the faculty, and many graduates who resided in the Boston area. Each year the new members put on a "play." I described it, by saying that Max, Bud, Sim, and I were putting on an acrobatic and gymnast act for which we had hired leopard skins in true vaudevillian fashion with which to gird our loins. "We are the Gluteal Brothers, Maximus, Medius and Minimus, while Sim is our assistant and wears a costume padded with balloons which break at appropriate intervals and is advertised as our Aunt Polly, O'Myelitis. It promises to be a great show." (Anterior Polio Myelitis = Polio.) And it was. Bud stood on Max's shoulders and jumped down on a springboard which was resting on Sim's belly. I was on the other end of the board and Sim would have been ruptured if the board hadn't been three-fourths sawed in two and there hadn't been a concealed support to take the shock.

In Cleveland more serious things were happening. The first lawsuit against the Clinic had been filed—for thirty-five thousand dollars. It was on the anniversary of the disaster, and of course was just the beginning of the parade. At about the same time, the Clinic celebrated the performance of Dr. Crile's twenty-thousandth operation on the thyroid.

On June 9 came my grades—A's in both chemistry and physiology and a letter of commendation from the dean. And also there was a notable social occasion. Dr. Cushing's daughter, Betsy, whom we all knew well, married Jimmy Roosevelt, the son of Franklin D., who then was the governor of New York. I wrote, "It was a lovely affair, Governor Roosevelt attending with his bodyguard. They had lots of tents and things in the garden, and there was much good food which saved us buying a supper, and dancing in which I indulged with Sally Baldwin [a Clevelander] who blew in for the ceremony. These younger girls are beginning to look pretty good after all—some solace at least for all our recent losses at the hands of marriage."

In Cleveland too, in spite of the depression, the socialites continued to gather. Mother wrote me:

The Will Mathers gave a wonderful party the other night. A garden dinner party. Dad said he was glad Louis XIV wasn't alive, as it would have given the poor old soul an inferiority complex—and it certainly would.

We sat at a table in the Tea House. I felt as if I had been hurled back to the Medici period. The get-up resembled the great paintings of the Louvre—a great U-shaped table covered with golden brocade and great epergnes of fruit and high candelabra.

High Roman flares illuminated the garden, and soft lights high in the great trees brought each individual leaf into relief against a bright moonlit sky. An exquisitely gowned pretty girl in Grecian costume played the harp and after dinner we wandered from the formal garden to the wild garden where pieces from the Cleveland Orchestra, hidden behind rhododendron bushes, played a symphonic program and two wonderful dancers gave interpretive dancing, their many and gay costumes being enchanting in that lovely setting.

I sat beside Mr. Horace Andrews at dinner—an old friend of my father's, and now well along in years and quite deaf. Just when the tones of the harp were sweetest and when everyone was just breathless from the enchanting poetry of the whole scene, he leaned over to me and roared, "I should think she'd scrape all the skin from the ends of her fingers, wouldn't you?"

In September of 1930, Max Eddy, Dutch Wells, Count Costikyan, and I—the group who in our senior year at Yale had been together in the Bones and in our Harkness rooms—all met in Cleveland and drove north to go moose hunting in Quebec. We drove in my family's Dodge touring car, and just outside Erie a car full of old ladies backed up into our path on the main Route 20 road. To miss it we swerved off the road, across a lawn, and before we could stop hit a wooden house which rattled but didn't collapse. We damaged the front wheel and had to replace it, and a stern-looking carpenter came and estimated the damage to the house at ten dollars. The accident put us only a couple of hours behind schedule. I wrote to my father:

> Mattawa House
> Mattawa, Ontario
> September 10, 1930
>
> In the Dodge agency at which we stopped, I found that the head had been operated on by you, Dad, the chief mechanic had met you, and another man knew Dennis Crile [my cousin]. We couldn't have gotten better service.
>
> We are going into Moosehead Lake, about 30 miles from here. Things look pretty good and John [our guide from Keewaydin Camp days] has done a good job on the outfit.

As I remember, in spite of continuous rain for five days, we had a great time. There was no prohibition in Canada and there was plenty of good ale. There were no moose, at least none that we shot at, but we killed a loon and I think we killed and ate a deer and a lot of ducks.

After returning to medical school, I wrote home:

September 22, 1930

Dear Mother and Dad,

Another summer is over and in retrospect it seems to me that it was the best yet. The Clinic with its opportunities afforded the most interesting work I have ever done [I was working in the research laboratory with Max] and home, after a year of Medical School, was like an oasis in a desert of dormitories.

Max Eddy, who had stayed with us and worked with me most of the summer in research, wrote to Mother, "This summer I almost fell in love with an abstract thing which you gave me by the chance to live with the best the world holds in personalities, a home and a medical career. I cannot even try to thank you."

Medical school was a breeze. I had worked summers in my father's research laboratory and had spent my life exposed to Latin in the names of butterflies, in prep school courses, and in scientific jargon at my father's Clinic and at home. I had learned from Keller and from my father not to memorize but to look for logic and cause-and-effect relationships, and to find a scientific explanation for everything. I enjoyed all the work at medical school, especially physiology, although even anatomy made some sense if one viewed it from the standpoint of how you would go about building a structure or a machine to do the particular job that each bone, joint, nerve, or muscle was called on to do. But the real excitement came when I saw my first patient.

I was in my second year, in a course in physical diagnosis held in the out-patient department of the Massachusetts General Hospital. Each of the students was given the task of recording the history and physical examination of one of the indigent charity patients— "teaching material" they were called.

I have never seen, before or since, a person who looked like my first patient. His features were Oriental, his hair kinky and African, and his skin was yellow with large chalk-white completely unpigmented patches. This condition, known as leukoderma, is the result of local loss of pigment, but I didn't know that. "Leprosy" was my obsessive thought, and, of course, knowing nothing about medicine, I thought of leprosy as being highly contagious.

I soon found that my patient came from the Philippines, and that seemed to confirm my diagnosis because I knew that leprosy was common in the tropics. Gingerly I did the physical examination. Heart, lungs, abdomen all seemed normal. Then the genitalia. There were no testicles! I looked up at him with a gesture of inquiry. "Operation?" I asked.

"No, no," he said. "No operation. Me cut myself."

"You took them yourself?" I asked aghast.

"Yes, yes," he said. "One day I got very mad at my wife. She was very mad. I was very mad. So I get my razor and I cut off the balls, just to teach her a lesson."

I made discreet inquiries as to how this extraordinary act would teach a lesson to anyone but himself, but the language barrier prevented me from getting an answer.

"But what has it done to you?" I asked him. "You don't think of women anymore?"

"No, no. Everything is just the same. Zig, zig, zig just the same, but now no more babies."

Checking up on this experience, I found that this was quite likely to be a true report. Many adult males when castrated continue to be sexually active, the male hormone being supplied by the adrenals. Perhaps that was why eunuchs were so widely employed in the harems of the Middle East.

All of this was in the 1930s at a time when there was not too much social consciousness about the segment of the population that could not pay for private physicians. In fact, most of us had no social consciousness at all, at least I didn't. I remember going into New York in the Pullman cars of the old New York Central Railroad, whose elevated tracks ran through the slums of the city. From them one could look straight into the second- and third-story windows of the tenements inhabited at that time largely by Italian or Central European immigrants. The squalor was appalling, but I have no recollection of feeling any responsibility for this. It seemed to me that social or economic classes were facts of life that were built into the country and were accepted the way they were.

At Harvard, we medical students felt much the same way about the patients in the out-patient departments and on the charity wards of the hospitals. The people who constituted the "teaching material" were treated differently from the paying patients, sometimes to their advantage and sometimes to their disadvantage. If a patient happened to have a rare and interesting disease, he would be given every X-ray and test known to man and some that were unknown but in the course of being devised. These patients were always treated courteously and with respect. Women's breasts, for example, were never examined in a large women's ward without adequate screening. As much as thirty years later, in England and Europe I would often see unscreened examinations, and in Scandinavia and in Germany, I would see the ward patients treated by an almost military discipline, standing by their beds. All of the research and study was, of course, an advantage to some patients who as a result received superior treatment. But to many others, whose disease could not be satisfactorily treated, it meant nothing more than a long and sometimes uncomfortable period of hospitalization.

One of my most vivid memories of my second year of medical school, when we first began to see patients, was my surprise to find that the practice of medicine was so little concerned with mumps, measles, scarlet fever, chicken pox, and all the diseases I was familiar with, and was involved so deeply with so many diseases that I had no recollection of ever having heard about. One of the main courses in the second year was bacteriology, about which I said, "I wander around all day like Lady MacBeth, rubbing and wiping my hands to rid myself of the contamination of the billions of plague-producing bacteria which the slightest slip in technique scatters to the four winds. In Chemistry, the penalty for poor technique was a low mark. In this course it is pestilence and death."

Another chief course was pathology, which fascinated me and I thought was excellently organized and taught. Pharmacology I found boring and hopelessly taxing to my memory. There is no way in pharmacology that you can put things together—chemical construction, dose, side effects—and make a sensible memorable structure of it as you can with anatomy and physiology. The trouble is that pharmacology is manmade and the others came by evolution.

From Boston, I wrote home about some of my problems:

> Last night, about twelve, we went down to one of the famous Boston Deb. parties. This was the debut of a Cabot. You know the newspapers of this town have been grading debutantes like milk in Class A, B, C and D. They publish lists of names— classified—and with brief personal comments or remarks on the social rating of the family. This was a grade A Debutante, and as might be expected, her party was my idea of a grade X. We left at one o'clock in disgust. I've never seen so many unattractive girls, heard worse music, or been annoyed by a wetter bunch of fellows than at this exhibition of Boston's best. Anyway, it taught

me a lesson of never wanting to go to another. Do you remember the terrible, eagle-faced Isabella, of whom Uncle Mac is always speaking? Well, she asked me to dinner and horse shows Tuesday night; so you see I am getting to be a real figure in the society of this City of Boston.

Love
Barney

In spite of all these social activities, the economy of our family was going from bad to worse. Mother wrote to say that my father would be going for a last duck hunt at the Winous Point Shooting Club and that then he was going to give up the Castalia Trout Fishing Club and the Shooting Club because "what we save in just dues alone would take the whole family up to our island in Canada for a month. These times, from a business viewpoint, are terrific. A banker said the other day that the banks in town were busy trying to keep millionaires from going under."

My birthday, November 3, had come around, and my father wrote, "The year that has closed for you has been so fine that I would almost be sorry it is over except for the expectation that the coming one will still be a better one. Professor Weinberg of the Pasteur Institute is here and has taken the keenest interest in our research. He seems to attach great importance to its significance—among other things its implication as to spontaneous generation."

Mother wrote of a skit that came out in the *Los Angeles Times* entitled "The New Aristrocracy" in which they quoted Dr. Crile as saying, "It may really be a compliment to acquire a peptic ulcer; the great genius, the poet, the philosopher are always the most susceptible." The article went on to say that peptic ulcer is a disease of higher civilization peculiar to people of superior intelligence. In an era of universal education, when we are apt to be swamped with intellectual climbers, the article suggested that the claimant produce the X-rays of his stomach before he could be admitted to intellectual circles. Mother's letter concludes, "Other strange things go too and my poor little band of stocks has sunk and sunk until I expect to hear a grand gurgling gasp as they sink out of sight. Dad is so anticipating seeing you at the Harvard Yale game."

Regardless of the financial difficulties, my family was urging me to return for Thanksgiving and go on that last duck hunt with Dad. And Mother, always fascinated with all aspects of science, wrote that she had been reading a book by Lord Birkenhead entitled *2030* in which he spoke much of Einstein's contributions and said that "Physics was on the brink of a new synthesis, and restatement of fundamental ideas that would solve the problem of supplying the world with limitless amounts of cheap power because locked up in the atoms that constitute a pound of water is energy equivalent to ten million horsepower. It exists, but we don't know how to release it." Sadly, we soon would learn.

The earl also predicted stereo, color television, the abolition of epidemic disease (like smallpox), in vitro fertilization of egg cells, and rejuvenation of the human body. Mother wrote me five single-spaced typewritten pages of her summary of this book! She ended with a description of a dinner at the home of Mrs. Billings—a rich patron of the arts and a grateful patient of my father who gave so much to support his research. "Her table was aglow," Mother wrote, "simply gorgeous with old lace and old Ruby glass, of which she has the best collection in the world. [I've seen it and I believe Mother is right.] We had pâté de foi gras in jelly, partridge with the tail feathers flying, rosy goblets so large I had to pick them up in two hands, a lovely dinner and she is always a bewitching hostess."

For my birthday, my sister Peg sent me some nuts "the shells of which are strewn on the floor as thick as a swarm of locusts," I wrote.

> There is something fine and understanding about a sister who sends food. In your maiden days you used to give me beautiful jars and vases and equally enchanting knick knacks, all of which comply with the adage, "A thing of beauty is a joy forever," but lose sight of the fact that forever is infinite and the human mind is but a trammeled mite of finitude, totally incapable of grasping the significance of such abstractions as infinity. Hence give to me a lot of fun, for a week. . . . I like my fun where I find it and preferably in the present tense. We have been leading the usual Medical School life of a week of work and a weekend of all manner of evil, and it is really much more fun this year than last.

The "all manner of evil" probably referred to visits with Jane, for we did meet from time to time in New Haven, Boston, or Northampton, and toward the end of November I had a long letter from her which spoke not only of our visits but also of her delight in the cultural aspects of Smith College—the lectures by Norman Thomas on international affairs and one by a Frenchman on the League of Nation's staff, and also a concert by the Spanish pianist, Jose Iturbi. Jane wrote for four pages about these lectures and the problems they raised, and then went on to discuss another international relationship, that of Winston Churchill's son Randolph with Jane's sister, Kay Halle.

Jane said she was currently reading Winston's biography and that Kay and Randolph probably would be in New Haven for the Yale-Harvard game and that all of us should plan to meet there.

I don't think we ever did meet Randolph Churchill at the game, but he was on a lecture tour and on December 7, in Boston, I had dinner with him at the Harvey Cushings' house. He was nineteen years old, and was, I wrote, "like a fiery little furnace of irrational and beautifully verbalized enthusiasm. We all ended up in a pitched battle on the field of international politics and numerous other questions equally far above all our heads and nearly broke off relations with Great Britain."

The headlines in the *Herald Tribune* of December 14 read "Science Awaits Outcome of Tests on Laboratory Production of Life as Dr. George W. Crile Aims to Create Living Cell in Glass Tube." It is not difficult to imagine the controversy that arose. "If Dr. George W. Crile of Cleveland has really accomplished what is claimed for him in current newspaper dispatches he has established his place in a seat of honor sought for since the Middle Ages." Mother, in commenting on the controversy, told of the Guelph Treasure of biblical bones and relics that had just come to the Cleveland Museum of Art and added that "perhaps after the reported finding of a grave marked 'Jesus Son of Joseph' the Christian World will not mind so much an autosynthetic cell." My father, at the same time, was invited to give three or four lectures in Argentina as a guest of their surgical association. His fame was worldwide.

Although I have no recollection of this aspect of my life in medical school, a letter dated January 23, 1931, says that "eight of us got together hockey sticks and skates and traveled forth to Groton, where we played the Groton hockey team, defeating them in an overtime period, 5-4." The bacteriology course with the great Dr. Hans Zinser was over and I was happy to report not only that Zinser was one of the greatest teachers I had ever known, but also that he thought I was a good student and gave me an "Excellent." I added a plan that was doubtless disturbing to my mother: "The opera is in town and I am going to hear Tristam and Isolde. Maybe I'll go Saturday night too if plans come through and Jane comes down from Northampton, as she may do after her exams are over." I also told of a meeting of the Lancet Club, where a young economist who had visited Russia and worked there in farms and factories said that he thought the system was going to be a great success. "I have turned Socialist," I wrote my parents. "Why not condition the mind of man to strive for position and not for money, because the only reason we work for money is to gain position? After all, if this thing is a success, everyone will have comfortable living conditions, and as far as I'm concerned, a Ford is as good as a Rolls Royce and much more fun." That young Socialist had a profound effect on me, because to this very day I keep asking the same questions.

Winter had come to New England, and on January 30, 1931, I wrote to my family to tell them that Simmie, Dick Durant, John Trommald, Bart Quigley, Hall Seely, and I were going to go to Mount Monadnock in Jaffrey, New Hampshire, for a weekend of skiing. "We have a big Hay Ride on a sleigh planned for Saturday night, and Sunday we expect to ski and coast and skate or ride horseback. You get board and lodging for $4.00 apiece a day! I am taking Jane and maybe Ted Williams and John Briggs [Clevelanders] will join us."

All of us, of course, had girls with us and, although we were theoretically chaperoned because Hall Seely had his wife along, it would have been hard to get approval of parents for such a weekend at a hotel in New York or Boston. There was something about the word "skiing" and the aura of a good clean weekend of sports that made the parents forget or at least fail to inquire into the bedding arrangements. One of the reasons that the cost was only four dollars was that we all slept together in one big cabin, two to a bunk. Bundling they used to call it in the days of the Pilgrims. It was great fun.

My friends were beginning to fall about me right and left. Francis Sherwin, my old companion from Hotchkiss and Yale, suddenly ran off and married Jane's sister Margaret Halle. "I think it is good for both of them," I wrote Mother. "They are a great pair. Mag is a darn good girl and I think Franny did well. I never thought she'd have him."

By now my mother had given the name of Adam to my father's autosynthetic cell. In writing about the lecture and exhibit in Philadelphia she wrote that Dr. Telkes and Miss Rowland (my father's research worker and his secretary) went down to give a proper background for the debutante. "Dr. Telkes found the perfumes of ether a bit too potent—emanating from the precious lipoids and proteins—so had to entrust our precious Adam to the mercies of the porter. However, when the proper time came for the first dance Adam was fit, and over a thousand students and professors came to be introduced."

In February in Cleveland two things happened. One was a testimonial dinner for 250 people in honor of my father and given by his professional colleagues. The other was Mother's receipt of Groucho Marx's book entitled *Beds*, which had been sent to me by Jane. I forwarded it to Mother, not telling her who gave me the book, and she wrote, "I fear you will feel that your book 'Beds' laid me out. Not at all. To be sure I found it necessary occasionally to catch my breath and to pull myself up by my bootstraps from an unenlightened age into a modern one, but don't forget that the Victorian was an age of subtleties. People did not wear their characters on their sleeves. What I really want to know is what girl recommended the book to you! I confess, however, I laughed aloud in places and in places I found myself blushing to the four walls, and wondering just how litmus feels when it turns red!"

In March, Dad was invited to join Albert Einstein's party on a trip to New York, and the two of them had long talks about my father's theories. Einstein said that he thought the autosynthetic cell was indeed a "living thing" but he added that the word "life" had no scientific meaning. Einstein apparently was as tactful as he was clever.

By the time that spring began we were beginning to study physical diagnosis and to see some patients. This was really exciting, "I never learned so much in so short a time before in my life," I wrote Mother.

Mother's reply was all about Einstein, physics, and mathematics: "I myself am going back to millions of years ago when I swirled about, hungry for a mate, amidst the great ocean of primeval matter, as it transformed itself into radiation in order to produce the infinitesimal bit of inert ash on which I was born, as to whether or not I was imprisoned in a sparkling crystal, or blobbed about on a bit of green scum, I do not care, for I firmly believe that what separates the living from the non-living is only a process of complication." My father had converted her!

Spring was coming to Boston and I was beginning to really enjoy my work—particularly pathology and bacteriology.

March 15, 1931

Dear Mother & Dad,

The Irish box of green candies and fruits was as pleasing to the palate as to the eye. I am most thankful for my Irish heritage. [About once a week, Mother, without regard for the disasters that attended such a diet, was in the habit of sending me a box full of delicacies.] Wednesday night some of us went down to the Massachusetts General Hospital and heard a discussion on hypersensitivity by Zinser, Racheman and Roseman. It was the best thing I've ever heard and one of the most profitable evenings I ever spent. I can't tell you how much admiration I have for this man Zinser. He's the most energetic power-house of all vital activities, which include a boundless capacity for work, a wonderful and absurd sense of humor laden with practical joking and a thorough good sport. There are more tales of his private life than you could write in a *volume.*

The depression was deepening and my roommate Bud Yandell was running out of money and was trying to get a job at Huntington Hospital that would give him board, lodging, and laundry. "I thought a note from you might help him land it," I wrote my father. "I don't think you have to say much except that you've known Hays R. Yandell a long time and maybe a couple of remarks. Thanks a lot. Love, Barney."

Mother in her next letter said, "Sunday Dr. Lupton almost preached a sermon on Dad. The subject was 'What if Science Produces Life?' Of course he hitches his cell onto the tail of God. In fact he feels it is Millikan and God and Millikan and Crile, good company, anyway, however one interprets it." (Millikan was the Cleveland physicist who won the Nobel Prize in Physics.) Mother continued, "Lupton is a Unitarian and he went hand in hand as far as he could with science, and when it stopped the research was gathered into the bosom of the Father."

Mother went on to say that "your little investment [in stocks] netted $400. Isn't that fine. The Kensington [real estate property] is slowly getting on its feet. Mr. Martin telephoned today that he could distribute $500 apiece [to the four children] if we told him to do so. That will make $1500 that each of you will have had this year." In 1931 that was enough to put me through medical school. "I also feel as if I had made a lot of money," Mother continued, "for by losing so much last year we do not have to pay much of anything in income tax this year. But times are pretty terrible. Today someone came in whom I used to know, actually asking for $5.00 for food. She gives dancing lessons, but people do not pay. Meanwhile, she cannot pay her board or her grocer's bills."

Mother wrote also of a big meat company that had failed because people did not pay their dues to clubs and so clubs could not pay their bills to suppliers. Uncollectible accounts worth $35,000 were selling for $3,000, she said, and noted that it was wonderful that the Clinic had gotten through without red ink: "In fact they really will have put by one third of the cost of the new building this year. I am just too proud for words, aren't you?"

March 23, 1931

Dear Mother and Dad,

I had a good week last week, getting a lucky break on the gross Pathology oral and being asked about hearts, which subject I knew cold, and also getting back a 100 on a path. Slide quiz and another X in Pharmacology with a note of congratulation from Hale (who teaches the course) telling me I had the highest record in the class on the first three. There is one more Pharmacology quiz to go, so things look pretty good in that direction.

There's all the old examination hullabaloo in the air again— everything just as tense as a violin string and everyone starting rumors about what they will ask or what they have asked in previous years. Pathology, of course, is the most important course of the first two years, and so the excitement is proportional. No one gets any sleep and they develop weird symptoms of all sorts and go rushing about for stethoscopes to listen to their hearts. Bud got in bed last night and thought he was going to have a breakdown. Max has given up his exercise. Trommald hasn't had a date for four days. Simmons is in the library pouring over references he can't understand. And I will probably flunk the exam because I can't get excited or even work up enough enthusiasm to study very much for it.

Thanks so much for the pictures of the cell and the explanation. I have showed them about a bit and they excite much interest. It is a most striking summary.

Love
Barney

P.S. Did you send Franny and Mag a wedding present for me? They leave for Europe soon, and I ought to give them something nice.

In reply my father wrote: "Dear old Barney, I thought again and again of the news referred to by Bud Yandell," who, in thanking my father for his letter of recommendation, mentioned that I was leading the class in grades. "Whatever may come you have led the highest quality class of medical students for two years and these are the two most intellectual years. If fortune should be kind to you for two more years you will have choice of almost anything."

But things weren't all going smoothly in Boston. On March 29, I wrote that "The Pathology exam came and went like a tornado, leaving desolation in its wake." I used about one thousand words on the details of this disaster, telling how I had spent a lot of time describing a slide as a cancer of the breast and then had to switch my diagnosis to inflammation of the pancreas. I wrote up two or more accounts of each of the three slides that I was given, and in so doing ran overtime half an hour into the next part of the exam.

The first written question was about lesions of the eye in a hypopy-on ulcer, but I'd never read or heard of such a thing so "I spouted about six pages of uncoordinated and totally incorrect and unrelated information containing all the unassorted facts that I could remember of ever having heard about the eye." This went on and on and finally,

I got a stenosis of the writing center on the fifth question which was "What could cause a unilateral enlargement of cervical nodes and discuss the distinctive pathological features of each?" Tearing over the pages into the last question, I had five minutes left to classify and discuss the pathology of all nephritis with the suppurative types and give their distinguishing pathology and clinical features. My heart was now up to 140 and a systolic mur-mur was heard at the apex. Moist rales were marked at the right base posteriorly. The abdomen was negative except for a large mass appearing above the symphysis in the midline. The entire body was bathed in a cold sweat and there was a pronounced tremor which made the window panes shake. The history re-vealed that there was no family history of examination failure.

This description went on for another paragraph during which "the patient rapidly passed into coma and after several convulsive move-ments, died of respiratory paralysis. The autopsy revealed"—and there is half a page more of the findings including "metastases to all the organs where they were growing in caseous masses and in the form of small white mice." I concluded, "Anyway I hit the slides right and cracked the gross exam. I really don't care a great deal, as I know I know enough pathology."

I must have done well on that exam, because I was given an excel-lent in the course for the year and in six of the seven other courses. In the minor course of neuropathology I received a passing mark. From then on, there would be far less science and theory and much more emphasis on the clinical aspects of medicine. But first came Easter va-cation. In fact, to my astonishment, I had just gotten permission to go to Bermuda with my friend John Trommald for the break: "Dad ap-proves of it with no reservation so go to it and best of luck. Am depos-iting April check today." The telegram was signed by Mother.

In 1931 there was no air service to Bermuda. John and I had a cabin on the *Fort St. George.* Aboard we met a Mr. and Mrs. Babcock whom we liked very much and asked to join us in a bridge game—a recreation at which I am ashamed to say we used to spend too much time in our gathering room in the dormitory. We mentioned a tenth of a cent a point and Mr. Babcock, who was the son-in-law of Reynolds, the tobacco king, shook his head and murmured that that was a bit steep. We instantly offered to play for nothing, but the Babcocks relented and consented to wager a tenth of a cent. They were very amusing, telling us first that they had three children, then that they were on their honeymoon. And so it went, we soon catching on and starting a game of competitive lying which passed away the rest of the trip most delightfully.

We thought that Bermuda was very expensive. It cost us one hundred dollars apiece for hotel, meals, bicycle rental, and everything for three days on the island! It was jammed with people and our hotel room had nothing but a double bed, so we put the mattress on the floor and took turns on it. Sometimes, during the midnight hours, when I was asleep on the floor, I had dreams that my friend John was not alone in his bed.

We knew many of the college people who were vacationing there and there were lots of girls that we knew. It was too expensive to eat at the hotel, so we turned adventurers. The only way we could afford to eat was on our personality. So at dinner time we dressed up most immaculately and went around to one hotel after another and strolled into the dining room, sat down with any acquaintance, politely declined all proffered invitations to order, but nibbled daintily at hors d'oeuvres, remnants of salads and sandwiches and whenever eyes were turned away slipped great rolls into our pockets. John followed a troop of New York debs for three days because every noon they all ordered club sandwiches and most of them, being on a diet, ate only half, which left us a hearty sustenance. There was dancing at other hotels and always a date with someone. I had a different date every night. The island was run over with girls. You had to beat them off. I got so sick of dates and girls that I hoped never to see one again. (A wish that was not fulfilled.)

In spite of the girls we bicycled the island from end to end and loved it. The ocean shores, especially along the inlets and bays, reminded me much of Timagami, with steep sloping rocks and many tiny islands. The natives were most extraordinary, blacks all speaking English with an Oxford accent and with the most perfect choice of English and a most variegated vocabulary. Before we left we hired a boat and spent a day on the reefs, fishing. But we didn't catch a single fish or even get a nibble.

At home it was spring and the trout fishing had started at Castalia. My father's mind was temporarily abstracted from its preoccupation with the autosynthetic cell, and he wrote that "Friday at 12:30 Mother and I started by motor for Wheeling where I gave a lecture and we swung around by night and the next day to Castalia where I helped to open the season, and I caught three fish in an hour. The birds were out en masse, the fish sporty down in the mill race where the big fish lay. Well the float is gone, leaving only four stakes, and sure enough here lay three great fish."

It was good to hear from Dad about something besides The Cell. In spite of the fish, however, his mind was on other things. On April 23, my mother wrote that he had given a public lecture for the Academy of Medicine, that the hall was filled with twenty-two hundred people and more than five hundred were turned away. "Tuesday Dad was presented with the Cleveland Chamber of Commerce Medal for public service." And, "Did I tell you that the Knob is open and that Dad and I went out there last Saturday and spent the night. The woods were carpeted with wild flowers, the day was actually hot, and Mary Bell and Jack hovered over us as if we were their grandchildren. We were all alone and it was wonderful. I read aloud to Dad late into the evening of the days of Nero. His hair stood on end before I finished and he agreed that our modern age is puritanical in contrast."

But Dad's obsession was not over. In the next letter he wrote:

Dear Barney,

By mixing some thyroxine, iron and calcium with the liver lipoid, protein and electrolytes, we are now getting better cells and they show a slight respiration. So we see the possibility of building up a better animal.

There will be a rather bitter controversy ahead, to which I will look with joy. It will consolidate our work—and speed up our program. The external structure of the new building is now completed and the entire building should be ready by July 15th.

Lots of love
Dad

Mother too continued with her obsession and on April 28 wrote, "Our funds and yours are at low ebb! Keep out of cards and away from girls. Both are expensive." By this time we had stopped playing bridge. Too many of us were flunking out as a result of the wasted time. But neither I nor my friends paid much attention to Mother's sage advice about women.

The clinical studies were starting, and I wrote, "In Medicine we go over patients—mostly the chests—and I find that I am no earthly good at it. I swear that I don't hear or observe a tenth of what I should. I have consolation that others are about as bad, but it is clear enough that it is a long road ahead before one can learn to observe and interpret physical signs."

Mother told of the opera week just finished—men in gloves, women decked out in all their finery. "The hall was crowded and little Pons created such a furor that people stood in their seats and bravoed or clapped. It is a strange thing that opera can come here for a week and that that great hall can be filled to capacity—ten thousand people—with seats ranging from one dollar to seven dollars"—ten to seventy in today's values—"and during a depression like this. Of course, I do think a lot of people like Madame Klein [my former French teacher] all year put by savings for the opera."

I wrote to Mother that Bud and I had been elected to the Boylston Society that picks twelve of the first twenty men in the class. Twice a month there is a meeting and a scientific address and discussion.

By the middle of May 1931, the total of the lawsuits based on the Clinic disaster was three and three-quarter million dollars—more than all the assets of the Clinic, the Criles, the Phillipses, and the Lowers, all of which were named in the suits. Along with it all came anonymous letters, one of them saying that "Dr. Crile wouldn't give a thought to what the anniversary of the disaster meant to others, but instead would probably be out playing golf because he wasn't a Christian anyway." Mother went on to say that "Ed was so nervous the last few days that he would have exploded if one struck a match near him, but Dad keeps his philosophy and keeps his eyes on the stars. In the meantime the cataphoresis treatments seem to aid in relieving pain, even in poor tragic Grace Mather." This was the first use of electrical currents that my father had devised to relieve pain and which now are widely used in pain centers. Mother went on, "In the less than 10 years since the Clinic Hospital opened we have had nearly 9,000 men visiting the Clinic to see operations—really to visit Dad's clinic. One thousand, one hundred and fourteen of them were foreigners from 50 different countries."

There were some celebrations in Boston before we all packed up and went to our homes. I remember that there were more violations of Prohibition than in the past. There also were many great singing parties in our rooms or on the lawns of friends. Max Eddy was one of the world's best basses—he could have been a pro. Dick Durant had sung tenor with the Yale Whiffenpoofs, and Dutch Wells was a natural baritone. I was a natural nothing, but knew all the words. It was great fun, for those were the days before TV, and everyone liked to gather around a piano which Yandell, with an inimitable beat, played by hands and feet and entirely by ear. On occasion I would still resort to my ukulele. And Bart Quigley, a professional actor in the summertime, would on the slightest provocation put on a monologue.

By this time many of us had gotten involved with girls that later on we married, but all of them weren't here in Boston, and most of us felt pretty free. Boston, with Wellesley and Radcliffe, attracted many girls, and Northampton and Vassar weren't far away. I remember one who had come down from Canada—the Governor General's Daughter, we called her—and that spring she occupied much of my time. I never saw her again.

Gradually the load of young women to whom I felt somewhat responsible became lighter. A letter from Tommie told of her engagement to a friend from Yale—Fletcher Nice. Toto also seemed to have strayed away. Jane was home that summer, but during the week I was busy at the Clinic. In late August, I went on to the elaborate Long Island wedding of Lloyd Smith, my old Bones friend and former editor of the *Yale News*.

At home I worked again in the laboratory and wrote a chapter, "Iodine and the Thyroid Gland," for my father's forthcoming book on *Diagnosis and Treatment of Diseases of the Thyroid Gland*. It was my first published work, and I was gratified when two reviewers, one of them from England, selected that chapter for commendation. Then it was back to Boston for another year of medicine.

Right after the second year of medical school, I took the National Board Medical Examination, and got a mark of 91.33, the eighth highest of the 679 who took the examination. "I feel like celebrating your success," my father wrote, "You scarcely know how much this means to me, for it tells me you have the ability to take successfully your full part in this highly competitive field—for the great rewards are only at the top—and around the top there is always lively contest. I am proud of you. Dad."

The next day he wrote again, repeating the praise and saying, "Of all things to take first place in pathology, the hardest subject, is a triumph and must be the greatest satisfaction to you. I give you equally good credit for your paper on Iodine and the Thyroid Gland."

In spite of my father's elation, I don't think that high marks in medical school necessarily betoken success in a medical career. Some of the most successful surgeons in our class were nowhere near the top scholastically and some of those near the top never amounted to anything. For example, Max Eddy, who kept flunking out of medical school and took six years instead of four to graduate, ended up as head of his hospital's surgical department, and was a respected member of the revered New England Surgical Society before Bert Dunphy, also one of my classmates and ultimately the most successful surgeon of them all, was even elected to that society. Incidentally, it is interesting that in 1931 nine of the eleven top men in the National Board Examination were from Harvard. One was from Michigan and one from McGill.

In the third year of medical school, the clinical work started and suddenly everything seemed to come to life. I began to appreciate what my father had told me since I was six years old: "Look for the meaning of things and their purpose—everything is there for a purpose and if you once find it you'll never forget it. You must visualize the inner process responsible for the symptoms and rationalize every symptom of disease."

However, I was still having a hard time with my parents. I liked to drink beer on Saturday nights, and sometimes sips from a bottle of bootleg Scotch were available. I still was a virgin and I never had so much to drink that I got into trouble. My father stood firm against liquor, but was lenient about my relationships with women. My mother, on the other hand, saw nothing wrong with a drink now and then, but absolutely forbade any involvements with the other sex. If I had taken my parents' prohibitions seriously, my life would have been ruined.

After Jane finished up at college she took a trip abroad, ending up in a spot on the Dalmatian coast, which then she called Ragusa but now is known as Dubrovnik. It is an ancient, walled city with a sheltered harbor on the island-filled coast of the blue Adriatic. There she was wont to go sailing with a Yugoslavian youth. The details of these voyages Jane never related, but it seemed to me that in some respects she was a little different when she returned from that trip.

Then too, Jane spent much time in the winters of those years after college with a friend, Bub Hanna, whose family had a huge and luxurious plantation in the stylish winter resort of Thomasville, Georgia. I thought that she probably was gone for good, for her friend was handsome and attractive. What happened I never knew, but by summertime we were back together again on weekends in Cleveland. Still, of course, since I had another year of medical school there was no talk of marriage.

During the year, she would come on for occasional weekends, and we still went up to New Hampshire in great bands of couples to cohabitate in ski bungalows. There also were local girls in Boston who came and went, but I never became involved. The Cushings continued to be most hospitable, frequently asking my friends and me to Sunday lunch where Mary and Betsy, quite attached to their famous lovers or husbands, would smoke cigarettes with us and their mother and then, when the steps of Dr. Cushing were heard approaching, would extinguish and hide them or pile them on our ashtrays. All of us were fond of the Cushing family, each member of which was fascinating in his or her highly individual way.

In spite of the social and intellectual life of Boston, I was still thinking of home.

September 23, 1931

Dear Dad,

I didn't have an opportunity of telling you as I left how much this summer at the Clinic has meant to me in every way. But I do want you to know how proud I am of the Clinic and of you and how much I feel with you in the joy of achievement you must have had at the opening of the new building. I always think of the lines in the "Defense" paper which I here misquote "To perpetuate in brick and mortar the ideals they (he) have always held."

And so again my regrets that I was unable to be home to share your triumph Monday.

Barney

Vanderbilt Hall
Boston, Mass.
September 30, 1931

Dear Dad,

This term we are taking Medicine all day Monday, Wednesday and Friday—in the out patient department in morning—taking histories and doing physicals and attending bedside clinics with Means [a marvelous and very famous internist] in the afternoon. Tuesday, Thursday and Saturday we have dermatology and syphilology in the mornings and a Cabot clinic Tuesday afternoon and a Christian [the famous Dr. Henry Christian] clinic Thursday. So time is full.

Today was the first day of Medicine, and Trommald and I were turned loose on a woman suffering from ureteral stone, ovarian deficiency, some gastric distress, hemorrhoids, headaches, nervousness, generalized pains and obesity. She had had ten operations and spent her entire life in bed. So our history took nearly three hours to get and we missed lunch in working the darn thing out. I have never seen such a one-piece museum of female pathology.

Love
Barney

About this time, my parents were deeply concerned about my brother Bob who had not been doing well in school and who had lost a lot of weight. Tests and X-rays revealed no cause for his illness, but they decided, quite rightly, that he should take a year off. They sent him to the southwest with one of the curators of the Cleveland Museum of Natural History (which my father had helped found) to collect animals for his studies on the relative size, function, and weights of the brain, liver, thyroid, and adrenal glands. Bob loved it. He had a healthy and productive year, and came home with normal weight and energy, and went on with his schooling. Several years later, when an X-ray was taken for some other cause, he was found to have such extensive calcification of the lymph nodes in his abdomen that he was declared ineligible for the draft. Was it tuberculosis of the lymph nodes, of the same type that killed two of my father's sisters, or was it some other infection? We never knew and he never had any more trouble.

Cleveland was suffering effects from the depression, as my father wrote:

November 1931

Dear Barney,

Financial conditions in Cleveland apparently have grown worse, but happily the Clinic is keeping its income above expenses. . . . Yale did finely in Chicago [football].

Love
Dad

The depression was apparent in Boston too, because I wrote to my parents:

Tomorrow afternoon Wells, Eddy, Yandell and I plan to go out and play touch football at Wells' old prep school somewhere around here. None of us can afford to go to football games this year. Poor old Bud's bonds are out of sight and Dutch has had nothing but salary cuts since he started work.

In spite of the hardships, I wrote home: "This is the best year I have ever spent. There is absolutely no routine or drudgery and everything is new and interesting. I don't see how anyone who has ever had a taste of Medicine could ever be interested in anything else."

In this same letter I told my father of a complicated case in which there was a goiter and intermittent attacks of nervousness and fast pulse. I asked him about diagnosis and treatment, and he answered as, in retrospect, I would have predicted: "You described your case perfectly. I do not think it could be hyperthyroidism. If you could rule out the mental factors it would be a nice case to do an adrenal denervation."

More and more as he grew older, my father was trying to find the solution to all obscure problems by denervating the adrenals. I had not yet become aware that this might represent a change in his ability to make sound clinical judgements.

About this time Mother wrote, almost jealously, of the experience of a friend, Dr. Fulton, in Tanganyika, who "got nine leopards, five lions," and so forth, and his daughter, "who is a beauty and is 23, got a lion at 70 yards—in one shot. He, like everyone else has just one desire—to go again." In those days there wasn't a thought about conservation of wildlife.

As an example of how widely my father's reputation had spread, Mother wrote about a friend who had been on a trip around the world:

When in Kandy, Ceylon, she bought a tortoise-shell cigarette case for Dad. While buying it, she got into conversation with the jeweler and he asked her from what part of America she came, and when she said "Ohio" he said, "Do you know Dr. Crile?" She said, "Why he operated on me." With that he dashed over to her and shook her hands so enthusiastically that she said "Why, do you know Dr. Crile?", and he said, "Oh no, but I've read about him. I think he's the greatest surgeon in the world."

Mother also mentioned another example of my father's fame: "Dad and I were invited to a reception at the White House next Thursday. I am sorry we cannot go, but in these days I would not spend money even to go to a reception at the White House." But my father went to a "gridiron dinner" in Washington where, among the celebrities, he was introduced.

Excerpt from a letter from Mother dated November 16, 1931: "I don't know anything about more law suits, but collections at the clinic are terrible. Dad came home so happy over his visit with you and the wonderful word he received in the Dean's office that you led your class the first two years."

In spite of the depression, we seemed to be having a good time in Boston. I wrote home saying, "Friday night we went to a law-school dance which really amounted to a gigantic Yale reunion of everyone in all the graduate schools of Harvard. As a result it was a perfect party. Saturday night we all went over to Henry Woodbridge's, a friend of

Dutch's for supper. All of our crowd were there, and we had a quiet enough evening with lots of fun just sitting around, singing, talking and what not." I had not mentioned to Mother that Jane had come for the weekend, but she found out because in the next paragraph I told about driving her up to Northampton to visit her sister and driving back to Boston in a terrific fog, "at a snail's pace with Jane leaning out the side to watch the curb and shout which way the road went."

In my mother's letters there was much about the polio epidemic which had hit Hotchkiss, and forced a temporary closing of the school. It is easy to forget what a threat and terror that disease was before the advent of the vaccine. On December 4, she wrote that all the banks in the West were "busted" and it was the same in the East, and that a lawyer told her he didn't think there was an insurance company in the country that was solvent in the sense of having liquid funds. A physician friend of Dad's had given his lawyer power of attorney. The lawyer had speculated and lost everything in the doctor's estate and had in addition embezzled $75,000 of the funds of the bank. The doctor had come to my father and said he hadn't a cent in the world and that his wife was in New York with no money to get herself home.

In 1932, one of my father's real estate properties, the Kensington—the returns from which had been used to educate all of us children—had suddenly fallen victim to a tax dispute in which a payment of $115,000 was demanded by the government. Today that would be $1,115,000. Of course my family didn't have it. A settlement for $50,000 finally was arranged and slowly paid off.

Unperturbed by these financial disasters, for he still had his somewhat reduced salary from the Clinic and my mother had a little independent income, my father remained happy in what he thought was my success. He wrote that "Harvey Cushing sent word by Dr. Haden that you had a certain standing which gave Harvey a kick, but you may be sure it was as nothing compared with what I got out of it." Dr. Cushing was a loyal friend of my father's and a true foster father to all of us who came down to Harvard from Yale.

My next letter home told of an experience encountered in the study of psychiatry:

Bud and I were locked into a small room with a schizophrenic for an hour. Every question we would ask him he would reply by asking us the same question. He became very insulting and finally began to slap Bud's face. When we tried to get out we found the door locked and no one around to open it, so we had to beat him off for about ten minutes until the nurse came. Another patient whom we had over there has become convinced that I am the cause of all his trouble and insists that because I wrote things down that he said in a book I am plotting against him and am the reason for his being held in the hospital. I don't dare see him anymore. Thank God psychiatry is over, as I was beginning to get not a little bored with the terminology and with the display of adjectives. We have now to work up and write up a case for our final exam and my patient is nothing but a darn liar. She won't tell the same story twice, and while I talk to her all the other patients gather around and listen and make crazy remarks, none of which is conducive to the conduction of a rational analysis.

Next I tell of a dinner with Max and Bud and Sim and his father and a friend, in which we had ten quail sent to Bud by his Texas father, fifteen lamb chops, twelve frankfurts, one pound of bacon as well as peas, potatoes, etc. (and the next day seven pounds of steak), all of which we cooked ourselves and found to our surprise to be delicious. Small wonder that at present only two of these six would still be alive. "We had a poker game in the evening, and I hit a grand streak of cards, and using my education of sophomore year at Yale, ended up the big winner" (probably about five dollars as we played for a tenth of a cent a point).

I wrote the family, "We have now become masters of the art of gynecology and are starting off on laryngology. As soon as we half understand what a course is all about it is over." I also mentioned that I'd had dinner at the Cushings. He was retiring from Harvard and was wavering between going to Johns Hopkins or Yale, and that Dr. Cutler probably was going to come from Western Reserve and become professor of surgery in Cushing's place. I also bemoaned the fact that most of my former girlfriends were getting married and my nonmedical male companions were going that road too.

The news from Cleveland's economic front got even worse. In January 1932 my father wrote, "For all last year we had 3% fewer patients through the Clinic and 5% fewer operations than in the year before, but the financial returns were much below. We will just about get through January whole, likely in the red, but not much. Real estate is more drab than ever. The research is coming on finely, and tomorrow we will perform the 140th adrenal operation—adrenalectomies and denervations. This work is all right. We now have in patients under 45 years of age, 1297 operations on the thyroid without a death." He closed, "The suits still hang over us as usual. I think I shall miss them when they are gone. Best of Luck, Dad."

My father was still collecting animals for his research on the "kinetic systems" and Mother wrote of an expedition to Detroit to harvest from the zoo a lion, a bear, and a baboon which they chloroformed or shot and brought back to Cleveland for dissection and weighing of the organs. "Fuller and Phillips skinned and then turned the carcasses over to the vultures of the Clinic. Bob went in for adrenals and kidneys and thyroid glands. Ruedman pounced on the eyes, and those of the lion were larger than golf balls. Gardner scooped out the brains. Ed [Lower] not wanting to be left out took his choice bits [he was a urologist], and so it went. It reminded me of the struggle among the natives, the wild beasts and the vultures in Africa."

In the same letter, philosophizing on my father's research, Mother wrote, "Wouldn't it be fun to get the adrenal glands of a comfortable lady, born and bred in the comfortable autocaptivity of luxury and ease, and contrast her apparatus [adrenals etc.] with that of the Pygmy lady who has to catch the bird that she eats, or hit it with a poisoned arrow, or the harassed and driving Jew against the smug and comfortable Buddhist priest?"

I wrote home to say that Max and I had

reinstituted the old custom of bowling. It is the greatest game in the world but too expensive and darn unsatisfactory as I get worse at it all the time. Laryngology is a joke. I can't see through my head mirror, to say nothing of being able to observe the nasopharynx through a tiny mirror. We all don gowns and nice new mirrors and look like the doctors in the yeast ads—and probably know just as much. Well, things are certainly looking as bad as ever, aren't they? No one is any better off though, and if things do collapse and the world falls into ruin, we'll all be hungry and naked together, and the doctor will be way ahead because people will still get sick and we doctors can live on the surgical specimens we remove, if worse comes to worst. Pathology was always my favorite subject anyway.

Then I described our outpatient work at the Boston City:

The system at that darn hospital is so rotten that when you give an infusion you have to boil up your own apparatus and then sit and run it under pressure instead of having it go by gravity. Like the building of the Pyramids, that institution has a wealth of slave power and very little equipment.

We saw the resident surgeon butcher a poor old Negro with [intestinal] obstruction, for which a cecostomy was done.

In those days the residents were not supervised by the staff, and they gloried in their privilege of independent operations. In fact, training programs like the Cleveland Clinic's, in which residents did not have "full responsibility," were severely criticized.

He was distended to begin with, and by the time they had explored him for half an hour he was bloated. Then for 15 minutes by the clock they took great handfuls of intestines and tried to wrestle them back in, to no avail. It reminded me exactly of your shock research. Finally the man died on the table, and that gave enough relaxation to get the guts back in, especially since the ether was kept on even after respiration stopped. Miraculously, he revived and was endowed with ten hours of life before he died for good and all. I forgot to mention that the tube slipped out of the cecum and spilled intestinal contents all through the peritoneum. I picked up a point or two about surgery in that operation—on the negative side.

I performed my first major surgical operation in official capacity Friday, when I opened an abscess in the neck under ethyl chloride [local freezing]. The outpatient is a lot of fun, as we dress all sorts of wounds each day and have an opportunity to follow them along. I am impressed with the efficiency of the nonspecific protein therapy of furunculosis [boils], carbuncles, etc. It seems that the antibodies or some resistance factor must be definitely raised in response to these injections. I wonder if it would be worth while to use this preoperatively on the thyroids or other patients who are in the hospital long enough preoperatively for it to have effect. I think it would be worth running a series this summer to see if we get less serum, infection, etc. I've got some other, more complicated problems I want to talk over with you too.

I went on to tell of our experience in urology at the City Hospital where we were treating "thousands of cases of gonorrhea, giving anterior permanganate washes"—injecting a stinging, burning solution of potassium permanganate into the already inflamed urethra, a treatment which it was later shown caused a striking increase in the number of strictures of the urethra. This complication often necessitated complicated reparative surgery. I concluded, "I am beginning to have a feeling that morality is not on as high a plane as the ministers would care to have it."

I then went on to tell of going to the Woman's Free Hospital to get a follow-up on a patient with a suspected cancer of the bowel.

A young lady there said she would write me the report as soon as it came in. A week later I was at the Copley dancing, when a friend came over and brought with him a gorgeous blonde literally poured into a clinging dress of shimmering blue satin. She was exquisite from top to toe and one of the loveliest creatures I have ever seen. She seemed vaguely familiar, and as I groped for her name she came towards me. I was about to confess my stupidity with apologies and ask her if it could have been at her chateau on the Riviera that we had met when she volunteered, "You know that Miss Jackson whom you were asking about *did* have a cancer of the rectum."

I continued on a different topic: "It may be of interest to you to know that Jane is wintering with the Hannas in Thomasville. It looks as if this is getting to be 'serious business.' I am going to spend a lonely summer if John continues with Toto and all of this continues." I went on to ask my father what specialty courses he thought would be most valuable for me, neurology, gynecology, X-ray, or orthopedics.

"I think it would be a good idea for you to take gynecology," my father replied. "The next choice would be neurology."

Mother wrote, "Dad has a chance to get an alligator that was in a fight and lost a leg, for $25. Wouldn't it be fun to go in after his adrenals?" She mentioned that her nephews, the McBrides, who were in school in the East, would be coming home by bus because it cost only $18.00 round trip compared with $20.85 for an upper berth in a train one way. She also told of a visiting friend, General H. L. Gilchrist, who knew Dad in the war, and told her that Dad had brought a whole carload of unexploded shells back with him from a trip to the front where he had picked them up as souvenirs. I still have many of these polished brass shell cases, even one of the huge cases of the German Big Bertha shells, but the explosives have by now been removed. "Providence alone saw you through that trip, Crile," the general is alleged to have said. "Isn't that a typical tale of the way Dad goes after things?" Mother commented.

She also spoke of my father's obsession with his research and his writing. "We had a wild time getting Dad off to Washington. He has so much chemistry and explosives in his head he simply cannot be trusted with a pencil in his pocket. Every time he stops, he sits down and writes and, of course, the result is he writes the same thing over and over again. Well, finally he began to cut out some and then began the process of patching. We spent a week at it, and would no sooner have it finished, we thought, than he would telephone for it to be sent to the Clinic and it would come back all rewritten again." This obsession arose, probably, because my father had never had any formal training in chemistry and more or less invented it as he went along to make it match and explain his theories. He would have been a magnificent novelist if he had ever put his pen to fiction.

And more from me in medical school:

March 21, 1932

Dear Mother and Dad,

I know for certain that I will never become a pediatrician. The other day my first infant came in and lay on the table squalling while the mother stood by looking as if she thought I was the kidnapper of Lindbergh's baby. I observed the little animal for a moment or so, drawing a complete blank on what to look for and trying to appear wise and expert for the mother's benefit. Then I completely ran out of anything more to do, so I decided I would have to turn the baby over.

Next came a long description of my unsuccessful attempt to turn the baby, of its bitter resistance, of my nearly dislocating the baby's shoulder in the struggle and of the mother's running forward and saying, "I'll turn him over for you, doctor."

I have been observing deliveries at the Lying-in-Hospital. My first sight was a real surprise because the baby was so blue that I thought it could never live, and when it started to breathe it seemed like a miracle. I am glad that I don't have to be born again. I think dying is a much easier and pleasant performance.

Betsy Cushing Roosevelt had a baby girl about a week ago, and I have never seen such a look on a man's face in my life as was on Jimmy Roosevelt's, when coming down in an elevator he saw Bud and me in white coats looking as if we were the chief surgeons of the Lying-in. He was terror stricken for he feared that perhaps we might have something to do with Betsy.

Mrs. Sanger of the Birth Control Movement came up to a Lancet Club dinner last week and gave us a most instructive talk. She is a most charming woman. (Her son, you know, was old Stewy Sanger, the end with whom I competed at Yale.) We had a lot of fun discussing everything from her experiences with the Japanese War Lords to football at college. After her talk, Sim, Max, Durant and I all piled into Sim's car with her and took her for the most hair-raising ride that she had ever had, down to the hotel. Sim's car has no brakes and it was a rainy night, but she was a darn good sport.

In April I was still on the obstetrical service in "the district"—the poor part of town where we would stay on call in a boarding house and go, when called, to deliver women in their homes. Our only training for this was observation of a few deliveries in the hospital.

Bud and I had a great time of it and I consider it to be the highlight of medical school. My first baby was darn near born while I was in the kitchen—the head *was* born in fact, and the placenta came somewhat tardily while I was in the drug store telephoning the house officer for instructions. Yet the family think I am a great doctor even in spite of a third degree tear.

The Italians are a wonderful people to work with and are intensely appreciative of what you do for them. They offer you meals or wine at every call and to them your word on any subject is the final arbiter. The women deafen you with prayers as the baby is being born and birth is an occasion for every friend or relative in the city to be present and watch with curiosity. Even the little children come in and, when they are tall enough to get their eyes over the edge of the bed, gaze with wonder at the perineum.

My father was in the East and visited me when I was on "the district." "I have rarely had such a kick out of anything as seeing you in action on your district service. You looked and acted like an old family practitioner. I have not the least doubt about your adaptation for the practice of medicine. You will get a great joy out of it." And he was right about that last remark.

In one of her letters to me, Mother told of the financial problem they were having with taxes on their huge Cleveland Heights house and large tract of land which had been evaluated at $208,000. That would be more than two million today. In 1916 they had paid only $80,000 for the house and land. On one of their downtown properties, the Ryder Building, the taxes were $22,000, the ground rent $20,000, but the property netted rental payments to my father of only $35,000. "Formerly," Mother wrote, "we had $45,000 a year out of the rear building alone—the garage—enough to cover taxes. Now we get $18,000 for it."

The depression seemed to have little effect on the social life of the Harvard Medical students. On April 17, 1932, I wrote my father and mother about a stunt that one of my favorite classmates, Bert Dunphy, and I played on his fraternity. He had agreed to provide a distinguished speaker for the annual banquet and had forgotten to arrange for it. We decided that Dunphy would be the speaker and that I would introduce him as Dr. Wyckoff, a distinguished British surgeon who was a friend of my father's and had had a productive career bringing Western surgical skill to India.

There was an epidemic of scarlet fever at the time, so Bert pretended to have a sore throat and to have gone to the infirmary. We next rented an outfit for the "Professor" to wear—a bushy black beard streaked with grey, steel-rimmed spectacles, a black hat and a sort of black cape and a venerable cutaway, a winged collar, and a flaming red tie. The Professor walked with a stoop, had a Parkinsonian tremor, and was quite deaf. My letter went as follows:

First we went to the infirmary, where the nurses stood back in amazement as the Professor went into a ward and raised the devil about the condition of the beds and the crowded conditions. He shouted for the superintendent and said he was going to report this shameful state of affairs to the authorities. All the nurses fluttered about and didn't know what to do. Finally he walked away swearing to himself.

We arrived late for dinner and the fuses had blown out so that the room was in darkness except for candles. The Professor looked like Mr. Hyde. There had been quite a bit of punch so the audience was more intrigued than critical. The Professor's deafness gave him time to weigh his replies and to disregard what questions he chose. At dinner the Professor limited his remarks to "Punjab, Punjab" which means "bottoms up" in India.

I introduced the Professor as a friend of my father's and a world authority on the relationship of the thyroid gland to pregnancy and the endemic goiter that is so prevalent in parts of India. The Professor was so deaf that he made no move to speak but joined in the applause. I shouted in his ear that he had misunderstood and that I had just introduced him, and said that he would tell of his adventures in India. Apparently the Professor again misunderstood, for he brought forth a tremendous manuscript and began to read a treatise on his work with 2194

Primipara in India in which he determined that the ratio of the L. Phototeric Iodides to the Amphiphototeric Iodide fraction was inversely proportional to the ratio of the Protopathic Phosphated molecule to the combined blood cholesterol. Several people began to take notes, but soon gave up. Many noticed that his paper was three inches thick.

After about five minutes I got up and told Dr. Wyckoff that we had not brought our notebooks, and would he please tell us about his adventures in India. The Professor grew furious and began to pan the U.S.A. He then ripped up American scientists and gave examples, including members of the Harvard Faculty. He called Dean Edsall a hydrocephalic with the biggest head that he had ever seen and nothing at all in it. "The only thing of value in his overbearing cranial cage is the salt in his ventricles." He said that "Dr. Cannon's first sympathectomy must have been on himself." Cushing was faulted because he charged by the hour, not by the operation. Zinser was described as a picturesque lab worker in a setting of flunkeys. And so it went on, the audience wide-eyed and disbelieving, but quite unaware of who was talking. Finally the Professor attacked the fraternity as a bunch of maudlin reprobate drunkards and neer-do-wells. "You Harvard hot shots are a bunch of lousy dollar hunters, you dirty bastards" were the final words. The audience was thunderstruck. Then the Professor grabbed one of the fellows, called him by name and shook him by the neck saying, "You Crummay, you won't ever amount to a —— and you ——."

He then got up on his chair and cursed and swore and even threw things before he was recognized. This was the same Bert Dunphy who in due course would be a distinguished surgical professor and author, as well as president of all of the most important surgical organizations of the country!

The evening ended in a similar fashion: "We stopped at a drug store to get ether to remove the beard. 'Will you have a large or a small can, doctor?' I asked. 'Heh?' he replied. 'I couldn't hear.' I repeated the question, much louder and everyone was staring. I went over and loudly ordered a small can of ether and a glass and a little ice. People were aghast. I explained that the doctor never drank anything but ether after sundown. So we hobbled out with our ether can, the people in the store being uncertain whether to be angry at or sorry for the old man."

The third year was coming to an end and there began to be thoughts about postgraduate training. The Clinic had an excellent residency program in the specialties, but at the time did not take interns. My father advised against the popular two-year program at the Philadelphia General Hospital where he said I would be wasting my time on obstetrics which I would not practice. He suggested that I look at Dr. Evarts Graham's service at Barnes Hospital in St. Louis. Later on I did, and was grateful to my father for his advice. In the same month of April, I was notified of my election to the honorary medical fraternity of Alpha Omega Alpha which, like Phi Beta Kappa, is awarded to the students who are scholastically at the top of their class.

The last course of the year was ophthalmology, which I enjoyed, and wrote that "It seems as though you were having a private peek into the inner secrets of metabolism, for there you see nerves and blood vessels lying naked for your inspection. It is almost unbelievable how much can be told of the patient as a whole from study of the eyes."

The year ended with a report that gave me "excellent" in ten subjects and "passed" in three. The three subjects in which I did not distinguish myself were dermatology and syphilology, gynecology, and G.U. surgery, all of them connected with sex. My father apparently wrote Dr. Cushing to thank him for his many kindnesses to me, and Dr. Cushing replied:

> July 1, 1932
>
> Dear George,
>   What a pleasant letter from you about our supposed kindnesses to Barney. Barney as you know stands easily at the top of his class and has the world at his feet, and you should be proud of him, as you and Grace doubtless are.

My father was a brave man. After spending some time in the summer vacation with the family on our island in Canada's Lake Timagami, he drove home with Bob and me, and as usual recorded on paper his impression of the journey.

> Once, Barney slowed down to what he thought was ample, namely 65 miles an hour, to make a sharp curve on rainy asphalt. The swerve of the car was somewhat more than at any other time. In this case the car executed a swerving skid, just this side of a complete circle—the car naturally emitted a loud screech and numerous snappy sounds incident to crystallization of steel

throughout the car. On the whole we did not lose materially in time, which after all, was all that mattered.

The very heavy darkness had a curious effect on the drivers; namely, the very resistance suggested by the black wall seemed to call for more speed and power. It was this that steadily stepped up our pace. In the midst of this column of darkness a blacker spot was seen. It quickly appeared as model T Ford with no tail light. The Ford moved uncertainly from side to side, confusing Bob who was now driving. On which side Bob passed the Ford there was no agreement.

My father had not only unlimited tolerance towards the behavior of his sons, but also a splendid sense of humor. He ended his reminiscence with the comment that none of us identified both Ashtabula and Conneaut. This led to the explanation; namely, "the gap in space between Ashtabula and Conneaut was filled in by the afterglow of passing Ashtabula just as the whirling bit of coal makes a complete ring and the same with the comet's tail."

In the summer of 1933, Yandell and I lived mostly at the Knob and wrote our "Sanitary Survey" of East Cleveland—all about matters of public health, water supply, sewers, education, etc.— a procedure that was a medical school requirement. We had good fun doing it, my father's secretary typed it up, and eventually we were given full credit for it. Then I worked again in the research laboratory, operating on rabbits and dogs for experiments, mainly on peptic ulcer, and continuing, through contacts with the staff and residents, to enlarge my medical vocabulary. I also did some writing for another book that my father was producing.

On the first page of the eight-by-eleven, two-inch thick collection of letters and memorabilia of my fourth year at medical school that my mother collected for me, my father wrote:

Dear Barney,

Here is another of Mother's creations, and as she read it to me this morning I got such a kick from the memories of that fine record you made that I asked to inscribe in it to tell you what a happy year for Mother and me solely on your Harvard record— all else [referring to the depression] was lost. You know the old adage—the boy is father to the man.

Dad

The book opens with a telegram from Albany, where I had been forced to stop on my way to school. "Recurrence of fan-belt luxation cured by specialist. All well. Barney." It was answered by my father who said he was glad that I had the service of a specialist and went on to say that the short vacation that Bob and I and he had had together in the Crile-Garretson cabin on Lake Timagami had been the highlight of his summer. Back at medical school, as a result of the maturation of the students and the decline of the economy, things had changed.

Dear Mother and Dad,

Upon arrival at medical school I found it an entirely different place with Dick and Bud moved out to take hospital jobs, John Trommald living in a different part of the building, Hopkins living at home, everyone's schedule taking them to all parts of Boston. There is no more of our delightful club-life of years past. There is no time for it anyway. The first day I was at Children's Hospital I had two cases to work up, was on call at night, had complete histories of what the parents and grandparents died of, thought of, voted for, favorite flowers—pages of the most irrelevant data—all to be transcribed longhand in florid style and complete physicals and lab work to be done. I got in at two-thirty. [In those days in teaching hospitals the medical students and interns did all the blood counts and urinalysis and collected all specimens for blood chemistry tests.]

Things have been quieter since then, and I am usually back by supper time or ten in the evening at latest; but you have to spend all your spare time in the library looking up literature.

It is a great course, the cases are good, and the Children's is a darn nice hospital to work in. I am going to try to trade off a month of surgery at Brigham Hospital in Boston for a month of pediatric surgery with Dr. Ladd, who is a fine fellow and a good surgeon. This will give me something I never again will have a chance to get.

I cannot ever express to you how much I enjoyed my summer at the Clinic or how valuable it has been to me. [I watched and scrubbed in on a number of operations.] Our hospital is without doubt the most efficiently organized and thoroughly pleasant place to work in that I have ever seen. In this beautiful weather, I also miss the Knob and think of your October rides.

Poor Bud has been up in that hospital all summer (where he was given free board and lodging), on call every night except Saturday and working like a dog on summer courses in the daytime. Max is fit and fine after a good summer at camp and is picking up real interest in the third year work. [He had slipped back a year because of his distraction by a beautiful companion.] Sim is a changed man since his engagement is broken, and has the appearance of a convict recently reprieved of a life sentence. Dutch has moved to Baltimore with the Consolidated Can Company and is characteristically living with a family from New Orleans with their daughters 24, 22 and 18, take your choice, all Baltimore Debs. With Dutch's passing from Boston, there pass also our contacts with what little we saw of Society, and now, there being no more a gang of trouble-makers up here and no more acquaintances at large in the city, I have retired to the hermitage of the library.

That letter must have made my anxious mother very happy!

An excerpt from her letter dated October 9, 1932:

Last week the fourth and fifth floors of the Clinic Hospital were very exciting places. Horace Dodge (automobile millionaire) was on the fourth. He, you know, has had a good many vicissitudes, including wives. His mother landed here one day to receive the message that her husband was being operated on next week for a lipoma (?). In the meantime the friend and doctor that came up with Horace had had such a good time in town that when they came to see him late one evening, they had to be put in bed in the hospital!

That same week Hearst arrived, taking a suite, and Marion Davies and her dog in a room next door. She is a darling little blonde and most bewitching as one sees her in her fetching pajama suits in the corridors. Their man and maid come in each day to attend to their wants. They ask for nothing extra, are utterly satisfied with everything, yet if you read the October Atlantic Monthly you will get a picture of how they live.

I cannot spell out his trouble or give the correct name, but it is something like diverticulum [a pouch off the esophagus]. Dad did a two-stage operation, about a week apart. He did the second yesterday, and this noon there is not a rise of temperature or a quiver anywhere; so Dad is very pleased.

Operations for diverticula of the esophagus were rare in those days, and although my father was famous as a thyroid surgeon he had not specialized in or even performed many operations for diverticula of the esophagus. The operation was a success at first, but later there was a recurrence of symptoms, never severe enough to require further surgery. The disease is perfectly benign, but interferes seriously with the ability to swallow.

And from my medical world I wrote:

> We are having lots of excellent cases, including dystrophies, meningitis, encephalitides—everything but chickadees—brain tumors, epilepsy, lead poisoning; it is a veritable neurological museum over there and I am certainly glad of this opportunity to get up on the central nervous system diseases. This year is really more darn fun than anything I have done except last summer. We don't have anything to do with infants and the children are all a pleasure to work with and keep life plenty amusing.

I went on to say that the new head of surgery, Dr. Elliot Cutler from Cleveland, was well thought of by the students because he let them do more than they had done before, assisting at operations and closing incisions.

> They say he runs around the hospital with a figurative broom in his hand and never stops sweeping. Bert Dunphy had his car parked in front of a no parking sign outside the hospital, and Dr. Cutler saw it from his office, seized a piece of paper, rushed out to the car and wrote a note which he pinned to the wheel. "There is a sign which says 'No Parking.' Your car is in front of this sign. Please remove it. Elliot Cutler" No wonder he does not have time for broader advances in surgery.

Dad wrote to say that his book, *The Diagnosis and Treatment of Diseases of the Thyroid Gland*, to which I had contributed a chapter, was out, and that "Our famous patient went through both stages perfectly. He is a most cooperative patient."

In a memo dated October 4, 1932, my father related a conversation with a friend who said that the gynecology service at Roosevelt Hospital in New York, under Dr. Howard Taylor, and his son, Howard Taylor, Jr., was an excellent service offering a lot of operative experience and the use of radium in cancer. "This six months' service would be open to Barney after his training." That was a prophecy. Three years later, I would spend six months on that excellent service, but that would be when my residency in general surgery was over. Gynecology, abdominal surgery, cancer surgery, and neck or glandular surgery, Mother wrote, was what my father thought I should be trained in. "He says studying pathology or post mortems gives a rough hand.

He says orthopedic surgery gives a rougher one. He wants you to keep your feather-edge touch, to stick to straight surgery."

In a long letter dated October 27, 1932, Mother wrote about my father's dominant role in the establishment of the American College of Surgeons and the Society of Clinical Surgery, and then went on to say that when a friend asked Will Mather, one of Cleveland's and America's richest and most successful businessmen, "How are you?" Mr. Mather replied, "Just on the verge of bankruptcy." "That gives me great courage," Mother said,

> for things are certainly in a mess. The ground rent for the Hanna building [my father owned the ground] was not paid this quarter. They want a reduction of its interest rate. Their letter stated they did not know when they could pay the ground rent. Of course, if they do not pay we shall not be able to pay our interest. And so it goes. Poor Miss McNally [owner of a delicatessen] is in the hands of a receiver because she has $100,000 out in bills that people will not pay any dividends because Miss McNally and all those people cannot pay any rent. Isn't it a funny vicious circle?

Mother went on to tell of a lecture she had heard by a man who was an authority of Japan and apparently something of a soothsayer:

> He said that Japan is the most highly militarized nation in the world, and per capita the most capitalistic nation. He referred to the number of industries in which Japan had wiped out Europe and America by taking them to herself. He spoke of the group in ascendency as being the militaristic group and said on the 14th of November (when he meets with the United Nations to discuss her aggressions in Manchuria) if Japan can be conciliatory and humiliate herself far enough with apologies to satisfy Stimson, things might straighten out, but he seemed very doubtful and said that if the militaristic power continued, before five years' time Japan would be fighting the United States.

He was mistaken, of course. It took ten years instead of five.

Mother then wrote of Dad's part in the founding and programming of the Interstate Postgraduate Medical Society and ended, "I think it is so interesting to see all the fields Dad has touched, and with it all, so modestly, and yet he plays so big a role. It just breaks my heart to have him have any financial worries these days, but there are plenty of them. After all, though, the real things are being well and having an unbroken circle."

November 6, 1932

Dear Mother and Dad,

Now with the quarter century and a dozen obstetrical cases behind me [I was born November 3, 1907] I feel very old and wise. I shall be more so when I put the twenty dollars to work on buying surgical books. It looks like a million in these days and I cannot thank you enough.

I went on to tell of my experiences in home delivery, with some first-year medical students watching.

I was going along splendidly, swinging through the procedure like clock work, and had preserved a papyraceous perineum from even so much as a mucous tear, and the baby was safe on the table. The two first-year boys, holding the legs for their first delivery, thought I must be Professor Irving's right hand man and the Father of Modern Obstetrics. I deftly slipped the first tie on the cord and pulled it tight—just a shade too tight—and cut right through the umbilical arteries, getting two nice arterial spurters from the baby and a good venous drainage from the umbilical vein at the other end of the cord. At just this instant when blood was flying all over from the baby, the mother had her first postpartum contraction and about 400 cc. of blood, dammed up behind the placenta, was expressed in one tremendous sluice—like a flood—which came pouring down in torrents all over the bleeding baby and cord. There was a maelstrom of blood when currents from Mother and baby swirled together, and I stood in the middle of it, grabbing the stump of the umbilicus, like the boy with his finger in the dyke, while student nurses screamed and one of the leg-holders fainted, thinking the end had come for Mother and babe. I was glad of thyroid training, for blood no longer frightens me, and of course this problem was a moron one to meet.

The next day I had a 12^{1}/$_{2}$-pound girl which stuck at the shoulders and refused to be born. The resident worked on her for 15 minutes and called for a cleidotomy [cutting of the collar bone] before extracting it—dead. The next was a 4^{1}/$_{2}$-pound premature which I carried in to the hospital in a market basket, feeling like a cross between a kidnapper and a stork.

Needless to say, after those experiences I never delivered another baby in all the rest of my life.

My father was still seeing patients in New York. (It would be illegal today without a New York license.) He wired me, "Have you any excuse to be in New York this Saturday and go to the Yale-Princeton game with me? I arrive New York Friday morning. Hope you can make it." Saturday was November 11, my father's birthday, and we celebrated it with Max Eddy and my old roommate Count Costikyan at the Princeton game, to which we had driven in my old Ford. "A Gala Day," Mother wrote of it.

All of my father's friends were gracious to me when I asked them if I could attend their clinics, which I was doing to try to decide where to take my internship. Dr. Whipple, the famous head of Surgery at New York's Columbia Presbyterian Hospital, wrote:

Dear Dr. Crile,

I should be very glad indeed to see you on Saturday, November 19th, in the morning if possible. If you come early you will have plenty of time to get to the Harvard game in New Haven. [He knew what my intentions were.] We should like to have you attend Rounds if you can get here early enough. Unfortunately, they start at 8:00 A.M., but you can get here at any time.

Sincerely yours,
Allen O. Whipple

I had been looking over Philadelphia too, but their internships took two years and combined medicine and surgery. I wanted a straight service. I was deeply impressed with the Lahey Clinic, but like the Cleveland Clinic they offered no internships, only residencies. "I have spent a lot of time at the Lahey Clinic," I wrote, "Lahey, Clute, Cattell and everyone have treated me like a King. They do beautiful work, but their technique of thyroidectomy cannot compare with ours, as I see it." Later I changed my mind and from the time I started to operate, I used the Lahey technique and had a much lower incidence of injury to the recurrent nerve than my father had had. "Lahey is a great fellow and a great showman and has been darn nice to me. Cattell"—who later became one of my friends and most admired colleagues—"was telling me that with their technique a pole vessel never got away from them and not two minutes later Brrrr—the superior pole got so loose that it nearly dropped out of the neck and the blood was flying all over the room. Very amusing."

My father sent me a memo in which the New York service was disparaged, "There is not an outstanding, at least not a commanding surgeon in the Presbyterian." Barnes, on the other hand, he strongly supported, saying, "It is well organized, attracts an excellent type of house staff, and has a group of excellent juniors. The Head of Staff, Dr. Graham, is the most commanding figure in American surgery. He is especially outstanding in the gall bladder, upper abdomen and chest surgery." (The thing that had attracted my interest in Barnes Hospital had been the publicity that was given to Dr. Graham when he performed the first successful removal of a lung cancer.)

Late in November, I applied for internship at Barnes Hospital. I told my father that when I finished my internship and then my two-year residency at the Clinic I could follow his advice and take six months of gynecology with Dr. Taylor in New York. This I did and did not regret it, although in retrospect, as I note how gynecology soon became a specialty that was no longer practiced by general surgeons, I might have been further ahead if I had spent an extra year in thoracic surgery. It was in this field, especially that of cardiac surgery, that the greatest advances of the mid-twentieth century would be made.

In the same letter I said, "I started Medicine yesterday, and have already found out that my life of obstetrical leisure is over. The Boston City Hospital is a messy disorganized place to work in, but the staff is head and shoulders above everything else in the city, in Medicine. Minot, Castle [Nobel laureates], Locke, Jackson, Kiefer, Weiss—a most outstanding and stimulating group." Almost all of these young men became world famous. "We have to have our cases, history and physical with complete blood, urine, stool and sputum if indicated and any other blood work they may deem necessary all complete before we leave the hospital on the same day we get them, and they don't usually come in 'till two or three o'clock. Then besides the day is full of conferences and ward rounds and everything under the sun for the edification of medical students. I'm not on to the routine yet and things still go pretty slowly."

On the twenty-fifth of November, my father received a telegram from St. Louis: "George Crile, Jr. of Harvard Medical School has applied here for internship. Is he your son? Evarts A. Graham." My father replied, "You bet he is."

Dr. Graham wired me, "Pleased to consider your application for surgical internship. Personal interview unnecessary. Please have Dr. Worth Hale send me letter about you by Air Mail. Appointment will be made latter part of next week. Evarts A. Graham."

I wrote to my father thanking him for his influence on Dr. Graham and saying that it was needed because "Only two places were open and besides they were being applied for by Dr. Cannon's son Brad, another student who had worked two years at Barnes in the summer, and two of my classmates, both in the first 10 or 15 percentile of our class, as well as the rest of the country. If I get the appointment I will be perfectly happy, as I know that is just the thing for me to do."

On November 30, I had a telegram from Dr. Graham saying that I had been appointed intern in surgery.

By December 5 I had received all the bad news regarding the family's finances and wrote Mother,

Isn't it a darn shame Dad could not afford that hunting trip with Gus? I certainly hope that everything [regarding the tax dispute] got straightened out in Washington. If not I don't see why I could not mortgage my share of the Kensington and get enough money to help out, because after this year I will not have any more need for money. It seems to me that would solve all the difficulties. Medicine at the City is so darn interesting that I cannot wait for ward rounds each day. The visiting men are the best teachers I have ever had and keep you right on your toes every second with questions and problems about the cases. Furthermore, they have a most fascinating variety of every sort of case you can imagine. I am absolutely serious about the Kensington, and it seems the only logical thing to do. There is no point in my keeping it because I can live on a hundred dollars a month from now on.

My parents refused my offer and somehow or other managed to get along. A little later, my father wrote about Dr. Walter Cannon (whose son also had been accepted at Barnes and one of whose lectures I had just written about to my father), "Cannon's work and point of view [about the adrenal sympathetic system, fight and flight, etc.] is probably the most intelligent in this day in reference to the field he has worked in so hard and so long. How clear one can see the influence at the critical time of the Ether Day address." My father was implying, as my mother often had clearly stated, that the Ether Day address, given by my father in Boston in 1910, had given Dr. Cannon some of his pioneering thoughts on the emergency functions of adrenaline. It is true that my father had similar ideas, but in the address in question he had made no mention of the adrenal glands.

In this same exciting month of December, I had a handwritten letter from Dr. Cannon:

Dear Mr. Crile,

Mrs. Cannon asked me to invite you to dine with us next Sunday at 1:00 o'clock. I think she has also invited some "inhabitants" of St. Louis.

Yours cordially,
Walter B. Cannon

December 11, 1932

Dear Mother and Dad,

Today the Cannons asked me to dinner and we had a most interesting time. An aunt, Miss Cannon, is a somewhat radically minded social-service head of the Massachusetts General Hospital and there was much argumentation.

I went on to tell of Dr. Cannon's interest in my father's adrenal denervations and then said that, "Later in the afternoon—Mrs. Cannon, whose innumerable daughters are in Radcliffe, asked all the St. Louis girls in Radcliffe to come over and meet Brad and me. You can well imagine what a treat that was! I nearly decided to break my contract at the Barnes." In those days, when few women went to college, Radcliffe was considered to be a place where the girls were taught dangerous, antisocial and anti-male-dominant ideas.

Just before I came home for Christmas vacation, Mother wrote regarding my offer to mortgage the Kensington:

Nothing could have endeared you more to our hearts than your thought about the Kensington. Somehow the uncertainties of old age seemed to drop away. Dad and I looked at each other, our eyes full with the same thought in mind. The loyalties—is there any quality that so makes life worth living?

No my dear, I do not think we shall need that. It is not that we have not things on which we could borrow, but banks will not loan. Of course hundreds are just like ourselves, and we are rich compared to the actually hungry and cold. So we are just digging in and perhaps sometime again we shall be able to dig out.

Things remained difficult at home. My father was as busy as ever, including periodic trips to New York where he would see thirty or forty patients in his suite at the Roosevelt. "It made me sick to have him go on all alone," Mother wrote, "but the sledding is so thin he did not want the extra expense of taking anyone." Then she went on to tell of his departure, "At three thirty he called for the car, but when he got home he found he forgot to get money from Whipple [treasurer of the

Clinic]—so there was a hurry up call from him to meet him at the station with a roll of bills. And from the station I have just had a telephone call from Dad, saying he had forgotten to take his envelope of tickets off the bureau!" And so it went on, but somehow Dad always managed to get where he was going.

Just before Christmas vacation I wrote home,

> I feel just as I did in fraternity rushing week in college when I was all packed [prearranged admission] for Chi Psi. All the boys are steaming around pulling wires wherever they can to get appointments and those of us who have them are just sitting back and laughing. The situation is particularly acute this year because 80% of our class are headed for surgery, and most of them are trying for a very limited number of Boston appointments.

During my summers at the Clinic Hospital, I had witnessed many operations and had become interested in some of the patients my father had treated. The immediate results of the adrenal denervations had seemed to me to be spectacular, but gradually, as a reuslt of follow-ups such as were afforded by the following letter which came to me, I became more and more disillusioned with my father's theories of the "kinetic drive," or at least with his surgical approach to its control.

> December 27, 1932
>
> Dear Dr. Crile Jr.,
>   . . . If you happened to look into my case you no doubt already know that after I had been home from the Hospital about 10 days my condition began to change so that by the time a month was up and I returned for an examination I was in practically the same condition as before the operation. My pulse is about 96, my blood pressure 150, face is flushed about the same, hands are still warm and sweaty, still very nervous and worrying about my condition—in every way about the same as before the operation.

The problem was that my father's personality was so strong that all of his patients, while they were under his mesmerization, reported that they were cured. I was to learn that this effect rarely persisted.

During this period all of my problems weren't with my father. I was having some trouble with my mother too—or was it vice versa?

> Barney dear,
>   That was a silly conversation we had on the eve of your departure. I don't know how we ever got into it. I know it was stupid

of me to divulge eccentricities to anyone. However, inasmuch as we got into it I would like to clarify my two reservations.

The first is social—It is the tendency to be too easily satisfied. Experience widens only as adaptations are made. "Intimacies with none! friendliness with all"—is a good maxim for a man on the threshold of what may be an enlarging life.

I presume that when Mother said this, she was thinking of my relationship with Jane Halle, and I don't think I was very happy over her attitude. Then she went on to attack the only other vices that brought pleasure to my life:

To be ever alert, to be on the tip-toe of one's full capacity, takes constant character. I merely want you to run your mechanism in such a way that it will have the least wear and tear. I know you know that the more nearly normal amount of sleep you get, the more abstemious you are in smoking and even so harmless a thing as beer, the keener you will be, the better you'll take the fierce competition upon which you soon will be entering and the greater confidence you will inspire in your colleagues and your patients.

Mother ended this letter, "Bob is out day and night—once in a while one has strange qualms of wonder if one's children are bored of being with one." After that attack, this child was beginning to feel a bit that way, but I wasn't at all bored with my work. On January 2, 1933, I wrote, "I have the most extensive case of tuberculosis I ever heard of with involvement of practically every organ of the body, a case of erythema nodosum, one of obscure paralysis perhaps combined with systemic disease, and another hypernephroma." Medicine at the City Hospital was forever new and exciting.

In spite of some of our quarrels, Mother had not lost her sense of humor, and wrote that she had just finished reading aloud to Dad a book called *Sons*, which was about a Chinese family that "rose from the soil." Then Dad got the flu and went to the hospital. Mother came to visit, bringing roses that she left for him at the desk. A few minutes later the nurse brought in the roses and Dad said, "Oh roses, where did they come from?" With a most dignified manner the nurse said, "The card is here, Dr. Crile." "Oh, will you read it please. I haven't my glasses." There was a pause. In a hesitating, almost haughty manner, she read, in nearly a whisper, "To the Old One—from Pear Blossom." Dad just yelled. The nurse left the room.

By this time, the internship appointments were beginning to be made, and I wrote my father about one of my best friends, Bert Dunphy,

> For some reason, largely because he has no pull and has not gone out of his way to cultivate personal relationships with the house officers etc., Dunphy failed to get the Brigham. His record is outstanding, and he is among the first ten in his class. He has excellent judgement, is sound, reliable and conscientious as well as popular with everyone who knows him. In my opinion he is one of the best men in the class and would, of course, have never been left out if Blue Blood and Politics had not weighed too heavily in the balance.

At the time, I didn't fully appreciate why it was that Bert was having trouble. But years later, when Bert might have been made chief of Surgery of Cleveland's Lakeside Hospital, the same problem arose. That's the way it was, at that time. For example, when at the Cleveland Clinic, there was a question of who should be the next head of the X-ray Department and the next in line was a Catholic, I remember the discussion. I had strongly recommended an excellent radiologist in the department, but my friend had said, "You can't do that. If you appoint a Catholic as head of the department, it won't be long before you have nothing but Catholics in the department." Over the protests of my friend, the Catholic was made head of the department and subsequent events proved my friend right. The department is not only largely Catholic, but also one of the best departments in the Clinic. In retrospect, this religious bias seems totally incomprehensible.

Incidentally, Bert did get an internship at the Brigham. It was in Pathology, not Surgery, but that gave him his start. My father wrote Dr. Whipple, chief of Surgery at New York's Columbia University Presbyterian Hospital, about Bert, and received a nice reply that ended, "I regret very much that we cannot have Barney on our staff, but I am sure he will get the best kind of training in St. Louis."

In spite of my mother's warnings, I continued to use (but not to abuse) alcohol and occasionally to stay up late at parties. In a letter to her I admitted, "I have become such a social light of late that I attended Lydia Lund's debut several weeks ago, which was marked by a very delightful dinner with champagne and other marks of returning prosperity. Dr. and Mrs. Lund wanted particularly to be remembered to you and Dad. The dance, which I could not stay for, was said to be a great success." If I remember correctly, I think the latter was a white lie designed to placate my mother.

My father replied to my letter about the City Hospital by saying, "It sounds somewhat like a war hospital." Again, probably to Mother's horror, I wrote about a skiing weekend on which twenty-eight of us, "chaperoned" by the Woodbridges, went up to New Hampshire during which the snow melted and we were drenched in rain. "Nevertheless we climbed the mountain in the rain and although I fear the weekend was not productive of much rest or sleep it was at least a healthy one." I presume that Jane was my partner on that occasion, but I did not mention her in my letter.

By now the reviews of my father's book *Diagnosis and Treatment of Diseases of the Thyroid Gland* were beginning to appear, and to everyone's astonishment, from the journal *Lancet* in England came a laudatory article that stated, "One of the best [chapters] is the chapter on iodine and the thyroid gland by George Crile, jun. This admirable summary of the subject has a good bibliography and is written in a pleasing style."

In Boston, I was busy with Dr. Kiefer of the City Hospital in writing a paper on the thyroid. I thought Kiefer was the most stimulating teacher I had ever met. The paper, however, was not a great success. Attendance was voluntary and only two students were in the audience, one of whom was the next speaker. On that same night, Yandell read a long paper before the honorary Boylston Society on "Cannon vs. the Crile Theories."

Then tragedy struck and I wrote that "The left anterior quadrant of my car caught on fire and burned to the ground. The damage was $5.75, and I am going to send the bill to the insurance company. Pretty darn lucky we took fire insurance after all." In the same letter, I mentioned that the price of a pound of steak was twenty-nine cents.

Next I wrote, "I have started in X-ray at the Brigham with Sosman who is one of the smartest clinicians I have ever seen as well as standing at the top in X-ray, and personally he is the cream of the crop." And, "Life is not all weekends, Mother dear, despite your present state of mind as to my private life in Boston." And I then went on to write about the Boston City Hospital:

> The City Hospital has been a madhouse. The wards on which we work have about forty-five beds normally, separated from one another by just a screen and the two tiers of them all the way up the ward. Flu has broken out and about every other patient has had it or is getting it. A rash was removed yesterday with diagnosis of scarlet [fever]. We have had up to ten admissions daily on the service, three of the six house officers are in bed with flu,

there are sixty nurses in bed, three of six students are laid up. The hospital has run out of bed linen and there do not begin to be enough screens; and in addition to all this, we have had two or three deaths a day and sometimes four or five, and a host of mad, delirious, and manic patients. I have had eight cases in eleven days and have not been home before ten in the evening more than two nights since I have been back.

The best day of all was last Friday. It started off with a Negro girl having one of the most horrible and violent epileptiform seizures that has ever been witnessed. It happened in the middle of the ward without screens, where all the patients could see it. Several cases of angina on the side lines began yelling for nitrites. Ward rounds continued after this episode and things were quiet except for eight admissions and a shortage of cots until four P.M. when I was assigned to work up a 260 pound weeping ex bare-back circus rider who refused to go to bed. I do not blame her as the bed would have broken with her unless she lopped over the edges enough to keep her weight on the floor. She was blind, gave a history of probable luetic [syphilitic] treatments, had a large trace, in fact a huge trace, of albumin, and was loaded with sugar; gave a history of hysteria, epilepsy, mental deterioration, destructiveness, incontinence, alcoholism, morphine addiction, vernal and sulphonal poisoning on numerous occasions, smoked three or four packages of cigarettes daily, and had terrific asthma. And she had a fixed idea that she was being abused and maltreated and that she would not go to bed or stay in the hospital. She was given enough sodium luminal to knock out three normal people, and the job of getting a history and doing a physical, to say nothing of getting her to bed, was mine.

I took her out in the linen room and then we had a long and serious talk about life and she began to think I was pretty much on her side. But I could not persuade her to go to bed. After I was all thru taking the history, I had several times asked her if she had had operations, etc., and she had denied it, I asked if there was anything of importance that she had not told me. Finally, as an afterthought, she said yes she had had a cancer taken from her breast two years ago. Recovering from that shock, I said "fine" and persuaded her to get down to the bed and sit on it so I could see the scar. We gave her another triple dose of luminal, hoping to hold her in bed. This merely excited her. I asked to see the scar, and before I could get screens up, and right in the middle of the ward, on a cot, during visiting hours with the room filled with men, she murmured that it was terribly hard to take the clothes off over her head, and seizing dress, underwear, and all in her two hands, she ripped the whole business from stern to stern before I could so much as say, "My God." There was I with a naked crazy woman in the middle of the ward, and I rushed around trying to get screens, and there were none. Finally I got some and had her completely naked when a lady across the way with aortic disease unexpectedly emitted a series of shrieks and died right in the face of a girl across the way who was being treated for neurasthenia and in full view of the whole ward. The nurse pulled down my screens to cover the corpse and left me with the naked bare-back rider exposed once again. And so it went while three patients died in quick succession. My 260 pounds of loveliness being exhibited to the wondering gaze of the visitors on each occasion.

The luminal began to take a little effect and she lay down and rested. I sneaked upstairs to the Lab. Two hours later, I heard the most terrific racket downstairs, with shrieks and wails and expostulations and language not meant for a Sunday school. My patient had gotten up and was groping her way home with a great number of nurses and house officers impeding the path and clinging to her like tugs to a liner. I came down and she recognized me, and I talked her into sitting down and waiting. In the meantime, the family had come and said they wanted her committed. The husband made me promise to hide him and not tell her he was there. He weighed about 110 and was a barber, and a terrified barber at that for she was yelling that she would kill him. I went upstairs again. They notified the State Hospital for Insane to send over for her.

Half an hour later, commotion was heard again, even wilder than before. Weeping and wailing. The House Officer ran upstairs and asked me to come down. It seems that a nurse told her where she was being sent and that the patient did not approve. Now she refused to leave the hospital. Two attendants, three nurses, two house officers, and a neurological consultant and Simmons had been trying to get her into a wheel chair to put her in the elevator and she had thrown them all over the room. I came down and she recognized me and threw her two arms around my neck sobbing, "My Doctor" and pleaded with me not to let them put her in the chair because then she would be pushed right to the Asylum. She would not let go of me. Finally, I told her she had to leave the ward and had better get in the chair. No, that would never do, she stormed and wailed and had the wildest type of hysterical fit. So I said, "All right. I guess you win your point. You come with me instead," and I gave her my arm and she took it and she and Sim and I walked her into the elevator just as quietly as to a prayer meeting and down we went to the basement. And there were we in the tunnels of the City Hospital with a mad woman. The attendants did not show up. We did not dare take her back to the ward. We could not find any one. After about ten minutes the keepers came and we all paraded out and with the aid of two policemen and a driver, got her into an ambulance and said good-bye to her.

On return to the ward, a patient had delirium tremors and was fighting the Junior and the entire nursing staff and swearing at the top of his lungs. Another patient died horribly and we went home and to bed.

Medicine is beyond all doubt the most eternally new and fascinating play and work that there could be. The cases continue to be as interesting as ever and altho I have had little time for reading and am behind in everything, I feel I am learning fast.

Love
Barney

In a letter dated January 20, 1933, Mother wrote "We have had to make a second ten percent cut at the Clinic. Everyone took it with shoulders squared. Collections are so terribly slow there is no leeway on which to run, neither is there for us. I was just interrupted to learn that Aunt Mary Helen just had a telegram from Harmon [her son] that his roommate died of scarlet fever and that he was under observation." She went on to say, "I am so excited about Mrs. Lux, at the Clinic. She is returning home after fourteen months at the Hospital. She is the infantile paralysis case you know. She could not blink an eyelid when she came and now she is able to dress herself. We should write up these miracles. My how we need you—someone with a restless yearning pen."

In those days of polio, diphtheria, pneumonia, and scarlet fever, when there were no vaccines and no antibiotics, an epidemic could be an exciting event.

Two days after her wedding anniversary, Mother wrote, telling how Dad had brought her seven American Beauty roses, the symbol of their nuptials on February 7. She said that she was touched the other day to hear of his invitation to a men's dinner for February 7, and he said, "Well, I shall have to look up and see if that evening is free," and then he turned and said, "No, I can't. That is my wedding anniversary and I am so often away then, I think I should like to keep that evening for Mrs. Crile!" She went on, "It is a sort of comfort to feel that even if we do live the kind of life that to many might seem quite devoid of interest in the way of dining and wining and a mad run of entertainment, at least it brings great contentment to him and to me. I know nothing that to me is so thrilling as working on a book with Dad."

Financial affairs kept deteriorating. In February 1933 Mother wrote that she was at dinner when, just as soup was served, there was a telephone call for a guest who was one of the directors of the Union Trust Bank, one of the largest in Ohio.

He missed the soup and fish courses, and when he returned he was not smiling. The next day the Maryland banks closed and the morning's paper announced that only 5% withdrawals could be made from banks today. The Central United and Society for Savings, like the Cleveland Trust, are said to be safe, but the general feeling is that there may be a shakedown in Guardian and Union Trust. Anyway no one will be able to pay their payrolls on February first. [She meant March first.] Fishers will not cash checks; people cannot pay their bills. You have $4,000 in your savings account so I am afraid only $200 [5 percent] can be withdrawn from it, so go gingerly until I can tell you how things are. Well such is the situation. These days are certainly exciting—a most constructive research on one hand and the downhill toboggan slide on the other. But who cares? The world is here and all its beauty and interest and life is just as much of an adventure as ever.

I was still studying in the X-ray Department, and was still excited about it, and reported: "We ended up in a blaze of the spectacular, discovering a hair ball in a woman's stomach which weighed four pounds and was over 10 inches long and which had been diagnosed by Cutler and Co. as spleen. You have never seen such an amazing sight in your life as that thing was under the fluoroscope surrounded by Barium."

I had been working on a chapter on the adrenal-sympathetic system for my father's next book and had a letter from him that it was accepted. He went on to ask, "Could you broaden the title and context of the peptic ulcer chapter to include—Theories as to the Etiology of Peptic Ulcer—A Critical Review of the Literature?" The article on the sympathetic system would be published when the book came out, but I was never sold on the belief that peptic ulcer was caused by stimulation of the "kinetic system." I expressed my lack of enthusiasm to my mother as follows:

> This whole field is one so full of controversy that it is extremely difficult to know what to include. What little I have done on this paper is accurate and I have checked it over carefully. There is much that could be added on the line of hypothesis and speculation, but it is my feeling that it would be better for Dad to do this. I think my cue in writing is to stick to the facts until I reach the point where my speculations will be of interest to the reader.

The problems at home continued. Mother wrote that

> vegetables are wilted in the green grocers as the grocers have not the cash to get fresh groceries. Only three-quarters of the Clinic got down in time to get their checks cashed on the plan arranged for, so now the Clinic is giving them allowances. One sees the cash of children's banks being emptied and one does not need to ask why. Even Peg gathered up all the stray milk bottles—a load of them—and trotted down with them to Fisher's. They at least can be exchanged for milk for a few days' supply. We are really pretty fortunate as I happen to have $1700 in a liquid account. I am paying no bills—I may need the cash. Had I not been so utterly cleaned out of everything else, I could not have had so liquid an account.

And about my own finances, Mother wrote,

> Do let me know your situation. Last month you overdrew your account $12.00, but I put in $100 the other day, into what is a "liquid" account, that is one from which you can draw money. Here all the checks which were sent out to pay bills, if they did not go through the clearing house last week, have been returned, so now people not only have not paid the bills, but their cash is locked up and they cannot get it. The banks are full of milling mobs. It is very exciting, but quite scary. Today a mob of 3,000 surged in Public Square. No violence, but police moved pretty carefully.

She went on to talk of President Roosevelt's inaugural services and said that it had been a "thrilling day."

The effect of the personality of F.D.R. was reflected in a letter from my Aunt Edith Sherman, March 11, 1933: "The main thing is the people are all turning to Mr. Roosevelt, Republicans and Democrats alike—for the present he is their great hero and they are counting on him to straighten out the muddle. If there is a question of issuing new currency, and really there doesn't seem any other way, many people feel if that is the case that stocks will go up and for a little everything will be very rosy, and if he really knows when to put on the brakes all will be well." These observations came from a lady who was married to a man who would be president of a bank and whose whole family were congenital and hitherto devoted Republicans.

It was March, and my senior year was nearly over. I was taking Surgery at Children's Hospital and wrote home that I would spend the last two months in Surgery at Brigham and could not do any work or papers for Dad's book. "I refuse to be anything but 100% on that job when I am there, because that is the one group of people here that give me a challenge and make me want to be on my toes—not so much from leadership as from antagonism." By that I meant that although I was stimulated by Dr. Cutler I thought that he and his associates were not great technical surgeons. To impress them I spent an enormous amount of time on the thesis that I had to write, and I wrote it on "Mortality in Acute Appendicitis in Children."

The paper has been misplaced and I cannot quote it directly, but it showed that the most common cause of death in eighty cases of fatal appendicitis in children was a condition that occurred during or a few hours after operation. This syndrome I named "dehydration shock," for I was completely familiar with my father's pioneering work on shock and I too had worked on it in the laboratory. The children, many of whom had been sick and vomiting for days, were so dehydrated and their blood volume was so low that any anaesthetic or trauma would throw them into irreversible shock. I was very proud of this completely original investigation and conclusion, but I had forgotten that at that time the surgeon's rule was "appendicitis = immediate operation." There was no time allowed for delay to correct the dehydration. My suggestion, that to waste precious time in preparing the patient, was heresy. I wrote home that I had had a lot of fun because I think I discovered a type of death which they were not aware of and would be interested to see what the professors said about the paper. I am still waiting. I did have the satisfaction of hearing from my mother that she and my father "were delighted with it." The paper was graded by Dr. Cutler and received a B. It was ten or fifteen years before the surgical literature began to encourage a little delay to prepare the dehydrated patients for surgery.

By this time I was beginning more and more to challenge some of my father's statements about the origin and nature of emotions and the question of whether he or Dr. Cannon had priority in their publication. On March 15, 1933, I wrote:

Dear Dad,

Since I wrote you the last letter about the paper [my paper for his book] I have gone to the library and find that not in the Ether Day address, but in a paper before the American Philosophical Society in 1911, you state very clearly the Emergency Theory. It is Page 56 and 57 in "The Nature and Origin of the Emotions." I have been unable to find any work of Cannon's relating to emotion that antedates this, except his measurements of increased adrenaline in fear. In fact Cannon did not produce any emergency theory until 1914. Hence I have revised the adrenal-sympathetic paper in several places, and it is simple to see how Cannon got his idea from it, but I do not think it is before 1911 that you actually say it in reference to the functions of the various organs, including the adrenal.

In April of 1933, my father heard from William Randolph Hearst that he was having a recurrence of the symptoms that he had had before his operation, and at his request, my father traveled to Mr. Hearst's Casa del Mar in San Simeon, California, to consult. "I wish you were with me on this 250,000 acre ranch overlooking the Pacific Ocean," he wrote home, "It is well named [House of the Sea]. It is the most amazing thing I ever saw in the way of an establishment."

On the train on the way back to Cleveland, he wrote again,

It proved that conditions were not favorable for anything but a consultation. The other perhaps later. I went up to the famous ranch "La Cuesta Encantado." Fearing I have not written it clearly enough, this means The Enchanted Hill. If there ever was Arabian Nights in reality this is it. Nowhere in the world have I seen such a creation. The ranch has its own seaport, about 50 miles of Pacific oceanfront, on 250,000 acres. On the very top there is the Casa Grande, and I rode horseback one day and it was amusing to encounter buffalo, camels, ostriches, musk oxen, even llamas, kangaroos, every kind of deer and antelope family and a fine zoo with lions etc.

At this weekend party there were a number of movie stars— each evening a movie on the screen. If Versailles were put on the campus it would not be much noticed. Altogether it is the most incredible creation one could imagine. For instance I slept in Richelieu's bed. All the buildings, furnishings, walls, structures were of monasteries, cathedrals and palaces of Spain and Italy. So it goes. This professional life has its hardships, but there are compensations.

Love, Dad.

It seemed that the depression had not yet hit California!

Mother wrote that Dad's consultation with Mr. Hearst was a secret: "A squib came out in the paper that Dad was in California for a meeting and was visiting Mr. Hearst on his way home for a day or two. That is a Controlled Press." Mother went on to say that there was great concern over the banks closing but that the Clinic gave a 75 percent salary in the middle of the month, adding that they cannot of course amortize their loans, but have kept up the interest.

My interest also was being sustained, but it pertained not to banks but to women. Spring had arrived in Boston, and I wrote to Mother:

> Friday night Quigley and I are having a novel experience. Neither of us had ever been out with a nurse, and Quig had told me the other day that he thought he would have to give it a try. A little student nurse at the Peter Bent Brigham came up to me the other day and blushingly said she knew no one in Boston and would I go to the Children's Hospital nurses' dance with her. I said, "Sure, if you'll get someone to take Quigley." So Quig and I are being taken to the dance and are on the lookout for a thrilling evening with the student nurses under the vigil of their Mother Superior and midnight curfew.

I thought that this news probably would reassure my mother, because it was not Jane that I was dancing with. But a week later she wrote me a warning, "As for the nurse, it just makes me think of tanglefoot fly paper. One foot in nearly always finished the fly." My father too must have suffered, for it was he who had told me, in respect to my associations with nurses, "A good sheepdog does not kill in his own flock." In the long run I found that there was some wisdom in his warning.

At this time in Boston one of the wild aberrances of surgery took place. Everyone began to do total thyroidectomies on patients who had heart failure. By this they hoped to decrease the metabolism and the demands on the heart. The idea started at the Beth Israel and soon metastasized to the Brigham and Massachusetts General. I wrote home to say it was enthusiastically embraced by cardiologists Levine and White, but I was skeptical and feared that "the heart muscle would, from one point of view, be weakened in direct proportion to the metabolic decrease elsewhere and the patient would be no better off than he was in the beginning, the heart having suffered from decreased metabolism as much as the rest of the body." This was indeed the case, and the enthusiasm for total thyroidectomy did not last the year out.

In the next letter I expressed my continuing admiration for the Surgery at the Lahey Clinic, "I went to the Lahey Clinic again the other day and had a fine morning. I always learn about twice as much in a morning there as in a week at the Peter Bent Brigham Hospital. Sim is a house officer at the Woman's Free Hospital now and is feeling very important since one of the surgeons let him do a suspension of the uterus." Those were the days when charity patients were still "teaching material."

In spite of the hard times our nonmedical Yale friends kept getting married—this time it was Joe Lowes who had roomed with Dutch Wells. "The younger generation (the ushers at least)," I wrote to my father, "with their Yale background bore up with remarkable fortitude and, in fact, I don't know what would have become of the party if we had not had some medical students there to assist a half dozen enthusiastic aunts who got too intimate with the punch. It was a reversal of the usual order of things."

Mother was beginning to express concern about my father's travels—"to Oklahoma City next Monday, then to Memphis, then to Nashville to peddle his denervation. It certainly is a thriller. I went to Erie and Zanesville the other day, thrilled to be on the road again. The thing that makes me maddest about this old depression is that I cannot trail Dad. These are the years when I should, and when I look forward I am just terrified the way the years are galloping on." Dad was then sixty-nine. "I am frightened not to make the most of each moment. I know the trips are less full of stress for him when I am along to pick up the threads." That was before the days of air transport and when a trip to Oklahoma was a long train journey.

Mother was so involved with my father's theories that she even viewed the president from the perspective of the adrenal glands. "I am awfully interested in Roosevelt and have got a hunch that his infantile paralysis has impaired his adrenal drive. In other words, like cases with a cross lesion of the spine, he can take strain and stress apparently without emotion. If this is true it explains why he can be so intellectualized without being unduly emotionalized. It is almost superhuman the way he takes this turmoil and seething emotional period." Mother went on to conclude with a compliment to me on a piece I had written and suggestions I had made about Dad's book:

I loved reading your analyses last night and getting the "writer's opinion." It all sounded so grown up, a far reach from lisping Barney. I don't know which I love the most, the snuggling of them in my arms, the feeling of their dependency, or the helpless feeling in seeing them weaned from dependency and the pride in seeing them strike out for themselves. It's all a great adventure and you have always given me a "kick" all along the way.

> Loads of love, old man
> Mother

On May 14, I wrote her:

Dear Mother,

I feel I should be in the woods somewhere today, to pluck you a garland of Spring flowers, but I am afraid I would not know where to look for woods, to say nothing of flowers. In any case, I have not forgotten you, in spite of my apparent failure to properly commemorate the occasion.

Last night we put on the Aesculapian Club show amidst great festivity, mirth, and song. The show was an old-fashioned melodrama, "The Dead Sister's Secret," and was produced in very elaborate fashion under the able direction of Quigley. We had real scenery, costumes, a make-up man to fix us up—everything. I took a minor part because I was busy this month with surgery, and Sim and I were Mr. and Mrs. James Glue—two "swells" who visit the bar-room scene in the second act. I wrote several unprintable lyrics. Then a lot of verses describing the fight and ending up with our sorrow over the event, "The show must go on," etc.

> "If perchance you should see from your seats below
> The gleam of a tear in our eyes,
> And learn that the laughter you've heard in the show
> Is an empty and mocking disguise,
> You'll know it's the heart of the cast that you've seen,
> You'll know of our serious half,
> You'll know, thru our tears, that our motto has been
> To laugh—clown—laugh."

Everyone was very enthusiastic over the show and Quigley's reputation is made in circles of Boston Medicine.

The letter ended with a serious description of the training program: "I saw and assisted Cutler do the worst hysterectomy that I have ever dreamed could be done." Dr. Cutler was primarily a brain surgeon but fiercely contended that all surgeons should be prepared to do all operations. "He had just got through doing a rather good (perfect, as he put it) job on a pituitary adenoma and he was modestly stating, before the hysterectomy, that he could shift with perfect ease from one end of the body to the other, but by the time the operation was over, he was talking more and more about the pituitary and less and less about the pelvis."

I still have a vivid memory of these operations. Dr. Cutler accidentally removed most of the vagina with the benign uterus, and the next day the pituitary patient died.

On May 21, 1933, my last letter home from medical school told of my shame when a visiting professor quizzed me about a patient from whom I had taken a complete and careful history. The man had a cancer of the colon and was old, arteriosclerotic, senile, and demented. I told the professor that the patient had had no pain. The professor then quizzed the patient, and the "old man put his hands over his stomach and rocked back and forth and groaned and said that for the last year he had never had so much as a moment that had not been in unbearable agony of torturing abdominal pain. Such is the life of a clinical clerk." The letter ended with a request for three hundred dollars to pay my term bill, other bills of forty-eight and twenty dollars for my National Board Examinations. I then suggested that "we sell some of my stocks which are up a little and get the money in that way. Would you do this for me by June, so I can pay these bills as they come in? Thanks a lot. Thank God, I shall not need any more money after this year." Little did I know what the future would hold when women would come into my life!

As my senior year ended, I had a personal letter from Dr. Cutler of the Brigham, congratulating me on being the only member of my class to have been graduated magna cum laude. Dorothy Murphy, the secretary of the dean, also wrote congratulating me, and giving the list of the thirteen men who were graduated cum laude. I was happy to note among them my special friends Dunphy, Lium, Low, and Yandell. My father too received letters of congratulation from surgeons and from the dean. But my letter from Dr. Cutler contained a warning that was to foretell the future:

June 19, 1933

Dear Barney,

My warmest congratulations to you. It is dangerous to start too well in life, for such honors as you have achieved will be a sword of

Damocles over your head since everyone will now expect that you will always do exceptionally well. However, don't worry. It was a good spur, and I am sure you will live up to the highest traditions of your school and will be a decoration to the alumni. Best of luck.

Ever yours,
Elliot Cutler

The best thing that happened to me in connection with my graduation was the letter that I received from my father. All of his letters to me were handwritten.

June 2, 1933

Dear Old Barney,

This is my final note in the most happy exchange with you in the four years at Harvard, happy for me because of what you have done.

Whatever Harvard may do, I give my own decoration which when you see it you will not wear, but it will carry my sentiments for your future.

Long ago when I was perhaps a little younger than you and possessed of the sentiment of youth, I had made a little symbol for myself and never showed it to anyone. The material for this symbol consists of silver sutures taken from the wounds in my capacity of assistant to Dr. Frank Weed.

When I had accumulated a sufficient number of these silver sutures, I took them to a little jeweler across the street from 380 Pearl Road and directed him to make for me a diminutive book— on one side there was etched a scalpel—the other a feather pen.

I have had reasons to regret the symbolism of the pen and book for I have been tormented with the urge to write. And so I now cast it off to rid me of the spell, and with this warning I offer it to you while in its place I will someday save some kind of raw material and cause it to be etched on one side a horse [my father's favorite recreation was horseback riding] and on the other a gun and rod.

So in the words of the poem "Here's a toast to the man that follows me!"

Dad

So ended my last year of medical school.

5

Internship at Barnes Hospital

I HAD THREE weeks of free time between the last class of medical school and the beginning of my internship in St. Louis. Two weeks of this I spent at my father's island at Timagami in Canada, with Jane and my sister Peg and her family. Exactly what happened between Jane and her friend, Bub, that made this possible I never knew, but she happily accompanied me to Canada. It was one of the best vacations of my life.

The main cabin where we cooked and ate and sat around the fire in the evenings was the same as it had been years before when my father had had it built. Some additional "sleeping cabins," consisting of nothing but beds and a wash basin, had been added. There was no electricity or running water. But who cared about those comforts? My considerate sister had assigned Jane and me to adjoining cabins at some distance from the parents and children.

In the daytime there was fishing and exploration of the waterways and portages to nearby lakes. As a result of my training at Keewaydin Camp, which was just across Lake Timagami, I was an expert paddler, and Jane, being a natural athlete and having had some experience in canoes, quickly picked it up. She already was a near-champion swimmer and diver.

There was a poignant aspect to the vacation, for we knew that after it our paths would separate. I knew I was in love, but with things as they were, there was no way that I could marry—at least until after the internship. Moreover Jane was still seeing her friend. We talked the matter over, admitted that we loved one another and that marriage would be pleasant, but decided that since for the present it was impossible, we had better go our own ways, without definite or permanent commitments. We decided that we would be "geographically monogamous"—faithful to one another so long as the other was available. So it was. Jane made still another visit to Thomasville, and I began to build for myself a new group of relationships in St. Louis.

St. Louis was completely different from Boston and from the standpoint of surgery it was vastly superior. In Boston, general surgeons did gynecology, orthopedics, hare lips, tonsillectomies, almost everything except neurosurgery, in which Dr. Cushing had cornered the market. On the other hand, Barnes Hospital, in St. Louis, under Dr. Graham, was at that time the world's most specialized surgical service. Not only did they have gynecology (Dr. Crossen), orthopedics (Dr. Keys), neurosurgery (Dr. Sachs), urology (Dr. Caulk), and surgery of the ear, nose, and throat and of the eye as specialties, but they also had thoracic surgery—for Dr. Graham had taken an early lead in surgery of the lung, and plastic surgery pioneered by Dr. Vilray Blair and his successor, Dr. Barrett Brown. Much of the cancer surgery of the head and neck was performed by the specialized and skillful plastic surgeons who were then able to correct the deformities that their treatments made. There even was a pediatric unit where much of the children's surgery was done. General surgery, for which I was headed, consisted of surgery of the abdomen, rectum, breast, thyroid, and hernias. All the rest was done in the specialist departments through which I would rotate.

Besides Dr. Graham in general and thoracic surgery, there was Dr. Brian Blades in thoracic and an extraordinary group of vigorous, young or middle-aged men at the peak of their careers. Dr. Glover Copher was the senior member of the group—quiet, conventional, meticulous, and skillful. His thyroidectomies were much longer, but they were done carefully and well. Warren Cole was there, working closely with Dr. Graham in surgery of the gallbladder. Nathan Womach, who later was to become a professor of surgery, was an excellent surgeon and an inspiration to his house staff. Perhaps the best of the young surgeons, from the technical standpoint, was Dr. Walton who was not, however, a dedicated scientist nor a spectacular speaker, just an excellent surgeon.

In St. Louis we lived in comfortable rooms in a section of the hospital reserved for the residents. Since only one or two of the house officers were married, we all lived in the hospital and ate in the doctors' dining room. There were no women either on the staff or in training.

The intern was the low man on the totem pole. It was his job not only to take the histories and do the physical examinations, but also to draw the blood, collect the urine, carry the specimens to the laboratory (about a quarter of a mile away), do the blood count and urinalysis, and record it all on the chart before the next morning. In return for these labors, and certain semimenial obligations such as typing the operative schedule on Sundays when the secretaries were off duty, the intern was allowed to third-assist at operations and to suffer the criticisms of the staff on the way he had recorded the examinations of the patients.

We also, on the charity patients, had the privilege of being first assistants to the residents and assistant residents, and occasionally, under their supervision, to perform a relatively minor operation. I remember one of my first ones, delegated to me by Dr. Bill Byers who was then an assistant resident and later would become a renowned plastic surgeon. The patient had what everyone thought was a pilonidal (hair nest) sinus that comes from ingrown hairs in the region of the low back over the coccyx (tailbone). These cause a hair ball to form under the skin, and when this becomes infected the abscess is treated by making a small incision and removing the offending material. I started out on the simple operation, but found no hairs. The draining sinus from which pus was pouring extended downward past the coccyx and forward into the abdominal cavity. Bill and I were lost, but it would never occur to us to call for help. That would be a sign of weakness. On and on we followed the sinus until we came to a pus-filled space lying just in front of the sacrum. It was filled with hair, teeth, and skin.

Dr. Byers and I had heard of presacral dermoid ("skin-like") cysts—a congenital anomaly, often found in the ovary, but occasionally anywhere in the midline of the body, and we knew that they contained parts of a different person. That is why ours had teeth, hair, and skin. But we had had no experience in removing such a thing, nor would anyone go about doing so from an incision made in the back if they had known what it was. We worked away, removing as much as we could, and remarkably the patient did well. I have little confidence, however, that he remained cured. In the 1930s it was the charity patients' job to let us use their bodies to learn on. The patient expressed no resentment and we felt no guilt.

Most of the private patients were in private rooms in a remote wing of the hospital. One of their private physician anesthesiologists was so particular of their feelings that he often anaesthetized them in their rooms with nitrous oxide, and with a parade of interns, orderlies, and nurses, wheeled the bed and the anaesthetic machinery all the way to the operating room several hundred yards away. However, most of the anesthetics were given by excellent nurse anesthetists, highly trained. Because of the pioneering experiments in chest surgery, they were expert at putting tubes into the trachea to assure an open airway. It was one of the world's best anaesthetic departments run entirely by nurse anesthetists under the direction of Dr. Graham. These women recognized me because I was the son of the surgeon who first used and arranged for the training of nurse anesthetists.

The charity patients lived in huge wards of thirty or more, supervised by a head nurse. These nurses were powerful and able, and to interns they were both scornful and condescending. They were dedicated professionals in their forties or fifties and under them was a hierarchy extending down to the lowliest little student nurses who had just graduated from high school.

My first letter to my father from St. Louis contained many suggestions as to how to improve the Clinic's medical exhibit at the World's Fair in Chicago, which I had visited on my way to St. Louis. I then told of my delight with being on the plastic service with Drs. Blair and Brown, and ended with a P.S., "I want you to know that I am not going to forget the mystic emblems of the gynecologic silver and that you, through it, will always be the star I shall steer for."

On July 15, 1933, I wrote in more detail, saying that the patients on plastic service had complicated problems and were referred from all over the country.

They do practically everything in the head and neck from cancer of the neck with radical resection [in which my father had been a pioneer—the operation is still called the "Crile dissection," and in 1987 the Journal of the American Medical Association would republish his paper on it under the title "Landmarks in Surgery"], cancer of the antrum, mouth, fractured jaws, impacted teeth, thyroglossal duct cysts, cleft lips and palates, burns, and all other congenital or acquired deformities. I never dreamed that plastic work could be so successful or skin grafting so perfect. Brown is a going man, and follows his cases like a hawk as well as doing all postoperative work on Blair's.

You operate until three o'clock without lunch, make rounds, and write postoperative notes until five, and perhaps sit with a few patients while you give glucose or other treatment, 20 minutes for supper, and at six o' clock find there are anywhere from two to six new cases to be worked up for operation in the morning. You don't get to bed till two, and you are up at seven. The hospital is spread all over. The labs are poorly equipped. When you take a Wasserman you have to carry it about a city block to the lab.

I went on to gripe about the paper work that we had to do, said that it was the depression that made it necessary, but added, "It is compensated for by the high quality of the work being done, the quality of the cases, and the fact that this is a darn nice and extremely smart staff and resident group." I didn't even mention that the salary of an intern was much higher than in Boston hospitals—twenty dollars a month, as I remember.

Continuing about the service I wrote, "I am still discouraged with myself in the capacity of intern as I do not seem to be able to remember all the things I should remember. Fortunately, there is a darn nice and very able assistant resident on our service (Bill Byers) who keeps me out of serious trouble. Blair is undoubtedly the weirdest man I have ever known. He is as absent-minded and erratic as any I could dream of, and I can never understand a word he says or figure out what instrument he will use next." I still remember some of Dr. Blair's operations. He was a pioneer in plastic surgery, and, among other things, he was doing some of the first breast reconstructions after mastectomy. At that time there were no plastic implants, and after a radical mastectomy the only hope of reconstruction lay in building up the wound by transplanting huge chunks of fat and skin and sometimes even muscle from other areas. Most of these attempts were such disasters that for twenty years or more I was discouraged from even thinking of reconstruction. One poor woman had flaps moved from abdomen and side and back, and all of them sloughed and had to be replaced by skin grafts placed right over the deep fascia or skeleton.

Although I was on the plastic service, on weekends the interns rotated through emergency call.

I thought I was to have a nice peaceful day of rest today, as we had no operations, but I was on emergency call and spent the entire day in running all over the hospital giving various treatments, admitting emergencies, an acute abdomen, a fractured arm, sewing up a wound into the prepatellar bursa [of the knee], every darn thing you can imagine. Then I found I had four cases of my own in the evening and here it is 12:30 and still some things left over to clean up in the early morning before the schedule starts at 8:30.

A week ago Sunday, I went swimming with a Smith girl whom I used to know when I was in New Haven, and Saturday night a lot of the boys had a party over at a local fraternity house with beer and songs etc. which was good fun.

I have been spending large parts of my afternoons giving salt baths to a 230-pound burned woman. She was covered with grease the first day and burned everywhere except on her round and slippery behind, and could not move, it was so painful. So I had the job of getting her into the tub. The only place I could grab was the greased parts, above mentioned, and you have never seen such a funny sight in your life as the journey from the side of the tub, ending with slipping hands and plopping buttocks, nearly shattering the base of the tub.

In my next letter I told again how good the plastic service was, but said that I missed the "esprit de corps" that I was used to at Yale, Harvard, and at home. "The departments squabble quite a bit and the chief grudge is against the executive force led by the superintendent. I don't give a damn about any of these things, however, so long as I get a bed that I can pile into, 3000 calories a day and plenty of good cases. Once a week I get homesick for a green vegetable and go like a deer to a salt-lick to get some. When the students get here (fall term) all will be rosy again as then they do all the stenography, orderly and technician work that we are now doing." Despite these complaints, I remember the plastic surgery service as one of the finest surgical services I have ever seen and Dr. Barrett Brown as one of the best surgeons.

My father, on August 14, wrote, "We have sold the church [property], our very best asset and this will keep us temporarily, at least, out of bankruptcy. It will enable us to pay off a part of our loans, to pay off a vast accumulation of back taxes, overdue principal payments, temporary loans to pay current interest, complete payment on the family lot. The latter is a great comfort to me as heretofore there was the prospect of being buried in a grave with a mortgage on it—'In Death as in Life.' The Clinic income has not yet increased one cent, but the continued fall is almost arrested." My father's remarks about the mortgaged grave were not made too seriously, because he had no belief in the existence of an afterworld. "Strange thing about banks," he went on to say, "There is no rush to draw out the money, and of the $29,000,000 drawn out but a small amount is deposited in the solvent banks, much in the postal savings, much is hoarded. There is a lack of confidence in everything, apparently, in the national finances." And he ended, "I am perfectly pleased with your service. Give my greetings to Vilray Blair. Love—Dad."

As an example of the value of money in those early days, I present the following Cleveland Clinic Hospital bill, patient #129564:

Room and board, 7 days	$35.00
Operating room and anaesthetic	20.00
Special nurses' board	2.00
Special night nurse's supper	.33
TOTAL	$57.33

In addition there was a $150 charge for a thyroidectomy.

In all this period of financial worry, my father still had about 2,500 acres of land in the country southeast of the Knob, but for that land there wasn't a chance of finding a buyer. Small-farm agriculture had left northern Ohio, and there was not yet any demand for residential land. It was lying fallow and would continue to do so until after my father's death when the estate would be declared bankrupt and Don Farinacci, the lumberman, would buy much of the land for lumber and then resell it. But even in the face of impending bankruptcy and with no market at all for rural land, my father had a scheme. Mother wrote:

> Dad is very anxious to put a lake in the property next to the Cloverdale and Petrus farms. We should like to sell the Chamberlin Gas Station which is really a little out of contact with the rest of our property, and put that money into making a lake, with a view to selling all that property across the Prouty-Adams road later as that property is really near Painesville and is the most salable property we have—but it could be far more salable if the sites faced on or overlooked a 12-acre lake, deep enough for swimming and stocked with fish. Dad is excited as a bee about it, and it gives him a new source of radiation. [Referring to his theory that the brain radiates energy.]

My father was endowed with great imagination and energy, but to conceive of building a huge lake at that time and with no money must have been as much an indication of the aging of his judgment as were some of his theories about the brain and radiation. However, Mother never had a doubt about the integrity of his mind or the correctness of his theories. She didn't even admit to his handicap of rapidly failing eyesight due to a combination of glaucoma, cataracts, and retinitis. She concluded the letter about the lake by saying, "Did you ever know anything like Dad? A box of red roses has just come in—August 22nd—the day we announced or rather *were* engaged."

Right after that letter about Dad is a letter from Dr. Blair:

August 25, 1933

Dear Dr. Crile,

It was a pleasure to have your son assigned to me for his first hospital service and we are all very much impressed with him. Not only does he show a broad training, but stamina and initiative and is utterly unspoiled. He certainly earned the name of George Crile Jr. and I think it is not improbable that sooner or later he will unwittingly put you in the position of signing your name George Crile Sr.—

With kindest regards, I am

Very sincerely yours,
V. P. Blair

[P.S. in the handwriting of Dr. Blair's secretary:] Every patient with whom I have conversation after they leave the Hospital mentions "that nice Dr. Crile."

Dell O. Cooper
Secy.

Mother wrote about the Halles—Jane and her father—who had taken to the air—an unusual adventure in 1933. Mr. Halle had bought a plane and at the age of sixty-three had learned to fly it and had arranged for Jane also to learn. "Meanwhile Mr. Halle climbs in his new plane to the stratum above, peering down through the cumulus clouds and laughing mockingly at upper Euclid as he loops around the Terminal Building." Mother went on to tell how my father— dreaming into a future and of a lake he would build—"sees eels and shining trout flashing in the lake; he sees wood ducks and mallards swooping down for luscious frogs; he sees waving wild rice and bashful water lilies, bathing children, boating, houses snuggled about the lake, and a way out for the House of Crile." My father had a great imagination and my mother a great pen.

My father was a friend of all the great surgeons of his day, but with some the friendship involved a little rivalry as in the case of Dr. Lahey, whose rapidly growing clinic in Boston was a competitor of the Cleveland Clinic, and whose personal international reputation as a thyroid surgeon was rapidly surpassing his. "Dear Barney," Dad wrote, "Lahey was here Friday and he gave before the Academy a lecture on Problems of Gastrointestinal Diseases. It was beautifully done. Really a model for propaganda." The choice of that last word was indicative of the underlying thought.

Barnes Hospital
Saint Louis, Missouri
September 26, 1933

Dear Mother and Dad,

I have not quietly passed out of existence or even contracted sleeping sickness, but have been busy averaging eighteen hours of work a day for two weeks now. We have had a whole flock of emergencies coming in night after night and I am dead tired. Students come back Thursday and then I shall write all about everything.

Love,
Barney

In the next letter I reported that in the National Board Examination I was given a 98 in surgery "which was, I believe, the best mark given." I received only an 87 in obstetrics and concluded, "I guess I shall have to go into surgery instead of obstetrics."

Mother wrote that Dad's problems with his eyes continued, but that it did not discourage him from operating. His associate, Dr. Tom Jones, had been trained in both surgery and radiation therapy as a cancer specialist, and he was one of the best technical surgeons I have ever known. However, Mother wrote, "Lately, you know, instead of turning his cancer cases over to Tommy Jones, Dad has been doing them himself, and he and the boys are very excited. Lately he has done two big cancers of the intestine with beautiful results." The situation here reminds me of the allegedly true story about the senile surgeon who in the course of repairing a patient's hernia somehow managed to cut off his penis. The problem is that not everyone is able, as he gets older, to realize his deficiencies and take the steps necessary to avoid accidents. A fixed retirement age may be an unwarranted penalty against many well-preserved people, but I certainly believe that from the age of sixty on, the performance of all people in responsible positions should be reviewed annually.

My mother at this time was not worrying about her husband's retirement. She had taken over the management of the Kensington property which had been given to the children and had sent us through school. "I am enclosing a letter that came for you, and the Kensington Statement. There is no money in view, I fear, as what is on hand does not cover taxes already due. Send me tenants. Woods is manager at $60 a month. Meanwhile I am running the hotel. I confess I hate it but it saves money just now. Loads of love, Mother."

My father's research and his enthusiasm for its discoveries continued and on October 9, 1933, in the *New York Times* were three columns under the headline: "CRILE ADVANCES LIFE-RAY THEORY AS MEDICAL BASIS. Says Wave-Lengths, as in Radio, Emanate From Body and Set Its Course. He Now Looks to Applying Physical and Chemical Laws in Medicine." In small print was a typical example of my father's imagination which was anticipating such tests as electroencephalography, "By 'listening in' to the short-waves and the long-waves, transmitted by the various organs, he would hear the 'symphony' played by the living organism and would determine the rhythms of the 'dance of life.'" Along the same lines, in a letter to me, dated October 17, my father said he had heard good things about my work in St. Louis but warned, "I have only one word of caution—don't use up the margin of your sympathetic system." By this time he was applying his theories to everything in life.

I answered and reassured my father and told him, "Saturday Dr. Graham took me to the Washington University-Chicago football game, and we had a fine visit and a lot of fun. He certainly is a real chief and an inspiration to work under. During the past month we have done quite a bit of chest surgery—thoracoplasties, mediastinal tumors etc., and I have the greatest admiration for Dr. Graham."

Dr. Graham was a leader in thoracic surgery, for little of it was being done elsewhere. Technically, however, his younger associates were much more skillful than he. Those were the days of tuberculosis, and when there were large cavities in the lung that became filled with pus that could not be drained out, the patients, mostly young women, were subjected to thoracoplasty, an extensive operation in which sections of many ribs were removed in order to collapse the chest wall and obliterate the cavity in the lung. I still remember a lovely girl in her twenties, sick and feverish from her infection, on whom Dr. Graham roughly, as was his way, collapsed the chest with considerable loss of blood. The patient never recovered consciousness. The temperature soared and in a few hours she died in a sort of toxic shock.

Dr. Graham also was removing the lung for patients with pulmonary cancer, but this operation too had a high mortality rate in his hands. I was discouraged from entering thoracic surgery, and as a result I missed the boat, for the greatest advances of the next three decades were to be in thoracic and cardiac surgery.

I rotated on through the service at the Shriner's Hospital for Crippled Children, where we operated on club feet, post-polio deformities, tuberculosis of the hips, and the whole gamut of chronic orthopedic practice. "The surgery is darn good," I wrote. "As for Assistant Residency, I have made up my mind, and even if they were to offer it to me or the position of surgical chief, for that matter, I would come home next year, as I know when and under whom I want to get my surgical technique." Perhaps my separation from Jane also entered into the decision to return to Cleveland, for I had found no one in St. Louis to take her place. However, it seems my life was not entirely devoted to surgery. My mother wrote a protest: "Barney dear, I was on the point of telegraphing when your letter arrived. I had begun to conclude that there was a new outbreak of sleeping sickness; and, instead, you are calling for your boots and spurs, stiff shirts and ties. Well! That's all right if you are meticulous about your foreign relations."

My mother's fears for my St. Louis Social Life were well founded. My next letter told of my

debut in St. Louis Society at a party given by the Bartletts [friends of my parents] for the 1933 debutantes. I set out in a borrowed car, got lost in attempting to find the house, got arrested for having no lights, had the car break down and had to abandon it and walk about a mile arriving about three-quarters of an hour late. All was well however, as they still were having cocktails. I met Dr. and Mrs. Bartlett and am much impressed with both of them. He was very nice to me, has, of course, the highest regard for you, Dad, and asked me to come over and watch his work, as I intend to do at my first opportunity.

The next letter from my father was not an admonition, but a warning:

October 23, 1933

Dear Barney,

I am glad you can find time to sleep and rest—What I always do is to be negative—sleep—and vegetate—omit anything that would disturb the nervous system—and keep on doing this until restored—for you have always been so completely immune against fatigue that you could not realize it as a fact that there is such a thing.

If you were to experiment for a time on omitting nicotine etc. [I smoked about ten cigarettes a day] until you are restored you would note a big difference. I am doing that at this time. [My father smoked a cigar after dinner and occasionally a cigarette during a lunch break.]

Dr. Higgins [one of the Clinic's urologists] smoked excessively, stayed up so excessively and overworked and took a lot of
alcohol—against my solicitude—that now he has a definite
tremor and has become much older than his years. Please don't
think of this as anything but a mechanistic chat.

In the case of Dr. Higgins, my father's prognosis was not accurate.
Charlie was very successful and would live to be ninety-four.

During my period on orthopedics and in the Shriner's Children's
Hospital, I was neither overworked nor over-interested and found time
and somehow enough money to take a horseback ride in the park,
"making an extraordinary appearance with my white trousers tied
down around the ankles and my white coat slapping in the breezes."

Mother, of course, put in her medical oar too. When I complained
about disinterest in orthopedics, she thought I was depressed.

Don't you think if you actually stopped all smoking for a little
while and really turned in early and got caught up you would
get over the dumps? If not I will send you some thyroid tablets—
givers of optimism. However, Dad suggests that inasmuch as
you are indoors so much and not getting the usual amount of
green vegetables perhaps you are beginning to feel the want of
them, and suggests Haliver Oil, so I am ordering a box. They are
so pretty and easy to take. So don't think we are crazy, but just
do it, as Dad wants you to, and it really is not a bad suggestion as
it cannot do any harm.

I have no recollection as to whether I ever received or took the vita-
mins which I think resembled cod-liver oil, but I am sure I didn't for
long because I have always avoided taking dietary supplements. I
have known people who got kidney stones from Vitamin C and two
of my good friends died of too much D in a polar bear's liver that
they ate.

My father continued to be busy lecturing and at the huge meeting
of the Interstate Postgraduate Medical Society, of which he was the
program director, he had sixteen patients on the platform for his dry
clinic. "It was absolutely convincing," Mother wrote. "They represented neurocirculatory asthenia, peptic ulcer, hyperthyroidism etc.
all treated by adrenal denervation."

Of the same Postgraduate meeting, Mother wrote that "Dad gave a
corking paper on gallbladder disease. He had splendid slides and
merely showed and explained his new technique and gave results. He
did not read"—of course his vision wouldn't let him—"which always

pleases me. I am simply amazed how few people read well, and you should hear the grousing. Elliot Cutler drew himself up in a most dignified stage-manner, spoke so deliberately and slowly and with such precision, but looked down, and the desk got his lecture, not his audience. The audience only heard when he looked up at the end of each sentence, and I was in the 12th row." Mother went on to tell how badly several others read and then commented, "Will Mayo one always hears—so my dear, learn to throw your voice forward. It is not done by yelling but by using the muscles of the diaphragm [something I am afraid I never learned to do]. Also learn to get your sentence in a glance, and if you *have* to read, look at your audience and not at your desk." Good advice.

I also received a good suggestion from my father which in time (nine years later) I would carry out. He told of a book called "Standing Orders" that he had planned but never written, and continued, "Would you like to take this book over, bring it up to date and collaborate with Alex [Bunts] and Charlie [Higgins] and bring it about?" I would bring it about, but without collaboration, and it would be published under the title *Hospital Care of the Surgical Patient* (Charles Thomas, 1943, and a second edition in 1946). At the time, I replied to my father's suggestion by saying,

> The book will be ideal training for me as well as a good thing for the Hospital to have the routines gone over again, critically. Treatments of all kinds have always been a weak point in medical school training, and I need just this to get up to date.
>
> I had a talk with Dr. Graham the other day and asked him to let me help him out in some research problems in my spare time this month. He set me on a study of gallbladder lymphatics helping Bobby Bartlett [son of my father's friend] and doing quite a bit of dog surgery, also learning about lymphatics, which will be a help when we tackle the breast problem.

I then went on to tell about a duck hunt with a Yale friend in which everything went wrong and I brought home none of the ducks that I had promised my friends for dinner.

And now at last, my father was forced to face up to the reality of the growing problem with his eyes. In November he wrote, "I told you I believe I must go to New York for a month and since this [operation for glaucoma] could be so devastatingly expensive to us and the Clinic [if the word of it got out], I am keeping this information to just you and Bob. The girls do not know anything at all. For you to be home without us at Christmas would raise too many questions. Would you think of accumulating vacation and hunt with Bob and Fuller [collecting specimens of adrenals etc. for the research]? Or would you spend Christmas with Elo? Send me a discussion about it. The hunting can be paid for by our Trust Fund provided the Museum is included. Love, Dad."

I assented to Dad's plans, saying that I hadn't even considered taking time off at Christmas. I added, "Do you think it will be possible to keep the entire procedure hushed up and not have comment made on your absence? It would possibly work like Hearst's diverticulum, the mystery resulting in greater exaggerations. However, I do not know what you are planning in this respect." I concluded by offering to come on to spend a week with him in New York.

On November 24, Mother wrote from New York that all had gone well in my father's operation for glaucoma. The procedure was conducted anonymously, under the title of Mr. Morgan, No. 600. My father was in the hospital for three weeks while my mother stayed at the Roosevelt Hotel and ate "at cafeterias and drug stores. My three meals today cost me ninety-five cents. I have learned how to go out in the subway, hobnobbing with all the Columbia students, and I come back by bus. It takes over an hour, but I like to sit up on top and see all the bright lights at night, and there are so many in New York that I never feel afraid." That was an extraordinary adjustment for a lady in her sixties who had never stayed for any length of time in New York or ridden on public transport. "Tonight on my way down," Mother continued, "I stopped off at Radio City. I felt tired and tense and strained as if I could weep if left alone, so I went in and saw a perfectly lovely movie—'Little Women.' I sat up in the top row, up among all the purple glow. It was enchanting, and the music was lovely—so beautiful and restful. It took me quite out of myself."

In those days no one thought twice about keeping patients in the hospital for three weeks. Ten days was about the minimum after an uncomplicated delivery. New mothers weren't allowed to get up for the first few days. Similarly my father was constrained in total bed rest. "The first days are hard," Mother wrote, "It is difficult to lie utterly still—stone still—on one's back with eyes closed and without even shifting the position of one's head. It begets a feeling of restlessness. No solid food is allowed for three days—no bowel movements. Sneezing is prohibited and to blow one's nose is immoral." She went on to say that his nurse, who had taken care of the king of Siam, was the "sweetest, mildest, fidgety-est Vermont maiden I have ever seen. She knows her business to the nth degree, is perfect in her nursing and so typical of the dear old Granite State, a type of that refined,

conscientious gentlewoman of New England that she intrigues me.
Dad teases her but she never unbends."

My only surviving letter to Mother during this period sends excuses for not having written and the comment, "It must be terrible lying inert in a dark room, unable to talk, sneeze or even listen—like a
potato in a basket."

On "Thanksgiving Eve, 1933" my father dictated a letter to me.

Dear Barney,

A potato's existence is certainly what this is. I only hope the
eyes will sprout. Just at present it takes quite a bit of faith.

It was strange to see the operation an inverted image—the
hands, the needle—the taking of the stitches—an inside view!

Dr. Wheeler, the ophthalmologist who had operated on my father,
said that the result to date was "100%." Mother wrote, "We are now
reading old manuscripts aloud, with a view to throwing out what Dad
does not want to consider including in his next new book [*Diseases Peculiar to Civilized Man*]. Of course I just adore this kind of thing. In my
next life I am going to arrange somehow to be Dad's medical secretary
and head operating-room nurse by day and his wife at night and the
mother of his children." In the world of Mother's dreams there would
seem to be little time for sleep. "When I stop to think of all that has
come into my life through him, and the privilege it has been to play
along in the shadow of so really great a mind and personality, I actually find my heart pattering with fright lest I might have missed it all.
What a Halle's comet I would have been. I remember seeing that as a
child—dashing through the heavens, a lovely trail, coming back again
sometime, someday, somewhere." Mother had confused the Halley
who reported the comet with the Halle who sired Jane. Mother went
on to describe how she spent an entire morning watching Dr. Wheeler
operate on patients with glaucoma and cataracts.

Describing my father's convalescence she wrote, "Suddenly from
the pillows this voice said, 'Grace, are you there?' I said, 'Yes.' He
said, 'Have you a pencil?' I replied, 'Why yes, why?' 'Get it quick and
take this down.' This is what I took down." Then followed a half page
of description of sharp pains that he had felt around his heart and of
their relationship to stimulation of the adrenal-sympathetic system,
and ended, "'Two hours after the first operation I had a good deal of
pain. Two hours after this operation I have none. I think this is a definite fact that the thyroid governs the activity of the sympathetic system." My father was persuaded by any event that his theory was
correct. My mother was so persuaded that she wrote, "Isn't it strange

that this [glaucoma] should be a Jewish disease too, particularly among Polish Jews? It must be just another form of breakdown from the drive through the sympathetic nervous system. I wonder what effect denervation would have?" Mother was so convinced of the genius of my father that later when I began to question the validity of many of his theories and of the supposedly good results of the denervations that he did, Mother was bitterly disappointed not only in my loyalty but also in my intelligence.

By now I was on the urology service headed by Dr. Caulk, who I said was a better talker than he was a urologist but still was an excellent urologist. "There are about 25 patients with prostates, carcinoma of the bladder, all manner of stones, renal tumors, diverticula, in short the gamut of urology. At present I have three patients hovering around the pearly gates with N.P.N. [a measure of kidney failure] varying from 50 to 90, temperatures 103 to 105 degrees, hemorrhages, chills, plugged catheters—you know the way it goes." Those were the early days of transurethral resection of the prostate, and the convalescences were exciting, marked by profuse bleeding, bladders so full of clots that it was up to the intern to suck them out through the often obstructed catheter. I didn't like that service at all. A little later I became further disillusioned with my ability to cope with the genital system.

"I did a hydrocele" (the sack filled with water that sometimes surrounds the testicle and makes a huge mass in the scrotum). I had never assisted on any operation in the scrotum before and had only seen one hydrocele operation which was years ago. "We thought this was a garden variety hydrocele, started opening up, made about five false-layer dissections, getting as many flaps to fool with, of course, discovered that we were dealing with a huge hydrocele of the cord and none of the tunica vaginalis, opened both sacs, got lost, took off the tip of the epididymis [that transfers the sperm], retreated in confusion, cutting all layers and flaps in sight, and ended up by getting it closed and dry. So far the result is perfect. Next time I am certainly going to keep those layers straight. The thing had as many as an onion by the time I got through." This happened in those absurd years when totally untrained interns and residents were allowed to operate on charity patients. In fact, the Surgical Boards demanded that the resident staff be given "full responsibility" for operations or the training program would not be approved. Fortunately, with the advent of Medicare and Medicaid, it is now illegal for an untrained surgeon to assume responsibility if a fee is to be charged, and hospitals certainly do not forego collecting fees in the names of the department's surgeons.

The first handwritten letter from my father after the operation was dated December 15, 1933, and read: "Dear Barney, This is to certify that the old owl has come out of the hollow tree and is somewhat dazzled by the light. Dad." My parents still did not directly mention the secret operation, and so far as I know the secret was successfully kept.

When convalescence was complete, my parents went to Cumberland Island, off Georgia, with Bob and Mr. Fuller from the Natural History Museum, to which Dad had made a large contribution. The museum was backing the expedition to collect specimens of animals for their collection and for my father's. Mother reported that Bob waded into an area filled with alligators and shot a nine-foot one in the head. "It leaped into the air whisking his tail round and round, and finally turning over and over churning the water. Bob got in more shots, finally quieting him sufficiently to get him by the tail and drag him ashore where we all awaited him." That was a pretty exciting kind of convalescence for my father. On the way back to Cleveland, he stopped in Jacksonville to give a medical lecture on the gallbladder.

My life was exciting too. I wrote from St. Louis, "Ten days before Christmas the G.U. service suddenly exploded and went completely to pot. We had three bleeding punches." In those days the primitive transurethral resections were often called prostatic punches for they punched out a hole in the prostate.

All needed glucose, transfusions, evacuation of clots etc. all at once and, of course, at all hours of day and night. We had a McCarthy resection also. The patient was Dr. Lamb and he of course, being the one everyone was most interested in, had the following complications. First, hemorrhage—severe enough to bleed him out to 2,500,000 red and 40% hemoglobin [about half of his blood]. Second, a prolonged shock—hemorrhage—sepsis, combined reaction which left him with a blood pressure of from 50 to 80 for three days. This resulted in anuria [no urine] and the N.P.N. rose to 77. This resulted in gastrointestinal inhibition and acute distention of the stomach. Next we discovered a mass in the pelvis, high white count and sepsis. A fasting blood sugar, accidentally taken, was 330 [three times the normal level]. Next came a convulsion, turning out to be an insulin reaction. An abscess then localized in the abdominal wall which was opened, and it was found that urine discharged, implying that much of the original reaction was due to extravasation of urine [from injury during the operation]. Of course during the first five days of this the patient never stopped hiccoughing for more than 20 minutes. When I left for Memphis he had not gotten pneumonia yet, but that and embolism are the only two complications left for him. I have never spent such a week and did not get over six, usually five, and sometimes two, hours of sleep a day.

By this time I was on neurosurgery with Dr. Sachs, one of the leaders in that field, and I had become very fond of my fellow intern and former Harvard classmate, Brad Cannon. After I spent ten days with Sachs, Dr. Graham shifted me to his service because he was going to be away at the time I normally would have been on it. I also admitted that "Jane came through town for a few days—just as I was switching services. It was great to see her again and we had a good reunion and incidentally settled a lot of problems, I believe, quite definitely this time. In any case, I am glad to report, Mother, that I do not think you will find me 'lovesick' next time you see me, as you diagnosed last fall. She has apparently given up Bub or vice versa, but has several others in the offing." As I remember, Jane had a college friend in St. Louis and had told her family that she was going to St. Louis to visit her. What happened was that the house staff had rented a little cabin down by the Meramec River which had nothing but a wood stove, a few chairs, and a few beds, and that was where our few-and-far-between staff weekend sojourns were spent. That is why on this occasion Jane and I were able to settle a lot of problems.

Things in Cleveland were on the upswing. "We have 133 patients in the hospital," my father wrote, "and are exceeding last year—not much, but definitely." Mother, however, was worried, "I still find myself in the night wondering if anything happened to Dad and debts were collected, if I would have capacity enough to have an earning power, say at the Clinic." In the next paragraph she wrote, "Then last week the crocodile came—ten feet of crocodile. To the touch he was cold and hard, his eyes green and glassy, his jaws bound. By Monday he was a real alive and hissing crocodile."

At my parents' home there were diverse types of entertainment. In spite of the depression, various social organizations kept using the enormous ballroom and other facilities for entertainment. "Within the last week we have had two parties at the house, Hariette Sherman [niece] and Dickie McBride's [nephew] set when we had supper for 100, games, and a George Washington cotillion, and for a party of Parent-Teachers League, of which Peg [my sister] is President of the Roxboro group. That means bridge and a style show and tea for 400. It was a terrible day. We had 800 galoshes to check, but Peg managed splendidly."

I wrote of my difficulties with Dr. Sachs, the head of neurosurgery to whose service I had been returned: "Brain surgery is of course extremely unsatisfactory and depressing, and although I guess Sachs is one of the best, the good results are far between. He is very difficult to assist as he criticizes us both for showing initiative and for lack of initiative. That is he does when things are going wrong for him. Dr. Graham removed a lung the other day for cancer, but the patient died that night. Several of the thoracoplasties have died recently, and all the mediastinal tumors that I have seen him do, so I am sort of discouraged with that branch too."

In the middle of all of my family's health and economic difficulties and of the Clinic's slow recovery from the disaster of the depression, my father kept collecting animals so he could study their thyroid and adrenal glands. On March 24, Mother wrote about a fifty-seven-pound chimpanzee that was "so tame that he was lonely unless someone was in the room with him all the time." He was partially paralyzed but "he screamed with delight, showing his teeth in a great broad grin whenever Ralph [the Clinic's Diener in charge of animals] came near him. He had the most beautiful thyroids imaginable." Mother went on to describe the adrenals too and then a four-hundred-pound tiger that arrived the next day—a circus tiger that had gone almost blind. All of these animals were anaesthetized and dissected in the Clinic's research building. It was very exciting, and an eleven-foot alligator was on its way! "The arrivals are beginning to fall into a different form of classification," Mother said.

Instead of classifying them on the basis of form they can be classified on the basis of energy, which is simpler. The extremely dynamic animals such as those who chase and those who are chased belong to one group which have larger adrenals and thyroids, that is a high energy system. Those who receive protection through armor, poison, quills etc. including the crocodile, belong to the more nearly balanced group which have adrenals and thyroids of about equal size, while those who have fled for protections to the trees where through orthogenesis and the rise of the hand they developed greater brain power, such as the primates and man, have larger thyroids than adrenals.

On April 1, 1934, all of this was published in the *New York Times* under the headline, ANIMALS CLASSIFIED ON BASIS OF ENERGY.

On Easter Sunday, I wrote my parents,

I received your Easter gift and nearly went to church today to have an opportunity to wear and exhibit it. Unfortunately, however, amongst the godless heathens composing the house staff of this or any hospital I could find no one who would go to church or who even knew where one was. So I contented myself with going down to the colored ward and working up an hysterical patient into a religious frenzy and watching The Lord take her body and soul to the Glory of His Own.

Yesterday Bill Byars and myself and two girls went horseback riding—a beautiful day, rather pleasant country, fair horses, but all in all just about good enough to make me a little homesick for the Knob. Today I am stiff and regret it immensely. Sometime soon I expect to take a fishing trip to one of the bass streams of the vicinity where there is supposed to be really excellent sport.

Gynecology here is excellent in that we have so much material, but the surgery that is done, or rather the things that are done in the name of surgery, are dreadful.

My trouble was that I was spoiled because I had worked with Dr. Tom Jones at the Clinic who in those days did all of the gynecology as well as most of the colorectal and abdominal surgery and was a superlative technician.

As spring came to St. Louis and I became accustomed and more efficient at performing the duties of an intern, there seemed to be more time for extracurricular activities. I wrote about organizing the "Barnes Hospital Bowling Team" and about playing baseball—house staff against permanent staff every Tuesday afternoon. "Dr. Graham played first base. Last time we beat them and won a case of beer."

By now beer was legal and we also had found an answer to the hard liquor problem. One of our friends on the assistant staff was working in the pathology laboratory where large demijohns full of alcohol used to preserve specimens were stored. There were two varieties, the regular 95 percent alcohol (the remaining 5 percent being water that boils off with the alcohol) and the 100 percent alcohol, used for special purposes. We were accustomed to taking small quantities of each of these with us when we would go out in the evening, and sitting in a cafe where we had ordered orangeade we would ask our partners whether they would prefer to add an ounce of the weak stuff (95 percent) or the strong stuff to their drinks.

By this time, my companion had become Brad Cannon, whose friend was the head nurse on the children's ward. Her best friend was one of the head nurses in the private section. These St. Louis nurses—not the student nurses but the regular nurses and supervisors—were extraordinarily able and energetic women who were accustomed to assuming great responsibility. I admired them greatly and so did Brad, with the result that during that spring we spent most of our spare time as a foursome. I felt that I was not parting from my father's advice that a good sheepdog does not kill in his own flock. These were not sheep, they were shepherds.

The women were fully mature—several years older than Brad and myself—and they neither had nor were they given any illusions about the future. They knew of Brad's and my relationships in Cleveland and Boston. We kept no secrets from one another and we had a marvelous spring, often visiting the little place on the river where Jane and I had gone and to which I referred, in my letters to Mother, as the river to which we went "to go Bass Fishing." To me these relationships were much more pleasant than the occasional ones in high society. I wrote to Mother, "Last night I went to hear 'Madame Butterfly' at the City's new Music Hall. It was very well done and I really enjoyed it, falling asleep only once, and for only a short time."

In scientific circles, the reaction to my father's unorthodox theories and widespread publicity was beginning to crystallize. At a meeting of the Philosophical Society there was an extraordinarily critical discussion, almost a condemnation of my father's paper. "Then up rose Dr. Heilbrun, a Jew," Mother wrote, "who started out that he did not see why Dr. Crile continued to give these papers on the autosynthetic cell when none of the biologists believed in it and that it was 'bunk.'" And Mother proceeded to condemn the critic for his behavior. Economically things were beginning to improve. My father wrote, "As a confidential bit of information my cash income from operations only last year was $108,000," which in today's values equals a million. And then Mother wrote of a visit by Dr. Cannon who had lectured at the Clinic: "He had much to say about the American habit of too much sugar. He enlarged on the subject showing how we take away the flavor of the food by sweetening it, but the next morning he forgot his theory when the cereal came along and before he was ready to eat it, it looked like a snow-covered Mount Etna."

The year at Barnes was ending. I have no notes and I wrote no letters that I can find that give details of those last months of service, but I have several clear, though undocumented memories.

I remember a patient on the private wing—an elderly lady who was in the terminal states of cancer, comatose at times, obviously dying, yet at intervals she was lucid. I had become attached to her and impressed with her bravery and her good sense. She had a child who lived out of town and was to arrive to visit her the next day, she told me, and said that all she wanted was to live long enough to see her.

I consulted all my friends and the staff and the books, and I rigged up a continuous intravenous drip of glucose to which I could add stimulants such as adrenaline which would raise the blood pressure for a while and restore consciousness. I let her sleep most of the time, and then when the daughter arrived I speeded up the infusion, poured in the adrenaline and had the satisfaction of seeing my friend awake, embrace her daughter and have an hour of talk before she fell back into irreversible coma. That was one of the satisfying things that I remember, but there were others.

Of course there were unhappy occurrences as well. I remember a young woman, also on the private service, who had had a minor abdominal operation, perhaps a suspension of the uterus, which aside from the risk of anaesthesia should have practically no mortality. At that time appendicitis was considered to be a very common and dangerous disease and, to prevent it surgeons, in the course of other operations, often did what were called "incidental appendectomies." In this case it could better have been termed "accidental," because the stump of the appendix leaked and the young woman died of peritonitis. From this I learned the lesson that the less surgery that is done the safer it is for the patient.

I have a vivid memory too, of Dr. Graham himself operating on a tumor that was very vascular and adherent to the bone and which he had to literally drag and chisel out of the pelvis. The bleeding was terrific. The pelvis was packed to try to staunch it, but in spite of transfusions of every kind of support, the patient died. Another lesson learned. Do not operate on inoperable tumors.

Dr. Graham was still one of the country's great surgeons, unsurpassed as an organizer, as an innovator, and as a stimulus to all who worked with him. On June 11, 1934, he replied to a letter from my father who had written him about how much I had appreciated my service with him, saying that he thought my father was "one of the great surgeons of all time," and that he felt it was a compliment that his son had come to him for training. He ended by saying, "We are just as delighted with Barney as he was with the work that he got here."

This letter was written just before the final debacle of my internship. I had never learned to type so that every five or six weeks, when it came my turn to type the operating schedule, it took me most of the day to do it. I thought it was a gross imposition to ask the interns to do this and made some complaints which fell on deaf ears. I then decided to take things into my own hands and arranged with my grateful colleagues to take over the typing of the schedules for the last three weeks of the year.

On the first Monday after the new arrangement everyone noted some absurd typographical errors on the schedule, but no one said anything about it. On the next Monday the schedule was typed up and down—spaced this way and that and spelled phonetically. It was nearly illegible, but I had a clear handwritten master copy that was available in the operating room to prevent serious mistakes. I was called to the office of the superintendent.

"Your typing of the schedule is a disgrace, Crile. You should be reprimanded."

"You haven't seen anything yet," I answered. "I've arranged to type it again next week too."

"But why do you type it that way? It makes it hard for everyone."

"I type it that way because typing is hard for me. I never learned to type. I don't know how to use a typewriter. You never asked me, when you appointed me as an intern, whether or not I could type. I never thought of typing as being part of the work of a physician. I thought secretaries did that. I'm sorry, and I'll do my best again next Sunday."

Next Sunday, one of the secretaries appeared. My battle was won and my internship was over.

6

Residency at the Cleveland Clinic
1934–1936

B Y THE STANDARDS of 1934, the salary of a resident at the Clinic was generous—enough so that, with my first month's wages, I was able to purchase and have leather-bound a copy of Darwin's *Origin of Species* which I presented to my father on his birthday. With it was a note saying that it was a privilege for me to be able to use my first paycheck to provide for him a bound copy of the greatest book that the world's greatest scientist ever wrote, and that Darwin's only rival in the realm of science was Crile.

After the year in St. Louis and the scut work that the interns there had to do, it was pleasant to be back in the familiar environment and well-organized hospital life of the Cleveland Clinic. At that time, only two years of residency after internship was required for the training of a general surgeon, and it was not necessary to rotate through the specialties like orthopedics or neurosurgery.

In 1934, there were three surgeons on the Cleveland Clinic's general surgical staff—my father, whose work now was almost completely confined to thyroidectomies and adrenal denervations; Dr. Robert Dinsmore, who had been trained by my father and whose work consisted mainly of thyroid surgery; and Dr. Tom Jones, who now was at the peak of his career and had become famous for the excellence of his operations for cancers of the rectum and colon. Jones also was skilled in the surgery of the upper abdomen and breast and in gynecological surgery. In those days the Clinic did not recognize gynecology as a specialty and there was no such thing as a vascular, a thoracic, or a plastic surgeon, although Dr. Jones did a little surgery in all of these fields.

Dr. Jones was my model, for he was the best technical surgeon that up to that time I had ever seen and he was also versed in oncological radiology—treating cancers of the skin and of the uterus by application or implantation of radium or of radon seeds, for the manufacture of which we had, under the direction of Dr. Otto Glasser, one of the first plants in the Midwest. We also had what in those days was considered to be one of the best radiation-therapy facilities.

Tom Jones's specialty, for which he had attained international acclaim, was the combined abdominoperineal resection for cancers of the rectum. This operation removed all of the rectum and lower colon and left the patient with an artificial opening in the abdomen. In the hands of the average surgeon who did perhaps only one or two of these operations a year, the usual mortality rate was between 10 and 20 percent. In the hands of Dr. Jones, who did one or two of these operations a day, the mortality was about 1 percent. It took the average surgeon three or four hours or even longer to perform the operation, whereas Dr. Jones often did it in less than an hour.

In 1934, there were no antibiotics and any surgery of the colon that involved resection of a segment of the colon and then suturing it together again was, by definition, dangerous, because when the bowel was opened the abdominal cavity was of necessity contaminated by its contents. If there were leakage at the suture line, the discharge of the feces into the abdominal cavity caused what usually was a fatal peritonitis. For this reason Dr. Jones tended to remove the rectum and lower bowel and establish a permanent colostomy even in patients whose tumors were quite high in the rectum or lower colon, and which today would be treated by resection and anastomosis that involves no colostomy. But in those preantibiotic days, Dr. Jones's way carried a much lower mortality because there was no possibility of a leak or of contamination of the cavity. Surgeons came from all over the world to watch Jones operate.

There was another aspect to Dr. Jones's practice that he never publicized or even wrote a paper about—that was the conservative treatment of small, low-lying cancers that could be treated by destruction and electrocoagulation without removing the rectum at all. This operation carried almost no mortality and involved no colostomy, and could be done without even admitting the patient to the hospital. Sometimes, of course, lymph nodes were involved and later would grow and cause trouble, but in the cases selected, not more than 20 percent had this complication and half of these could still be salvaged by the radical operation. Moreover most of the patients who had metastases in nodes were doomed to die of liver metastases, so leaving the nodes in made little, if any, difference in life expectancy.

Dr. Jones apparently was aware of these arguments in favor of the lesser operation, but he never presented them in public, and used them only when a colleague or close friend would come to him. Then he would explain it all, and if the patient agreed he would use the conservative treatment and save the rectum. If Dr. Jones had preached this doctrine to the profession and had used the conservative operation intensively, I am sure that he would have been exorcised by his colleagues just as I would be when, in later years, I questioned the necessity of performing radical mastectomies.

Dr. Jones was not only a great surgeon, he also was a good friend and an entertaining companion. He was of Welsh ancestry, had a marvelous sense of humor, and in the evening enjoyed a drink or two around the fire. He never married, and was never caught in a compromising relationship with a woman. How he managed this I don't know, because I'm sure there was nothing neutral about old Tommie.

The other general surgeon, besides my father, was Dr. Robert Dinsmore, also a bachelor who, until he got married, used to share a suite of rooms with Dr. Jones. Dinsmore was a dedicated duck hunter and sportsman, a gifted storyteller, and such a good politician that eventually he came to be President of the American Surgical Association—the honor society for surgeons.

Dr. Dinsmore did a good thyroidectomy by my father's technique, which involved no anatomical dissection, and he did a good modified radical mastectomy, also by my father's technique. He was very conservative, but never seemed to feel at home in abdominal operations, and never originated anything. Nevertheless, his complete integrity and pleasant personality won for him the respect of referring physicians and colleagues and even the love and affection of one our most attractive nurse anesthetists whom he eventually married. I felt that there was little that I could learn from Dr. Dinsmore, and hence spent as much of my time as possible on Dr. Jones's service.

My father, of course, was delighted to have me back, and by now he really needed me. His eyesight had deteriorated to the point that he could not read, drive, or even walk without stumbling over things. Yet he was still doing five or six operations a day, mainly thyroidectomies and adrenal denervations, and these he was doing almost entirely by sense of touch. The resident would make the incision and expose the gland, and then my father would step in and denervate or remove whatever was necessary, and the resident would complete the closure.

In retrospect, the conviction that made my father continue to operate could be criticized because it certainly caused accidents that threatened lives of some patients, but there is another consideration. In the early 1930s, the Cleveland Clinic was still recovering from the financial disasters of the X-ray film explosion and the Great Depression, and it was barely able to meet its obligations. The salaries of the physicians had been cut, and every method of cost-containment had been used. The secret of my father's eye trouble and operations had been so well kept that referring physicians and patients knew nothing of it. He was still the greatest money earner on the Clinic staff. If he had retired in the early 1930s, I do not believe the Clinic could have survived.

As an example of the accidents that happened as a result of my father's glaucoma and cataracts, I remember a patient who had an extensive cancer of the thyroid, upon whom my father was operating and I was the first assistant. Alice Matley, who later would marry Dr. Dinsmore, was the anaesthetist. The cancer had invaded the tissues around the upper pole of the thyroid and made it densely adherent to all surrounding structures. My father was feeling his way through this, trying to disentangle the tumor from the surrounding anatomy and from time to time using scissors to cut adherent tissues. I was very nervous because I could see things that he couldn't.

"Look out, Dad," I said, "that's the carotid artery—" (the main artery to the brain and head). "Don't worry," he said and continued to operate. "Look out, look out," I repeated. Stimulated by curiosity, Alice, the anaesthetist, stood up to look over the drapes that separated her and the patient's head from the operative field.

Just as Alice stood up, my father's scissors cut. The blood, about a bucket of it, squirted from the severed carotid and hit her square in the face. We managed to control the bleeding, and luckily the patient survived on collateral from the vessel on the other side, but more often than not such an accident causes death or paralysis of the opposite side of the body.

On another occasion my father, in performing an adrenal denervation, accidentally cut one of the large vessels to the kidney, right at the point that it leaves the aorta. It was really an injury to the side of the aorta, and bleeding from such an injury is most difficult to control. My father couldn't see well enough to sew it shut and he wouldn't let his assistant try to. He just put in a big pack which temporarily stopped the bleeding. Packs can permanently stop bleeding from the ends of small arteries, because the blood in the arteries clots and prevents further flow, but this injury was to the side of the man's largest blood vessel. There was no way that the blood coursing down the aorta could be persuaded to stop long enough to clot.

The patient was transfused and returned to his room in fair condition, but during the next day he continued to ooze and at intervals to bleed briskly. The packs were made larger but the trouble continued. The patient was a physician and well aware of the difficulties. He was put on the danger list and his wife was notified and allowed to stand by. At about midnight of the day after the operation, I was on duty and received an emergency call. It was well justified, for when I got there the bed was flooded with blood and in spite of pressure that I put on the pack it continued to gurgle up out of the wound. I had to risk removing the pack so I could apply finger pressure directly to the hole in the aorta. As I was working the patient said softly, "Please call my wife. I wish to speak to her." She was just outside the room, and the nurse brought her to the head of the bed. "It has been a wonderful life—thank you—you have made everything perfect for me." Those were the last words he spoke. By the time I could find and block the hole in the aorta he had lost consciousness. In a few moments, in spite of our primitive (by today's standards) attempts at resuscitation, he expired. Since that time, I have been present at the time of death of a number of patients, but this is the only one whom I remember as making a significant death-bed statement—the way the characters in novels so frequently do.

At the Cleveland Clinic, the time it took the surgeons to do the standard operations was much less than in either Boston or St. Louis, and the volume of work done by each surgeon was larger. It was obvious that we were deficient in management of patients requiring specialized plastic surgery, but all other fields and specialties were well covered. I was happy to be home and confident that the Clinic offered an ideal situation for surgical training. There was one major difference. Here the residents did not perform the operations, they first-assisted the surgeon. However, they did that so often and they were so well instructed that when the time came, they knew exactly how to do them. For example, many years later when Tom Jones would suddenly drop dead, his resident, Rupert Turnbull, who was just finishing his training, would be appointed to the staff and take over much of Dr. Jones's practice. The Clinic's operative mortality in the major operation of combined abdominoperineal resection for rectal cancers would be, for that year, a shade better than it had been with Dr. Jones the year before.

In addition to the surgical experience, there were ward rounds on which the problems of care were well discussed, and there were weekly meetings of the surgical staff and also meetings of the sub-specialty staffs and fellows. Out-of-town speakers came frequently to give Bunts Lectures (named for the founder) and there was an excellent medical library. Moreover I was at home at least every other night, which was a lot more pleasant than the one or two nights a week that we had had free on some of the services at Barnes Hospital.

I remember how strange and lonely it was to move back into my room in that huge and empty house in which I had grown up, surrounded by family, servants and guests. Now there were just my mother and father, a cook and two maids. My parents still dressed for dinner every night and were served downstairs in the huge dining room. My mother was kept busy reading to my father—his mail, the news, and his own papers that he had dictated and needed final editing—a job at which Mother excelled. One skill that never left my father was writing or dictating about his theories. And although I tried to pass on to Mother my growing disbelief in the long-run value of adrenal denervation, and of the difficulties, from the scientific standpoint, of some of his theories, I soon found that this was met with by fierce antagonism and that it produced no results, except unhappiness for all concerned. I gave up discussing Clinic affairs with my parents, for strangely enough my father, who by now everyone in the family and many of his associates at the Clinic were calling "Chief," had convinced himself that the nerves to the adrenal could not be visualized and severed under direct vision, but could best be identified by palpation and then by severing them with a long scissors. This was fine so long as what was being palpated was a nerve. However, in perhaps 10 percent of the cases, they were small vessels, and in 2 or 3 percent, large vessels, like the renal artery, which would be injured. Since the Chief couldn't see to clamp these bleeders, I as his first assistant had a lot of experience and soon became pretty good at it.

The thyroid surgery wasn't so bad. The first assistant would make the incision and expose the goiter which my father could then feel, and apply clamps over which he could cut out what he wanted of the gland. After that, it was up to the assistants to stop the bleeding. Since he never had done an anatomical operation with identifications of the recurrent laryngeal nerves or parathyroid glands, the results were not much worse than before, and so long as there was not an extensive cancer to deal with, no serious accidents occurred.

Since the Clinic had a very limited emergency service, most of the residents were free from Saturday afternoon until Monday, which in the summer made it nice for me because the Halle farm was only about five miles away from the Knob. Jane and I, who were not going out with other people, could spend a lot of time riding horseback at her parents' place or at ours, or going on fishing trips to neighboring streams or dancing on Saturday nights at the Kirtland Club. Jane had become interested in photography and kept herself busy with taking and developing pictures for exhibits, and also in joining her father in flying lessons.

The Halle farm was ideal for everything. There was a "log cabin" that originally had been a log cabin, but by a series of additions had become a three-bedroom log house with a sleeping porch on which the three unmarried sisters, Kay, Jane, and Ann, slept. Jane's brother, Walter, and one of her older sisters, Margaret, were married and had moved out.

I had not as yet started to write medical articles, although I did collaborate with Dr. Dinsmore and write most of one entitled, "Thyroid Problems and End Results of Operations of the Thyroid Gland." Rereading this article today, I can find almost nothing in it that I still believe. Operations were advised for practically all enlargements of the thyroid gland and the radical advice given for the treatment of malignancies I now consider to be completely wrong. In fact, they were based on purely theoretical considerations because neither I nor Dr. Dinsmore ever practiced, as preached in the article, that "In early cases a radical operation is performed without regard for the structures of the neck." This is ironic, because I spent all the rest of my professional life trying to persuade the profession that in cancer of the thyroid it is almost never necessary to sacrifice the normal muscles and nerves of the neck.

My life was fully occupied with my work and my weekends. When winter approached and the Halles moved in town, their home was only a few blocks from ours. Both families continued to go to the country for weekends. Then, on November 3 came my twenty-seventh birthday. Jane's sister, Margaret Sherwin, asked Jane and me to dinner and to spend the night. She had graciously arranged for us to have adjoining rooms, but she did not plan to have her chauffeur drive my car into the garage and lock it in to protect it from an impending storm. This unpremeditated action resulted in my being unable to have the use of some essential articles that I had kept in the glove compartment of the car.

Jane and I made the best of the situation, but it was only two weeks later that she admitted that her expected period had not arrived. The next day the test was positive. I went to my father for advice, saying, "Dad, I want you to know that Jane is pregnant and I am going to marry her. The only thing I want to ask you is whether you think the baby should be aborted to avoid all talk of illegitimacy or do you think it's okay to carry it through?" My father thought a minute and then replied, "Please, don't tell your mother anything about this. Let me deal with her. But first I want to talk to Uncle Ed." Uncle Ed was Dr. Lower, cofounder of the Clinic, my father's first cousin and his most trusted friend and associate. The next day, my father told me that Uncle Ed had been all for it. The lights were green. I told Mother that Jane and I had decided to marry and would like to honeymoon in the Florida Keys in the hotel that she and Dad had stayed in when they were collecting alligators and that we were planning a simple ceremony at the Halle's next week. Mother did not jump with joy, but she made no objection. After all, she was a rather old-fashioned lady and remembered that in the seventeenth century more than half of the brides in both England and America were pregnant on their wedding days.

My next task was to ask Mr. Halle for permission to marry his daughter. This I did with some trepidation, for there was no way that I could think of that I would be able to support Jane and our child. I had saved a little money during my year of internship and the year of residency because I had no living expenses and had the income from the real estate that had put me through school and college, but I still was making only about fifty dollars a month and that wouldn't increase for another two years.

When I confessed to Mr. Halle about my financial problems and my desire to marry his daughter, he just smiled, congratulated me on my good taste and changed the subject. Unknown to me, Jane had enough independent income to make it unnecessary for us to worry, and fortunately Mr. Halle had enough confidence in my future to welcome me into the family.

On the morning of the scheduled wedding I received a communication from Mother's secretary, who through the years had gotten to know me well and was well aware of all my failings. The telegram, dated December 5, 1934, read:

Reminding you of your wedding today at one. Please attend.
> Miss Maloney

The Halles put on a perfect wedding. The Unitarian minister, Reverend Lupton, performed the ceremony. The only guests were my siblings, Jane's, their spouses, and my uncles and aunts. The Halles had no uncles or aunts that they associated with because Mrs. Halle had no relatives in this country and all of Mr. Halle's orthodox relatives had left him when he married a Catholic.

The Unitarian minister was a great solution. The service was short and sweet. Both of my parents were delighted with the Halles' good taste. My mother wrote of it, "Everyone present yesterday expressed utter satisfaction in every detail, even to the new model of the marriage service." (It had been greatly contracted.) And my father wrote, "Everyone asked about the wedding as people all do, and I was able to describe this new model in such a way that I think you would do well to have it copyrighted or patented." We didn't do that, but we stuck to the formula with the result that none of our daughters were married in churches or had huge receptions. I was so excited by it all that by mistake I went off with my Uncle Malcolm's hat. Jane was so unperturbed that you would think marriage was for her an everyday happening. We were chaperoned to the train by some of our friends who had heard of the event. The papers had been full of it for two days, talking about the union of two prominent families and showing a picture of me as an end on the Yale football team. Even the *New York Times* ran a paragraph about it. True to form, my medical school friend, John Trommald, to whom I had attributed the article that I had sent to a Boston paper about selling the state of Maine to Canada, had our wedding described in the *Boston Daily Record* under the headline CRILE TO MARRY RICH RESCUER. After announcing the marriage, the article went on to say, "The young doctor became excited during a Harvard-Yale boat race on the Thames, New London, back in 1928, lost his balance and plunged into the water. He could not swim. In an adjoining boat was Miss Halle, an excellent swimmer, who realized his peril and jumped in after him. This was the start of the romance between them that became known to hundreds of Harvard students who witnessed the rescue."

Our friends put us aboard the train for Miami. We found that they had stuffed our stateroom with a live duck, goldfish, turtles, and a library of books full of instructions for newlyweds. Also they had notified friends of mine in Cincinnati, where the train stopped, that we were aboard. Consequently, our honeymoon was rudely interrupted by a band of noisy people who boarded the train and molested us. In spite of all these difficulties, we made it through to Miami, changed trains to catch the one that in those days ran along the Florida Keys and over the channels and waterways all the way to Key West. It was to the Island of Matecumbe, about two hours from Miami, that we were headed. We were met at Islamorada by Mr. Butters, the owner of the Matecumbe Hotel, who had known my father when he had stayed there, and who now, in this off-season, put the almost empty hotel at Jane's and my disposal. I telegraphed my parents, "Delighted beyond words with everything. Swim and beach this morning, reef fishing this afternoon. Have a suite with five double beds! Forgot to tell Quiring I promised he would return Tiger's Skull to 200. Probably forgot other things too. Call Halles and say Jane shares above sentiments. Barney."

It was a good honeymoon, unmarred by the fact that the temperature fell until the water in our wash basins froze. There was no heat in the room, but we didn't stay in our rooms during the day and why would honeymooners need heat at night?

I have a distinct memory, but no record, of my feelings on that honeymoon and of what I took to be Jane's. She seemed to be a veteran and to be perfectly accustomed to living intimately with a person of the other sex. I, on the other hand, felt shy and embarrassed about such things as sharing a bathroom. However, Jane was so easy and natural about everything that I soon felt that she was a part of me and never again was uneasy in her presence.

The days were magnificent. Boats were available for a song and took us out to the famous alligator reef where so many years before I had dived with the barracudas in Captain Dunn's Diving Hood. Again, the water was crystal clear and we could look down on the coral twenty feet below and see the sea fans waving and the angel fish swimming and the great moray eels protruding from their holes. Once a shark swam by and again there was a big sea turtle that surfaced near us. The lighthouse still stood to warn the freighters that passed a mile away in the Gulf Stream. The reefs of the Florida Keys were just as I had remembered them as a child.

It was one of those rare calm days when the sea is glassy and the visibility perfect. Jane had never before seen the underwater world and was as entranced with it as I was. I had of course told her of my childhood experience in the diving hood, so when I said, "We're going to build one," she cheered. Jane was a near-champion swimmer and had no fear at all of either the surface or the depths.

With Mr. Butters as our guide we fished the reefs by the lighthouse, where we caught as many huge barracuda—up to thirty-five pounds—as we wanted. Then we caught a grouper which was bitten in two by a shark, and on the way in we saw two more sharks. Next we tried the Gulf Stream. I caught two small tuna fish, had four sailfish strikes and finally landed a sailfish six feet four inches long—a perfect beauty. It was so perfect a specimen we had it mounted. Before returning to Cleveland, we waded the mangrove marshes in a vain search for the rare crocodiles that inhabited that part of the Keys. We also borrowed a car to drive up and down the road at the side of which was a canal, in which the creatures were supposed to live. It was a great vacation, and we were sad that it had to be so short, but my duties at the Clinic were about to start again.

Although our search had been unsuccessful, my father made up for it by wiring us to please pick up and bring home with us two crocodiles that he had ordered in Miami. I wired back, "Delighted to have two friends as guests. Will they insist on using the lower berth or can we give them the upper? Leave Miami ten-fifty Monday. Barney."

Before we left Cleveland, we had rented a little apartment in a building on East Ninety-first Street just across Euclid Avenue from the Clinic. This area was no longer stylish, most of the well-off people who used to live there having moved to the suburbs, but it still was a safe, slightly ethnic, and pleasant place to live. Neither of us spent any time there, because I was at the Clinic all day and Jane's home was only five minutes away. We still had the dilapidated old car that I had always driven. Jane found furniture in the attics of her family's home and mine, and we were settled.

Housekeeping and cooking were novelties for Jane, for she like myself had been brought up in a home replete with servants. One of her first experiments with cooking had dramatic ramifications that were long remembered. We had invited my parents in to dinner to see the apartment and talk about our adventures in Florida. By now we had unwrapped all the wedding presents and put them to use. Among them was a lovely sterling silver platter on which Jane planned to serve something that needed to be warmed. She put it in the oven. Conversation over the cocktails grew interesting, and we were telling exciting stories about Florida when there was the smell of something burning. Jane dashed to the kitchen, my mother following. Dripping from the oven in long streams was molten silver. It lay in puddles on the floor. All that remained of the platter was its copper core.

Neither Jane nor I ever became over-interested in conventional indoor cooking, although we did learn to get along with the ordinary affairs of the kitchen. In the country, over the campfire, however, our art was superb. We did our fancy cooking on weekends and merely subsisted in between.

Letters and telegrams congratulating us on our marriage had poured in from old friends all over the country. The Roosevelts, Jim and Betsy (formerly Betsy Cushing), all my old friends from the Skull and Bones and from Harvard Medical School, and even a two-page handwritten letter from Dr. Graham in St. Louis: "I am sure that she is to be congratulated, and from what I know of your good judgement I am equally certain that you are to be congratulated as much." John Trommald threatened me with a lawsuit from "the Governor General's Daughter" with whom I had consorted when she was in Boston, and Yandell wired that this was "the greatest news I have heard since Tyzzer disproved your diagnosis of Ascaris" (roundworms).

Jane was having no difficulties with her pregnancy. Weekends we often went to the Halles, where there was a living room, kitchen, bath, and bedroom in "the Stables," where once the groom had lived. I was fully enjoying the surgical experience, first assisting—and when I was on my father's service he let me do parts of his operations. We spent weekends also at the Knob with my parents, and Jane and my mother got along splendidly, as I had been sure they would.

Soon it was time for the baby to be born, and right on schedule Ann arrived. I remember the anxious wait, walking outside around the tree-covered grounds of the University Hospitals and seeing an unusual sight, a flock of hundreds of sea gulls that, only occasionally for reasons that are not clear, congregate inland and fly about for hours. As evening fell and they swooped closer and closer to the now illuminated hospital, I was reminded of the sea hawks and man-of-war birds and gulls that we had seen in Florida, and I became convinced that this congregation was a huge flock of Placenta Hawks.

Apparently in the delivery room the time of conception had been calculated from the wedding day so that in spite of the fact that baby Ann weighed nearly nine pounds, she had been treated as premature. When the obstetrician, Dr. Bill, made rounds he took one look and is alleged to have said, "Get that elephant out of the incubator." From that time on neither mother nor baby had any trouble.

At the time of Jane's delivery, there was an epidemic of some sort sweeping the hospital. I can't remember what it was, but our doctors advised us to leave early. Almost without precedent, and in the eyes of the community with great risk, we picked up the baby and Jane left the hospital on the second day after delivery instead of remaining flat in bed for the usual ten days. That ten-day hospital stay, which at that time was thought essential, is just another of the strange customs that from time to time crop up in the minds of the practitioners of medicine. After Ann came, we moved permanently to the Halle stables, and I commuted back and forth—about forty-five minutes twice a day. That's something I never wanted to do again, but it was good for Jane and the baby to be next door to her family. When autumn came, we moved to an apartment about halfway between my parents' house and the Halles—an upstairs suite over the drugstore on the corner of

Surrey and Cedar. We were fortunate in soon finding an attractive and competent young woman, Mary Margaret, to take care of the baby and help with the housework. In retrospect it seems strange, but at that time I knew no one with a family who didn't have at least one servant.

In spite of all this activity, I found time to write my first independent medical paper with no senior coauthor. In it I reported a patient who had had a huge pulsating tumor of the sternum (chest bone), which my father had successfully removed along with most of the sternum—a very daring operation in that day. The tumor was a metastasis from a tumor of the kidney, and I had looked up the literature and found several reports of similar pulsating tumors of the same kind. "I shall be very pleased indeed to accept the manuscript on 'Pulsating Tumors of the Sternum' for publication in the *Annals of Surgery*," the editor, Dr. James Pilcher, wrote me, and I was very happy. Later, when it was published, Dr. Will Mayo, true to his gracious way, took time to write and congratulate me on the article. His letter ended, "I have special pleasure in writing to you, the son of my old and loved friend. To see the son following in the footsteps of his father in the profession which the father has loved so well and to the advancement of which he has contributed so brilliantly is gratifying. With kindest regards, W. J. Mayo." In March of 1936, the Muncie Academy of Medicine had asked my father to suggest the name of a speaker for their monthly medical meeting, and he had suggested mine. Sure enough, I was off to Muncie to give my first medical address, "The Medical and Surgical Treatment of Thyroid Disease." My wife wired me, "And let it be said of you his speech is a burning fire of bombastiloquence. Good luck and love." Apparently the telegram had the desired effect, for the president of the academy wrote my father a glowing letter of thanks and praise.

Medical meetings were beginning too. In June of 1935, I attended the meeting of the American Medical Association in Atlantic City and revisited the beaches which I hadn't seen since I had convalesced there from my childhood illness. Atlantic City in the 1930s, with its splendid tourist hotels and magnificent boardwalk, was a delight. I presume that Jane came with me, because we have pictures of the boardwalk in her scrapbook. Later in June there was another medical meeting. This one was the first meeting of the organization that was to mean the most to me in the practice of medicine. It was known as the Surgeons' Club and it had eighteen members. Its first meeting was at the Mayo Clinic and I was the most junior member by five or more years.

The concept of a Surgeons' Club originated in the second-generation surgeons of the Mayo Clinic. The Mayos, Dr. Judd, my father, the distinguished Dr. Finney of Baltimore, and other surgical leaders from the eastern cities had formed a visiting surgeons or travel club, which used to make annual visits to a clinic of one of its members, and sometimes would travel to watch surgery in other clinics or abroad. The society was small enough to be informal and to fit into an operating room or a home.

Our Surgeons' Club was patterned after that one and consisted of several sons of members of the original one—Deaver, Finney, Mayo, and myself. The others included Dr. Cattell, who became one of the best and most highly regarded technical surgeons in America; Ferguson, who was a scientist, a scholar, and a good surgeon too; Gray, who in his generation was the surgical leader of the Mayo Clinic; and the rest, each of whom became distinguished in his own way. They came from Boston, Philadelphia, Baltimore, New York, St. Louis, Chicago, Des Moines, Chattanooga, Pittsburgh, Cleveland, and Lancaster, Pennsylvania. Most of the surgeons were already recognized in their fields. I was admitted to the society solely on the basis of my father's qualifications. It was the greatest opportunity that could possibly have been given me, not only to learn from the ablest young surgeons of the country, but also for Jane and me to make lifelong friendships with the most delightful group of young men and women that I had ever seen assembled.

That first meeting in Rochester was a memorable one. For the first time I saw the Mayo Clinic and its associated hospitals and research institutes, and needless to say I was both astonished and deeply impressed. It was the biggest and best-organized medical institution that I had ever seen or dreamed of. And the work that was being done there by my friends and the rest of the surgical staff was of the highest quality.

The program consisted of operative clinics on Friday morning, followed at eleven o'clock by dry clinics (showing cases) and lectures. After lunch there was an afternoon of lectures by the staff of the Mayo Clinic, all of them nationally known figures, who addressed us on such subjects as the treatment of liver disease, management of patients with lesions of the colon, physiology of the colon, coagulability of the blood, the hormones of the anterior pituitary body, experimental peptic ulcer, care of the diabetic patient, and a tour and inspection of the Clinic and the medical museum. This was followed by an informal dinner. Saturday morning, starting at eight, there was another operative schedule followed by a tour of the Research Institute, luncheon, and then golf and a formal dinner.

The wives of Drs. Mayo, Priestley, and Gray were just as attractive and able in their own way as their husbands. Jane had a wonderful time with them. The meeting was a model of good teaching and good fellowship. For the next twenty-five years, except for the war years, the Surgeons' Club continued to meet annually at different places. At those meetings, I learned more and had more fun than at any other medical events that I ever attended. Gradually my friends would wither away and die and finally the club would give up and no longer meet. But it was great while it lasted.

In late November of 1935, my father and mother went off again to Africa to collect more specimens for research and to have the first real vacation that they had taken for several years. Again, part of the cost was borne by the fund with which my father had endowed the Natural History Museum and the museum sent along a naturalist and shared the collection.

They sailed to London on the *Ile de France* and from there boarded a 2,200 horse-power biplane run by Imperial Airways for Paris. In the book she would write for publication the next year, *Skyways to a Jungle Laboratory* (Norton, 1936, and dedicated "To The Chief"), Mother described the setting within the plane:

> We had the first seat in the first cabin, with a table in front of us and a small shelf of books overhead. The kitchenette and lavatory were between the two cabins. The chairs were roomy and comfortable, and each one had a pillow and warm woolen rug. A reading light was beside each chair, and the windows were shaded with pretty silk curtains. We rose so easily, so effortlessly, I hardly knew we were off. A hot luncheon of soup, meat, vegetables, and dessert was served.

The Imperial Airways people put them onto the Paris-Brindisi Express, which carried them comfortably for two nights and a day. Then aboard a three-engine seaplane, "The City of Khartoum," to eventually land, after some refueling stops, at Alexandria. From there this intrepid pair would fly in another plane over Cairo, the Pyramids, Luxor, Aswan, the rock-hewn Temple of Abu Simbel—all the while, of course, photographing the scenes from the air with still and movie cameras.

They would take a safari into the Great Rift Valley and in the shadow of Mount Kilamanjaro hunt, kill, weigh, and collect the adrenal and thyroid glands and the liver, coeliac ganglion, and brain of elephants, giraffes, lions, hyenas, and every creature that moved. The skins, heads, tails, and giraffe tibias (Mother later had a lamp made from one) were brought back to the Museum of Natural History. The four feet of a giant elephant were preserved (with bones removed) and one presented to each of their four children.

Mother recorded everything that went on in detail in her meticulous journal, as well as photographing everything as the adventure went on. In Alexandria, on the way back, my father became very ill with a temperature of 104°, gastroenteritis, and weakness. He was hospitalized for about two weeks. No diagnosis was ever made. When he was well enough, they got back onto a different Imperial Airways seaplane ("The City of Kartoum" that had brought them over had crashed). Then they were off for Brindisi and the Express to Paris and London.

Her book would end:

> Travel-worn and dusty, our shoes torn by the desert sands, still wearing our big safari coats, and the Chief his cap, we drove to the Hotel Carlton, where the handsome liveried Porter, bowing low, said: "Good evening, sir. I presume you have returned for the King's funeral!" (King George had just died.)

At the time, my mother was in her sixties and my father had just had his seventy-first birthday.

Before leaving on the African trip, my father had written us a letter with a word of warning about Jane's interest in flying and both our interests in diving: "It would seem to me to be just as well to defer the upper air and under water until Ann's consent is obtained by her father and her mother."

Neither Jane nor I felt that he was practicing what he preached and we would soon set off on an adventure of our own. It was just a year after our honeymoon in the Florida Keys, when we left Ann in the care of Mary Margaret and the Halles and headed south again to Key West with Dr. Ruedeman, head of the Clinic's Ophthalmology Department, and his wife. One of my father's patients, Dr. Porter of Key West, had offered us his comfortable fishing boat that had four bunks. We hired a man to run it and guide us, and off we went to the Dry Tortugas, one hundred miles west of Key West and not anywhere near anything at all.

The Tortugas consist of eight tiny islands, none of which rises more than a foot above the water. On one of these, in the year 1836, the construction of Fort Jefferson was begun. Forty million bricks went into it, and its walls—eight feet thick—towered sixty feet above the sea. Each cannon-mounted side of the Fort's huge hexagon was 150 feet long. Like the Maginot Line and probably like Star Wars and every other "impregnable" defense will be, it was rendered obsolete before it was completed. The explosive shell had been invented.

To the "Forgotten Fortress in the Sea" we putt-putted in our little motorboat and spent an enchanting week exploring the dungeons where Dr. Samuel Mudd, who set the leg of Lincoln's assassin, was for so long confined, and in watching the huge rookeries of sea birds that covered the islands and the men from the fishing fleets that were anchored in the channels. Also, and most exciting, we had brought with us the diving hood that on our honeymoon I had threatened to invent and build.

My invention had not been very scientifically carried out. When we tried to make the air-filled hood sink, we found that in our calculations we had squared our figures instead of cubing them so it took more than 120 pounds of lead to put it under. Remember, this was 1935 and diving apparatus was unknown in America except to the sponge fishermen of Florida's east coast. We had a telephone in the hood and it was connected to the surface by a rubber tube leading to a bicycle pump. We had a camera with us too, housed in a rebreather bag from an anaesthetic machine with a glass window on one end and the rubber end of a blood pressure cuff and a brass clamp on the other. Jane's first descent in the diving hood was described by her in the book that we would coauthor soon—*Treasure Diving Holidays.*

> When you take your first salt-water solo your heart thumps, blood pounds in your head, your mouth is dry. The hood pushes you down, slowly and irrevocably beneath the surface. There is no sound except the rhythmic hissing of the pump. The air smells thin and rubbery, like an anaesthetic and breathing seems difficult. You are irresistibly compressed by an invisible force. Your ears are full, ache, are resonant to the sound of your breathing. You drift down, down.

Jane did drift down to a depth of about twenty feet, took a few pictures, and then stumbled off the reef into deeper water.

> The hood came to life. It rose half off my head and lurched sideways. It blew out great blobs of air. Water rose to my mouth. In panic I tried to tilt the hood off my shoulders, but now it clung to me like Sinbad's Old Man. There was a leaden foot on my neck, and it was pressing me down into the sand. I fought my way free and started for the surface. A ropy arm clutched me

around the neck and I was dragged to the bottom by the dead-weight of lead. I clawed at the rope, slipped out of the noose, and with bursting lungs beat my way to the top. "What did you do to our hood?" Barney asked. "It tried to drown me," I gasped.

Luckily that monstrous hood and its cords and tubes and wires was so tangled in the coral that we, with no diving apparatus and without even underwater goggles, couldn't see or breathe well enough to untangle it. It's probably still lying there on the Tortugas reef. But we had the first good underwater moving pictures that we'd ever seen and we vowed to return.

After leaving the Tortugas, we went on up the Keys to Matecumbe where we had honeymooned. It was December and about a month after the hurricane that had swept through the Keys, drowning hundreds and destroying not only the railroad to Key West but also most of the buildings on the islands, which were so low that the rising waves and water had completely submerged them. Our friend, the manager of the hotel, and his wife had survived by getting into a bus that was parked by the hotel. When the water rose over the seats they stood up and breathed in the narrow air space until the water receded.

It was a great trip. We speared sharks and rays and electric rays that gave us shocks and ten-foot manta rays that towed our boat for an hour and then broke their lines. We caught tarpon at the trestles, king-fish, and scores of huge barracuda on the reefs, more sailfish at sea, and a little angel fish that we had hooked was swallowed by a 250-pound jewfish. We watched the endless processions of the sea birds. "An amazing sight," Jane wrote, "100 or more man-of-war birds, gulls of all kinds, pelicans, and terns all diving for baleo which were breaking water trying to escape from a school of jacks that was chasing them."

In another area, more inland on Cape Sable, Jane described

hundreds and hundreds of birds, curlews flying singly and in fours, white cranes, blue cranes, egrets, wood ibis, herons, blue herons, little green herons, great white herons, cormorants, geese, terns and gulls. On either side, as far as you could see, muddy grey stubble of trees, once verdant and now a lonely desolate reminder of a hurricane's ruthlessness, grey-white stalks and stubbles of grass on grey mud, olive grey muddy waters and silver mullet jumping sulkily out of the water. Suddenly ahead of us flocks of birds would be startled and they would fly off like flying white sheets, over grey water, winding up the river to the greyer water of White Water Lake.

Before leaving, in the shallow water of the Lake, we shot a porpoise for my father's collection, dissected it, and preserved and took home its thyroid and adrenals.

Then I was back at work at the Cleveland Clinic, where two significant events took place in that year of 1936. In June, Dr. Crile did his twenty-five thousandth thyroidectomy and a few days later, accompanied by much less fanfare, Dr. Crile, Jr., did his first. I cannot remember why this operation was scheduled in my name—perhaps I knew the patient personally. In any event, she was a young woman of twenty-two years and she survived. The anaesthetic was a combination of paraldehyde analgesia and local. There is no photograph of my operation, but an excellent one of Dr. Crile, Sr.'s shows thirteen people crowded into the patient's room, seven without masks and several without gowns. As usual in those days, when the operation was done in the patient's room, lighting was provided by a shaded bulb on a stick swathed in a sterile towel and held by a nurse.

By this time my old medical school roommate, Bud Yandell, who had taken a two-year internship, caught up to me and was a first-year resident on the Clinic's general surgical service and was getting ready to fall in love with and eventually to marry a Cleveland girl. Those were good years, during our training, for there were parties with Alex Bunts—neurosurgeon and son of one of the Clinic's founders and a contemporary of my sister Peg and who had gone to Yale a few years ahead of me—and with Perry McCullagh, of Scotch-Canadian ancestry—a lifelong friend and endocrinologist from whom I learned much about medicine and many unprintable limericks—and with many more congenial residents and younger members of the staff.

Gynecology still was a part of general surgery at the Clinic and I decided to apply for six months of it with Drs. Taylor, Sr. and Jr., at the Roosevelt Hospital in New York. As a result of my father's name, I was immediately accepted, my service to begin January 1, 1937. In the meantime I was scheduled for several other operations under my own name and continued to assist my father.

Some time during this year, I am not sure when or why, my father stopped doing adrenal denervations and instead began removing the celiac ganglion, which is the center of the abdominal part of the sympathetic nervous system. The results, especially in the treatment of hypertension, were much better than those of adrenal denervation and seemed to persist longer. Whether he was the first to perform celiac ganglionectomy or whether Dr. A. W. Adson of the Mayo Clinic preceded him I am not sure. Dr. Adson emphasized division of the splanchnic nerves that lead from the ganglion, and Dr. Crile emphasized removal of the ganglion itself, the "brain of the sympathetic nervous system" that lies near the aorta and the arteries to the kidney and is about the size of a penny. My father wrote in his book *Surgical Treatment of Hypertension* (W. B. Saunders, 1938) that he had come upon the idea while dissecting animals in Africa and, "I rehearsed ganglionectomy by operating on cadavers, and devised the plan of operation and certain special instruments which were required because of the depth of the ganglia"—(and of course also because he was unable to see it).

Regardless of who first thought of or performed a celiac ganglionectomy, it was, in those days, before we were able to block the sympathetic nervous system by the beta blocking drugs, a fairly good answer to some of the problems of hypertension. It was taken up quite widely throughout the country and used much more than adrenal denervation ever had been. Some of the patients with hypertension had prolonged and satisfactory response. At the time my father pioneered this operation, he was seventy-two years old.

On the whole there were fewer complications following the celiac ganglionectomies than there had been after adrenal denervations. I would do all of the operation except the actual cutting out of the ganglion, which my father did by touch, sometimes with his back to the patient and gesticulating with his other hand to the attentive audience of visiting surgeons. There still were hemorrhages when a major vessel was injured, but I had become expert in finding and ligating these so that most of the patients recovered. Towards the end of this period, in fact, it was I, rather than the patient, who was at greater risk. This is what happened.

The patient had had some bleeding which we had managed to control, but during convalescence he developed a hemolytic streptococcal infection of the wound and a hemorrhage. I was called, and found blood all over the bed and floor. The wound had been closed with wire sutures, but there was no time to send for instruments to cut them. I plunged my hand in through the drain hole, broke the sutures loose, followed the flow of blood down to the renal artery and was able to staunch it by pressure until we could get help, expose the bleeder, and tie it. During the course of this procedure the wire sutures had scratched and punctured the skin of my hand. The next day the hand was red and swollen and red streaks were running up the arm. Nodes in the armpit were swollen and tender. My temperature was 103° and I had a full-fledged streptococcal infection. Those were the days before antibiotics or any effective treatment. I had had an uncle who had a similar infection from a shaving cut in his chin and died four days later. It was a dread disease.

I had the usual treatment with immobilization of the arm and hot packs. My temperature went higher and I was on the verge of delirium. I still remember a dreadful dream that kept recurring with black figures of crows and witch-like creatures. An operation was performed and the areas were opened for drainage. Gradually I recovered, but my hand was not fit to take care of patients. Jane and I set forth again for the south and spent a couple of weeks in the Florida Keys, part of the time with Dr. Hartwell Harrison, a urologist from Boston who had married one of Jane's close friends, Gertrude Chisholm. Later Hartwell, at the Brigham Hospital, would be on the team that was the first to perform a successful transplantation of a human kidney.

After a couple of weeks, my hand was again usable and we returned to Cleveland for the rest of December and then packed up our bags, Mary Margaret, and baby Ann, and set sail for New York. By this time, odd as it may seem, Jane was again pregnant.

7

Fellowship at Roosevelt Hospital

IF I HAD had any insight into what the future developments of the surgical specialties would be, I would never have taken six months of gynecology. I was impelled to do so in order to keep up with Dr. Tom Jones, who was doing practically all of the gynecology at the Clinic. If I had had any notion that in a few years gynecology at the Clinic would be a specialty and that in a few more years thoracic and cardiac surgery would be general surgery's largest and most exciting subspecialty, I would have returned to St. Louis and taken a fellowship in thoracic surgery. But when I had interned there, Dr. Graham's successor, the able and skillful Dr. Brian Blades, had not yet been launched on his career and I had not been impressed, in observing Dr. Graham's results, that there was much future in thoracic surgery. So there I was in New York, in an apartment at 1 West Sixty-fourth, with Central Park across the street for Jane and baby Ann and nurse Mary Margaret to enjoy.

It was a pleasant six months, in which I had an opportunity to assist Drs. Taylor, Sr. and Jr., and other members of the Roosevelt Hospital staff and to perform some operations under their supervision. I wrote home that they "can't hold a candle to Tommy Jones so far as technique is concerned, but there is always plenty to be learned from working with and watching anyone of Taylor's experience." In spite of my disillusionment with the rather cumbersome technique of the gynecologists, their work was careful, their patients did well, and I learned a great deal about the fundamentals of gynecology.

By the end of April, Jane was well on her way to maternity. Word had come from my cousin, John Sherman, that he was about to be married, and my classmate, Bert Dunphy, had married. All my friends seemed at last to be settling down. Jane left me and went home to her family to have the baby and to find a new place to live. I wrote her from New York, indicating that I was getting tired of gynecology and could hardly wait to get home, but I said that I was enjoying my work with Dr. Taylor, Jr., "and find my admiration for him steadily increasing. He let me do a vaginal hysterectomy this morning which went OK and was lots of fun." Here for the first time I confessed in surgery to what Konrad Lorenz has called "Functionlust"—the joy of doing something like ballet dancing or ice skating. I closed by noting, "Incidentally I read in the paper the other day that the rhythmic movement in utero is the baby breathing."

Baby Joan was born uneventfully while I was in Atlantic City, speaking at a meeting of the American Medical Association. I am sure my talk must have been on the thyroid, because in New York the only research work I did was to look up the results of the treatment of endometriosis, and since nothing new was noted there was no excitement in the publication.

Although I was on the gynecology service at the Roosevelt Hospital, the head of Surgery was a great friend of my father. I have two reminiscences from that period. First, there was a distinguished Society Lady who was operated on by the chief of Surgery for a cancer of the rectum. He performed a combined abdominoperineal resection, removing all of the rectum and packing the area open, to heal over a period of weeks, and also making a large abdominal incision and establishing a colostomy, through which the bowels would move. Her convalescence was difficult, but by about the seventh day she seemed alert and interested in what was going on. When her surgeon visited her on rounds, I was a visitor. "Do you think you got all of the hemorrhoids out?" the Lady asked. Those were the days when patients asked no questions and were told no lies.

The other experience was with one of the members of the gynecology staff who was working with us in the Out Patient Department. These were "charity patients"—many of them black. To my surprise, he selected one of these and scheduled her for admission for a "suspension of the uterus," an operation that once had been popular and widely performed, but which of late had fallen into disrepute because it was done much too often. I asked him why he thought this patient should have a suspension when he never did that operation on his private patients. He replied frankly, "We just don't have enough patients in the hospital for the interns and residents to practice on, and maybe it will do her some good anyway."

A few years later I visited a hospital where a resident was removing the pancreas for an extensive cancer. I asked the surgeon who was helping him and who was a good friend of mine, why they were doing this radical and dangerous operation for advanced and incurable disease, for I knew that he did not believe in doing the operation on patients with advanced cancers. "They've got to learn to operate," my friend said. "The patient is going to die anyway." The concept of "teaching material" was a strong one.

Back in Cleveland, I found that the house Jane had been telephoning me about was just what we needed. It was about a block from my family's house and half a mile from the Halles. It had been built in the early 1900s and needed a lot of plumbing and repair, but it was only four minutes from the Clinic, it had a nice fenced-in backyard for dogs and children, it had a kitchen, a dining room, a living room, and an open, screened-in porch. There were four master bedrooms with three bathrooms, and in the attic, with a special "maid's stairway" leading to it, were two more bedrooms, a bath, and a lot of storage space. This, in the year 1937, we bought from the bank for ten thousand dollars, and we moved in. Jane, the housekeeper, had a full-time job.

At the Clinic, I wanted to brush up on general surgery, especially as practiced in the office, so I took a few months with Dr. Jones. Occasionally my father would have a patient with a problem suitable for transfer to me for operation. One of these had a cancer of the rectum. Although I had never done the radical operation for rectal cancer, I had assisted Dr. Jones on about a hundred of them and knew the routine. The operation went smoothly and took an hour and thirty-five minutes, only about half an hour longer than Dr. Jones's average. Both my father and I were delighted, and he referred a few more goiters to me to operate on. I also did a few celiac ganglionectomies, finding that it was not difficult to locate the ganglion by sense of touch, as my father did, and then to expose it and excise it under direct vision.

Just before the time when I would be eligible to be appointed to the staff of the Clinic, Jane and I, with my sister Peg and a guide that both Peg and I had known on Lake Timagami, set out for a moose hunting trip in Canada. We drove, picking up Tom Bell, the guide, along the way, and stopped at the cabin of a friend who was a fisherman on Lake Expanse—one of the largest lakes in the area—about ten miles across, as I remember it. We had dinner with the fisherman, trading him a bottle of Canadian whiskey for a bucket of the caviar that he harvested from the sturgeon of the lake, and the next day he towed the canoes that we had transported on the top of the car down the lake to the Winawash River where Tom said the moose were waiting for us.

It was a beautiful summer day all the way down the lake, but then, just as the water grew shallow and the power boat had to leave us, a black cloud appeared. The sun disappeared. The wind rose. We couldn't paddle against it so we sat and steered through the reedy shallows. The bow of our canoe ran up on a stump. Jane grabbed for its roots in the freezing water and held on while the boat swung around in the wind. Then down the wind we went again, tail first, bailing and steering as best we could.

Finally we were blown into an area where the bushes growing in the water were so thick that they broke the waves and there, half frozen and with the sun setting, we waited out the storm. Tom led us to the mainland where we were lost, but he knew that nearby was a lumber camp. He made a fire and we set up the tent. After a cold night Tom led us to the lumber camp. The episode was to set the style for a typical Crile holiday. I blame my father for all this, because twenty years before, it was he who nearly swamped our canoes in a storm on a Canadian lake and it was he who got us lost in the fog in the Gulf of Mexico. He established the precedent. We found our way to the cabin Tom knew of and there, hanging from the ceiling, was the heart of a moose that the last visitor had killed, and on the table, well preserved in the cold, was the beast's liver. We feasted, then we paddled up the river, past waterfalls at the base of which we caught a fine doré—the golden pickerel of Canada. We wandered through the swamps where for centuries nearly imperishable cedar logs had fallen so that they lay one upon another like jackstraws in a layer of logs three feet deep, all carpeted by thick green moss. It was a vein of coal in the making.

Then we drifted down the stream, a great horned owl winging silently ahead. The evening was breathless. Not a breeze rustled the forest. Complete silence until twigs began to crackle in the underbrush. I gave a shove with the paddle and ran the bow in the bush. Jane stood. Six feet away was a brown bear on its hind legs, its front legs bent like a begging dog. The pair looked at each other, eye to eye. The bear blinked and dropped to the ground. Jane shot and missed. She and I killed no moose either on that trip. We didn't really want to. We just wanted to talk to them, and we did. They answered our call and came down towards us, but always something happened or a real cow called and the bull went home. All but one, and that one was called down to Peg by a trick Tom used. When the bull hesitated in the alders, Tom filled his moose horn with water and let it run out of the small end and trickle into the lake. The bull could not resist the cowlike sound. He plunged out of the alders into the water and headed for the canoe. Peg shot him in the nose as he swam at her and we all had all the moose we could eat and all we could carry home. It was trips like this that put Jane and me in love with hunting and fishing. It was not for the game or the fish, but for the sights and sounds that we experienced and for the adventures that occurred in their pursuit.

I found that on October 24 I had been elected to the staff of the Clinic. I had a telegram from my father: "Congratulations on your unanimous election to the Staff of the Cleveland Clinic as surgeon. To this day I have long looked forward. As Chief of the Surgical Division I accord you all the rights and privileges pertaining thereto. Love to Jane, Ann and Joan. Chief."

And that was the end of my long period of training and the beginning of a much longer period of education in which it would be the patient, not the profession, who would teach me the truth about the practice of medicine.

8

The Prewar Years

🙣

M Y FATHER still had a large referred practice, and now I saw the patients with him in the Clinic and he began to refer them to me for treatment—especially the goiters. He still could not bear to give up doing the celiac ganglionectomies, and I still was unconvinced of their value and insofar as possible avoided doing them or writing about the operation. I was not engaged in any research projects, but in the years 1936 and 1937 I did write a number of papers, some of them case reports such as "Diverticula of the Jejunum, A Report of Four Cases," and "Exophthalmic Goiter in a Boy Two and One-Half Years Old." Some of the papers discussed problems like "Surgery of the Aged—Preoperative and Postoperative Treatment," "The Significance and Treatment of Delirium and Confusion Following Thyroidectomy for Hyperthyroidism," and "Hyperthyroidism in Children Under Five Years of Age."

There were two articles I had no business writing because I knew nothing about the subjects. One was on "The Treatment of Burns"— which I was delegated by the editor to write in spite of the fact that I hadn't seen or treated one since my internship. The other was "A Radical Operation for Malignant Tumors of the Thyroid" published in the country's most respected surgical journal, *Surgery, Gynecology & Obstetrics*. At the time of its publication I had never operated on a patient with a malignant tumor of the thyroid. My recommendations were for making a vertical as well as a horizontal incision in the skin to expose the venous system of the neck and to ligate and excise the jugular vein on the affected side along with the thyroid veins that drain into it. The rationale for this was purely theoretical, based on the fact that what was at that time the commonest type of malignant tumor often invaded the veins and grew into them causing local recurrences or blood-borne metastases. What the results were following such a procedure have never been determined, because so far as I know neither I nor anyone else ever did the operation. Perhaps the fact that my father was on the editorial board of the journal bore some relationship to why such a theoretical article was accepted.

On the corridor where we examined patients, I was not very busy because I had only the patients that my father referred to me and the few who came to the Surgical Department without asking for a particular doctor and were rotated between Drs. Jones, Dinsmore, and myself. I therefore had time to look up the results of our treatments, study the records, and draw conclusions, some of them fit for publication. For these sundry and variegated activities my salary was, as I remember, ten thousand dollars a year.

In those early years when I had time enough to go over the records and when there were no computers to lead me astray, I got in the habit of doing the chart work myself and not relying on statistics compiled in the Record Room. Very early I found that record clerks, regardless of their integrity and intelligence, were not trained in medicine to the extent that they could accurately interpret such data as the cause of death, whether there was a recurrence of the cancer, or whether there was a local recurrence of the cancer. In fact, much later I would write an editorial for *Surgery, Gynecology & Obstetrics* (April 1983) showing that the incidence of local recurrence after operations for breast cancer in our own experience had varied from the 6 percent that I had reported to 18 percent that was reported by our statistician.

The variation in these reports came from the interpretation of the phrase "local recurrence." To me the appearance of tumor in an area like the axilla, or supraclavicular region, was not a recurrence unless the area had been operated on or treated by X-ray. In addition, the statisticians had been far more careful than I in reading the full autopsy reports and letters pertaining to patients who had died of cancers in some other hospital and the information about the local recurrence was in fine print and hard to find. This resulted in my having to correct my figure to 12 percent and this was the final figure for the incidence of local recurrence, agreed to by all. Since that experience, I have never published figures given me by a statistician and never published figures derived solely from my review of the records. I have reviewed the charts myself and worked with the statistician.

I had transplanted the Lahey Clinic technique of thyroidectomy to Cleveland, and from the first this more anatomical dissection gave better results, in terms of complications like injuries to the laryngeal nerves and parathyroid glands. In the celiac ganglionectomies that I did perform, under direct vision, there were none of the hemorrhages that had plagued my father using his sense of touch technique. More and more gynecology was being referred to me by the staff of the Clinic because they all knew that Dr. Jones was exceedingly busy. I just worked away, doing all the conventional things, trying nothing new, because at that time everything to me was quite new.

In the summer of 1937, Ted Williams, my roommate from the Yale days, accompanied Jane, her sister Ann, and me on a pack trip through Montana's Glacier National Park. We went by train, of course—two days of it—and as recorded in Jane's diary:

> The plains of Missouri were magnificent, alternating luxuriant wheat and corn fields, and miles apart, the farm units. Always a white farm house, a red barn and a windmill in a grove of trees. Montana was a desolate contrast to the previous abundance and fertility. Here was no vegetation except occasional scrubby fields of winter wheat, no trees, ramshackle houses bare against a barer background. But there were little gophers standing up on their hind feet, waving their tails at the train. An eagle attacked one of our friendly waving gophers.
>
> Five full-blooded Black Foot Indians, white feathered, white buckskinned and white moccasined, dripping with beads and scalps, met us at the Glacier National Park Station, Chief Lone Wolf and Chief Wades in Water. In front of the large rambling brown and log hotel was a great and wonderful white skin tepee with primitive colorful drawings of deer and moose; I long for one for a hat.

That was our introduction to the Wild West. We took a bus to Mc-Donald Hotel, and as Jane put it, "fled into our woods clothes, set up trout rods, took an outboard down the lake and began fishing. This was a sort of perpetual motion only to be interrupted by riding, eating and sleeping. A lovely wild deer roamed in and around the hotel and goats peered down from every crevice. One would soon be weary of these wattled faces."

The trip was spectacular—up to far above the timberline, high enough to cause one of our party to turn back and wait for our return. With us was a cook, a guide, a horse wrangler, and thirteen horses. We had comfortable tents to sleep in and a big tent for eating and meeting. We rode through the country for ten days, moving camp every day. Jane came home with a series of beautiful photographs and drawings of the mountains, the plains, the Indians, and the wildlife including mountain goats, black-tailed deer, and marmots (one of which I caught when it stuck its head in a hole to hide from us and left its tail sticking out). We also saw many tracks of elk and one night a bear came into our camp. The cost was eleven dollars per day per person and it gave us a great view of the high country of our West.

On the last day of the trip, about twenty miles from the hotel, disaster struck. Jane had abdominal pain. It was a typical attack of acute appendicitis. There were no helicopters then, there were no roads, there was no alternative to bouncing that appendix twenty miles to the railroad, and then there were no hospitals anywhere near.

Those were the days before antibiotics, when appendicitis was considered to be deadly dangerous. I wired my father. By the next morning, he had arranged for a doctor friend to meet the train, which he did, but by then more than two days had passed and Jane was better. We took the train back and as scheduled, I stopped off at the Mayo Clinic to spend a few days observing surgery. Jane and the others went home and all went well. That was as trying an experience as I had ever gone through. To prevent its recurrence, before we embarked on another long trip, we had Tommy Jones remove Jane's appendix, a prophylactic procedure that was popular in those days. Today I would never recommend it. Now we have antibiotics.

Back at home, it was great fun because Bud Yandell and his wife were still there, Bud finishing his residency. Also Max Eddy, my old friend from Yale and Harvard, had at last joined us and started his residency. Each day at the Clinic was like a Yale-and-Harvard-Medical-School reunion, and in town also were my old Yale roommates Boots Britton and Ted Williams.

In those days, there were beer parties at the Knob with singing of the old songs, for that was before television came along. Everyone knew and enjoyed all the words. Yandell played the piano by ear so that if you hummed a tune to him once he'd play it with one hand and then repeat it with both and with banging of feet on pedals so that he sounded like an orchestra. Eddy was a professional bass singer. I couldn't carry a tune, a skill I inherited from my father, but I knew all the words.

There were picnics too, given by my father at the Knob or at the farm next door to it where Dr. Lower had his country place. All the employees of the Clinic were asked and bused out there—about three hundred of them. There were baseball games in the pasture, walks through the woods, climbs over the rocks, and swimming in the pond. Then there was a great fire, corn-on-the-cob and chicken, and a lot of happy and contented people who climbed into the buses and got home in time for supper. There was a real *esprit de corps* in the employees of the Clinic, and everyone enjoyed it, from the department heads to the janitors.

In addition to those huge parties, there were the smaller ones with ten to twenty people who congregated in the evenings of weekends at the houses of either the McCullaghs or his research associate, Ken Cuyler, or at our house at the Knob, because the Cuylers and McCullaghs lived only a quarter of a mile away from us. At those parties there was plenty of beer and no end to the recitation or singing of Old English limericks to the tune of "Tooroli tooroli eddy, Tooroli tooroli ay!" (That's phonetic spelling.) It was fun.

Often we'd bring along a live pig, which we would dispatch and clean and roast. In want of a pig, there were good fat steaks and always corn-on-the-cob and lobsters dripping with butter. Those were the days when fat-rich rare meat was supposed to make you healthy and strong. Anyway my friends enjoyed themselves to the full, while they lasted. I am the sole survivor.

In town, we had friends too. One of them was André Pacatte, who was then head of the local Berlitz School and later would be in charge of the system. Jane and I had been thinking of vacationing in France. I had been brought up to speak French, but Jane had studied it only in school. She went to the Berlitz School to learn to speak and came home with tall tales about her teacher. "Let's ask him to supper," I said. Happily, Jane agreed.

André and his lovely wife, Connie, an English teacher, arrived. André proved to be everything that Jane had described- and more. He had been born in France, had engaged in some sort of a war in Morocco, then he migrated to America, learned English, and started to teach in a western Berlitz School. Recently the company had moved him to Cleveland and put him in charge. His English was picturesque, to say the least, but his French was magnificent and pure. André began to boast of his prowess in forest and field. I told him of mine. There was a twelve-inch tree standing in our yard that we had planned to have taken down. Why wait? André and I took axes and together we showed our woodsmanship to our ladies. Down came the tree smack on the light and telephone wires to the house. That was the end of the formal part of the evening and the beginning of a lifelong friendship.

Jane too had friends who from time to time visited us, including the artist Fran Rich, daughter of the actress Irene Rich and Jane's roommate at Smith. Fran was a magnificent sculptress. Another friend was Jane Ickes, wife of the secretary of the interior. She was a good companion and through her we arranged for the Department of the

Interior to let us purchase a couple of beavers for our pond at the Knob. At first these were great fun, but then they began to cut trees and build houses and dams, and it was with the greatest relief that we heard they had moved downstream and were now cutting down our neighbor's forest.

On weekends in the summer, we would sometimes pack up and travel west a hundred miles to the Castalia trout streams where my father and I used to fish and which was no longer owned by the private club. Part of it was owned by Owens Illinois Glass and part by a sort of open club that almost anyone could join. Below the controlled areas, the stream flowed through farm fields and pastures, and we used to dicker with the farmers for permission to fish their waters, and would sometimes come home with two or three large trout that as fingerlings had slipped through the fences and grown up, downstream, into near record-sized catches.

Not far from the trout stream was the duck marsh where my father and I had come to shoot. This was still an exclusive and very expensive club, for the water of Lake Erie kept rising and flooding the marshes, and the club kept dredging and diking them to keep them attractive to the ducks. Next door to the Winous Point marsh, however, on one of the rivers that flow through the marsh, we found an island with a trappers' cabin on it, and this we rented for the duck season and went there with our babies and our friends. We would cook on the great woodburning heating stove, sleeping on the floor or on the four or five cots that the trappers used, and have a glorious time with the Brittons, our next-door neighbors, the Dan Moores, the Yandells, the Eddys, and any other of our friends who liked to camp and shoot.

It was about this time that an old friend returned from France. It was Dr. Henri Welti, who had come to Cleveland after World War I as the recipient of a scholarship that my father had offered to a young French surgeon to spend a year working with him. The money for his scholarship came from an award that my father had been given by the French government in recognition of his contributions to medicine in World War I. Dr. Welti and his wife were now successfully practicing in the American Hospital in Paris, where he had, in fact, removed Jane's sister, Ann Halle's, appendix a couple of years before. This renewal of our friendship with the Weltis was the beginning of another long-lasting Franco-American relationship.

My father was now seventy-three years old. As an example of his phenomenal "kinetic drive," my mother recorded the program of a meeting in Denver which she attended with him:

Yesterday was typical, an 8:30 meeting, a 10:30 meeting, a 12:30 lecture before 600 business men, a 2:30 meeting before a hall jammed with doctors, a 4 o'clock meeting, a six o'clock dinner, an 8 o'clock lecture. Sometimes I've even selected the slides for the lecture and told Dad—i.e. read the slides I selected on the way to the lecture. It was a tour of triumph. Sometimes I wish you could be along and see the adoration and adulation of the various groups all thru this great North West. Over and over again men have said to me they felt they were hearing something as important as a pronouncement of Darwin or Haeckel. Dad has the whole thing wonderfully in hand and I've never heard him speak so well or so effectively. Some men have been so interested that they have followed from Seattle to Tacoma to hear it again.

The only significant paper that I published in 1938 was "Successful Resection of the Head of the Pancreas for Carcinoma, Report of a Case." In it I concluded, "In a large percent of patients the tumor is localized and resectable at the time of death. Recent advances in surgery should encourage more radical attacks on cancer in this region." Although the resection of the pancreas was successful, in that I got it out, the operation could not be called a triumph. The patient died a year or two later with persistent disease and with jaundice resulting from complications from the operation. For the next twenty years, I persisted in attempting to cure cancers of the pancreas by surgery, but not a single one of the ordinary adenocarcinomas was cured. The mortality rate from the operation was about 15 percent, and as a result the patients who had radical resections did not live as long or as comfortably as did those who had palliative operations to relieve the jaundice. In 1970, I would publish an article in the same journal, *Surgery, Gynecology & Obstetrics,* which would shock many of my optimistic colleagues—"The Advantages of Bypass Operations over Radical Pancreatoduodenectomy in the Treatment of Pancreatic Carcinoma."

The debate about the treatment of cancer of the pancreas would continue, but the trend would be towards conservative surgery. In the history of the Cleveland Clinic there is not a single case in which operation has cured a patient with adenocarcinoma, the common type of cancer of the pancreas. The same is true in most other series. The Mayo Clinic originally held out for the radical operation, claiming several cures, but then they went back and reexamined the sections and found that most of the patients whose cancers had been reported to have been cured did not have the type of cancer that everyone else had been talking about. And so it was that in 1938 I embarked on one of my longest battles, one in which I was forced to change sides half-way through, and would live to see my original report condemned as a premature claim of success.

As the staff gained confidence in my ability to operate, my practice grew. They had watched me grow up and at first it had seemed to them that it would be impossible for me to be mature enough to operate on their patients. Also my father traveled more and left his practice to me. In 1938, he and Mother took off for the frozen north to investigate the thyroids, adrenals, and brains of whales, walruses, and seals. I thought at the time that there was a resemblance between my father's travels and those of Paul the Apostle. Paul's travels were instigated by the desire to spread religion while my father's were designed to further our knowledge of science.

I was happy for the extra work, even if it meant performing some of the celiac ganglionectomies that he had admitted for me. An aspect that had been hard for me in those days when my father was still operating was to hear a visitor from abroad telling Mother about his day in the operating room with my father, and how Dr. Crile (accidentally) cut the main bile duct and then repaired it. "Such a change of pace he showed!" expressing admiration. My father was famous as a fast operator, and my mother didn't realize that to cut the bile duct was an almost unforgivable technical error and was due to his lack of clear vision. "How marvelous," she breathed. I said nothing.

Home life was comfortable. Jane had an income of about ten thousand dollars a year. I had the same from the Clinic plus a little from the Kensington property that had put us through school. By selling a little capital our house was paid for, and we could afford a cook and a nursemaid. In those days every young wife thought she had to have a cook.

The work at the Clinic was becoming more interesting. I experimented with a then-novel operation for a cancer of the esophagus, at that time a universally fatal tumor, only one or two of which in the history of surgery had been cured by radical operations. Relying on my minimal St. Louis training in thoracic surgery, I removed the involved esophagus and brought the stomach up through the diaphragm into the chest, linking it up with the esophagus. For a few days things looked good, and I could have been on my way to fame and glory, but then the patient suddenly died. Dr. Jones too, was doing some thoracic surgery, and in two cases had successfully removed a single lobe of a lung for bronchial cancer, the first successful operations of that kind in this part of the country. I began to regret that I had not returned to St. Louis for training in thoracic surgery.

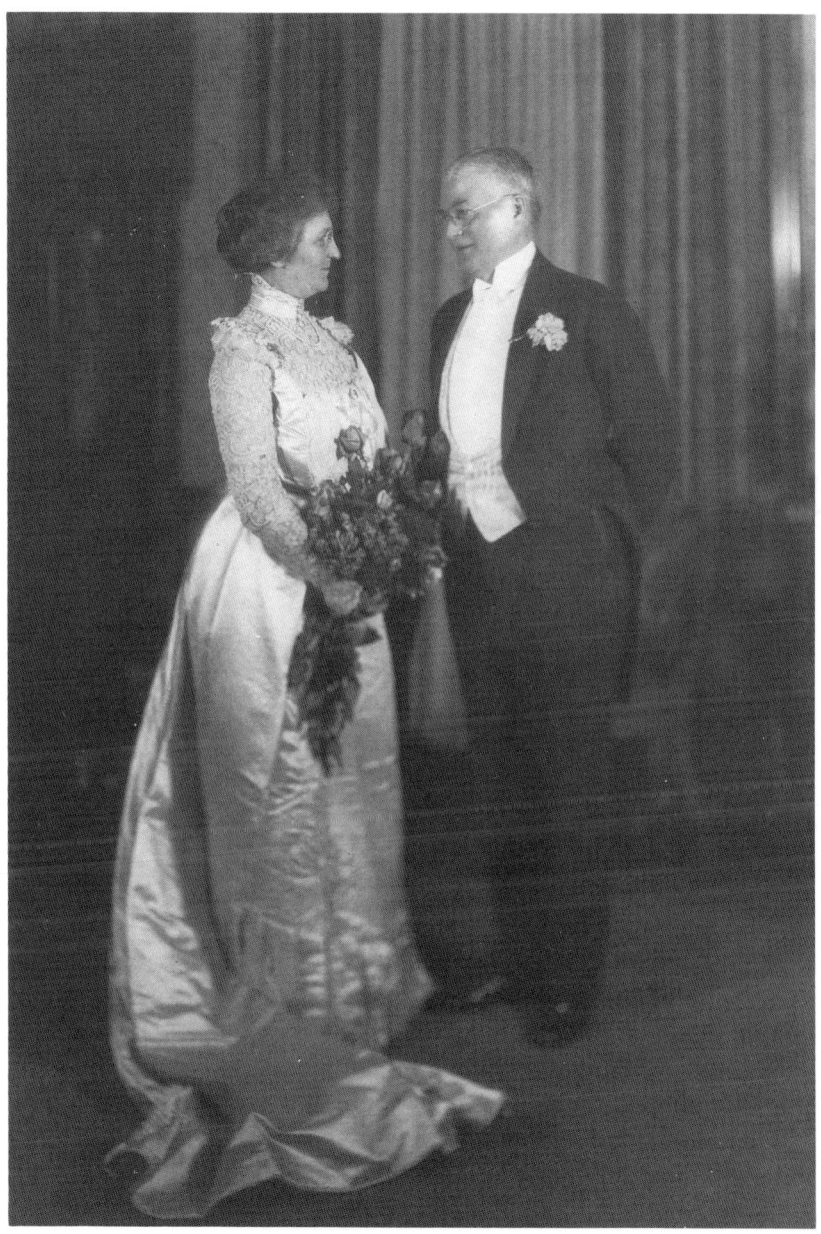

Dr. and Mrs. George Crile, Sr., on their anniversary, February 7, 1925. The Chief frequently gave his wife seven American Beauty roses in honor of their wedding date.

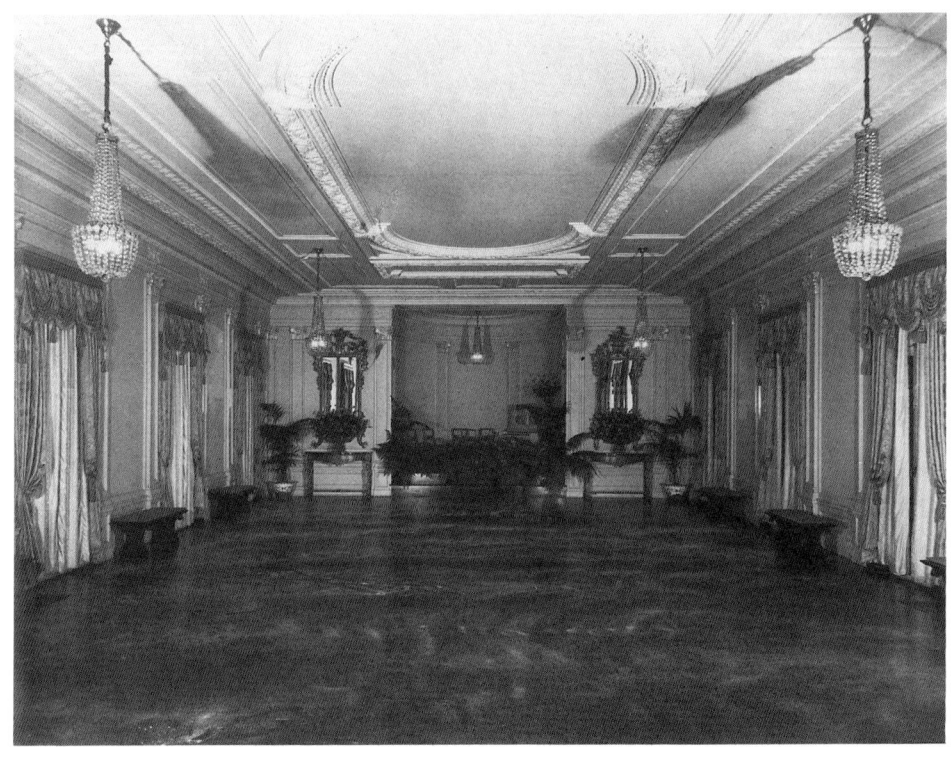

The ballroom at the Crile home on Derbyshire in Cleveland Heights.

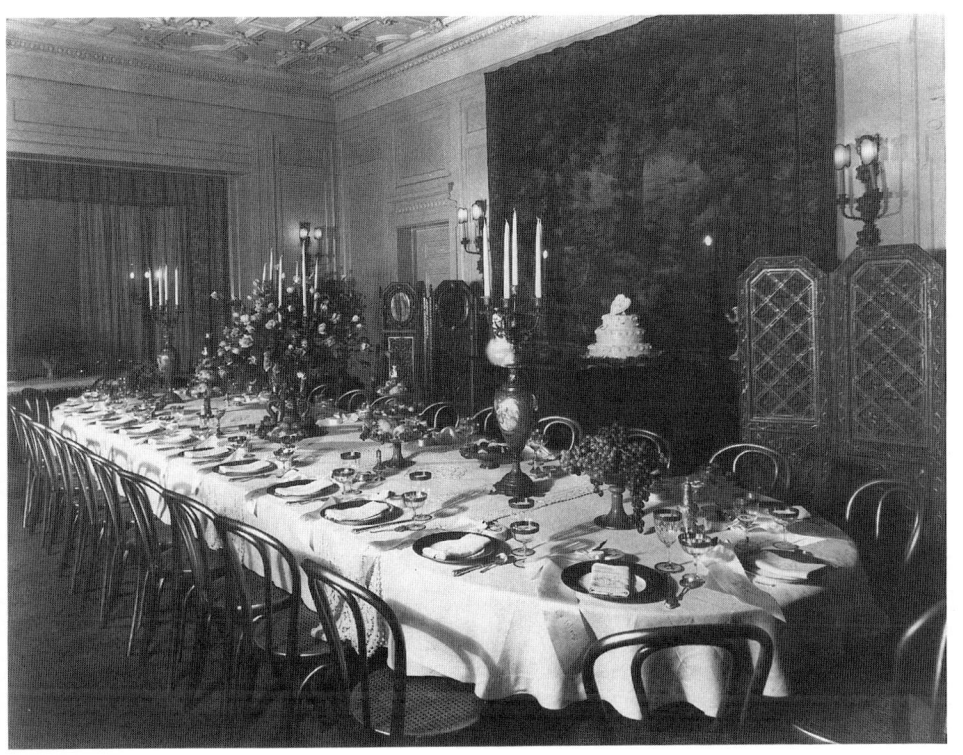

Entertaining on a grand scale at the Crile mansion.

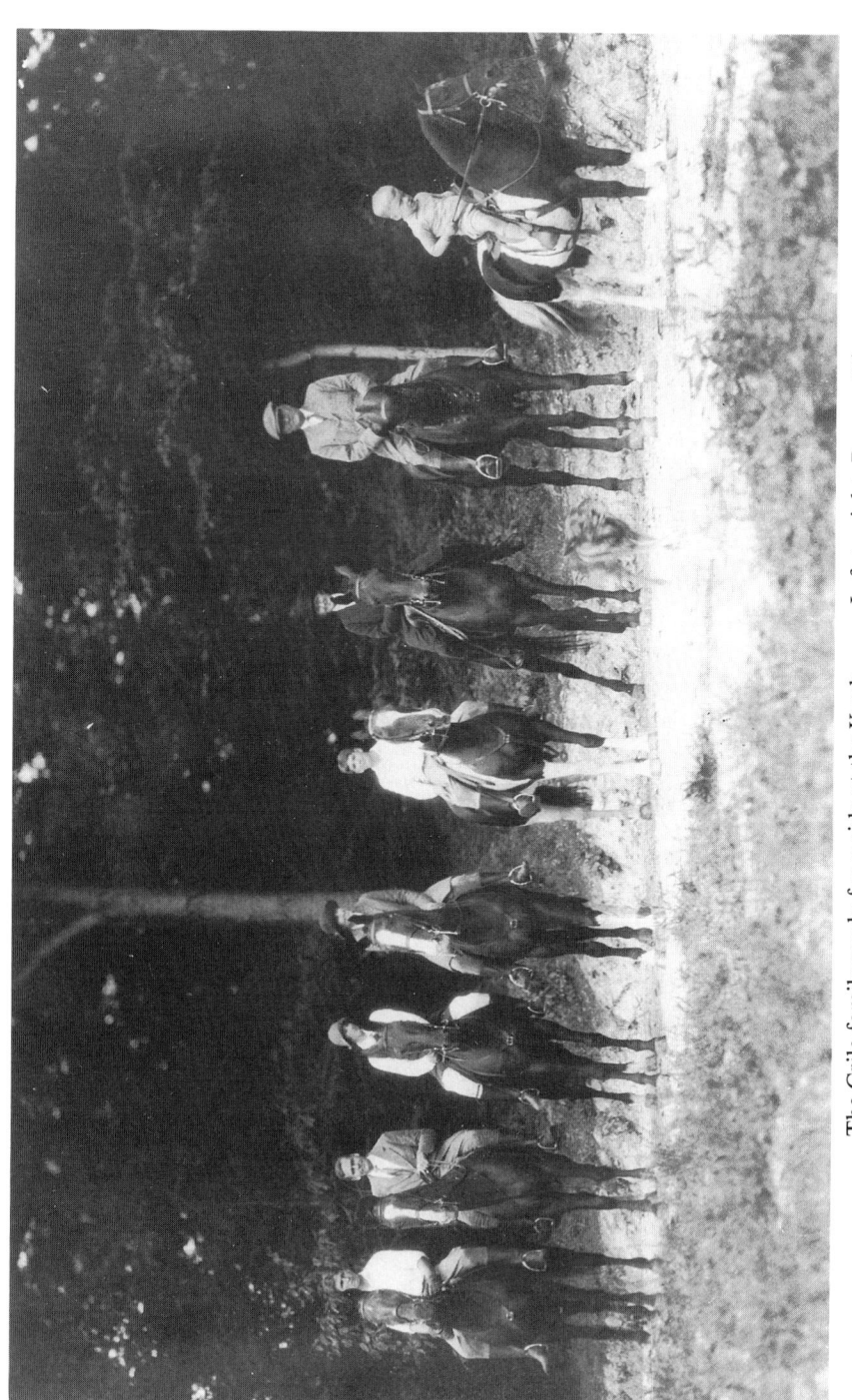

The Crile family ready for a ride at the Knob, 1927. Left to right: Barney, Hiram Garretson (Peg's husband), Elo, Peg, Bob, Grace, the Chief, and Dick Garretson (Peg's son).

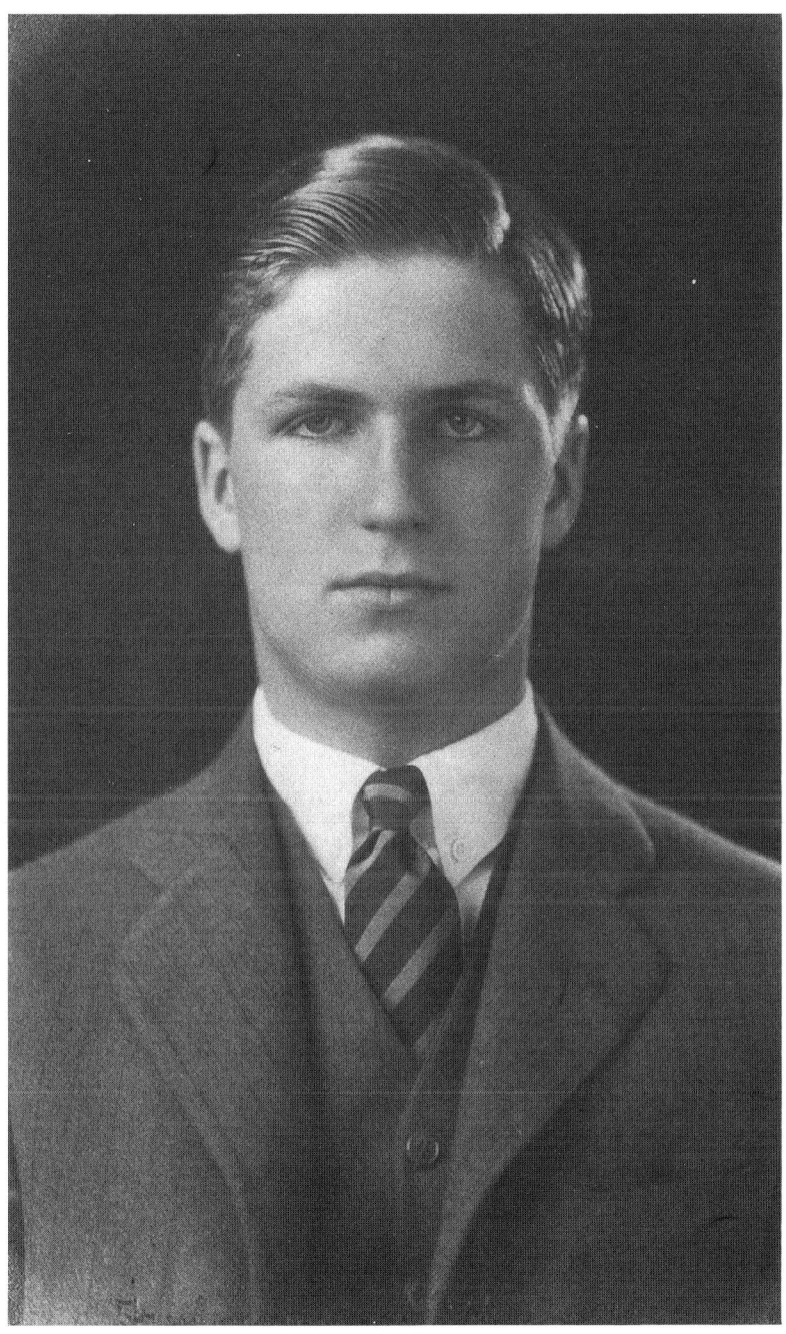

Barney at the time of his entrance to Yale, September 1925. His eighteenth birthday was two months later, November 3.

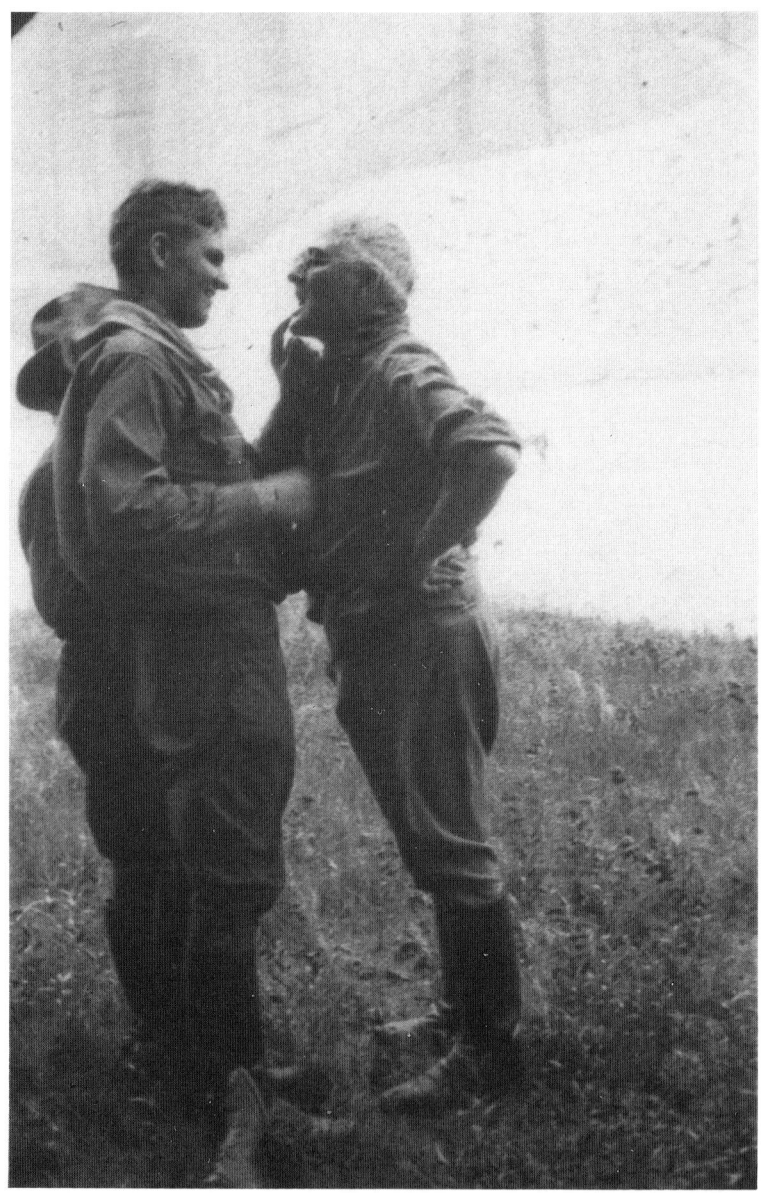

Barney removes cactus spines from the tongue of the Chief who had been experimenting on diet—one of the many highlights of a three-state family pack trip in 1926.

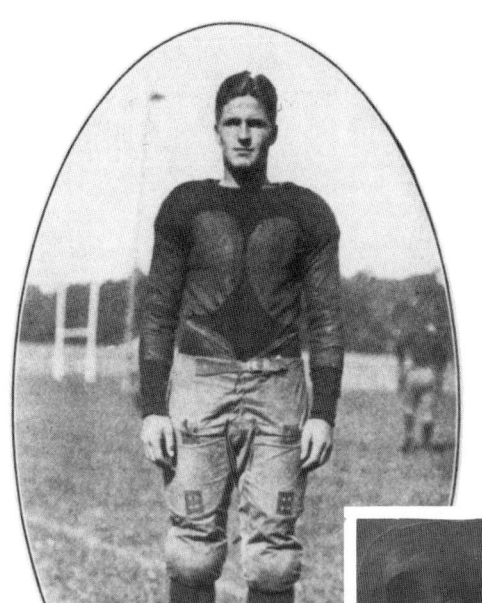

Barney on the Yale varsity football team, 1927.

Friends and fun during Barney's second year at Yale, 1927. Left to right: standing, Boots Britton, Ned Foot, and Barney; seated, Ann Ingalls and Mary Foot.

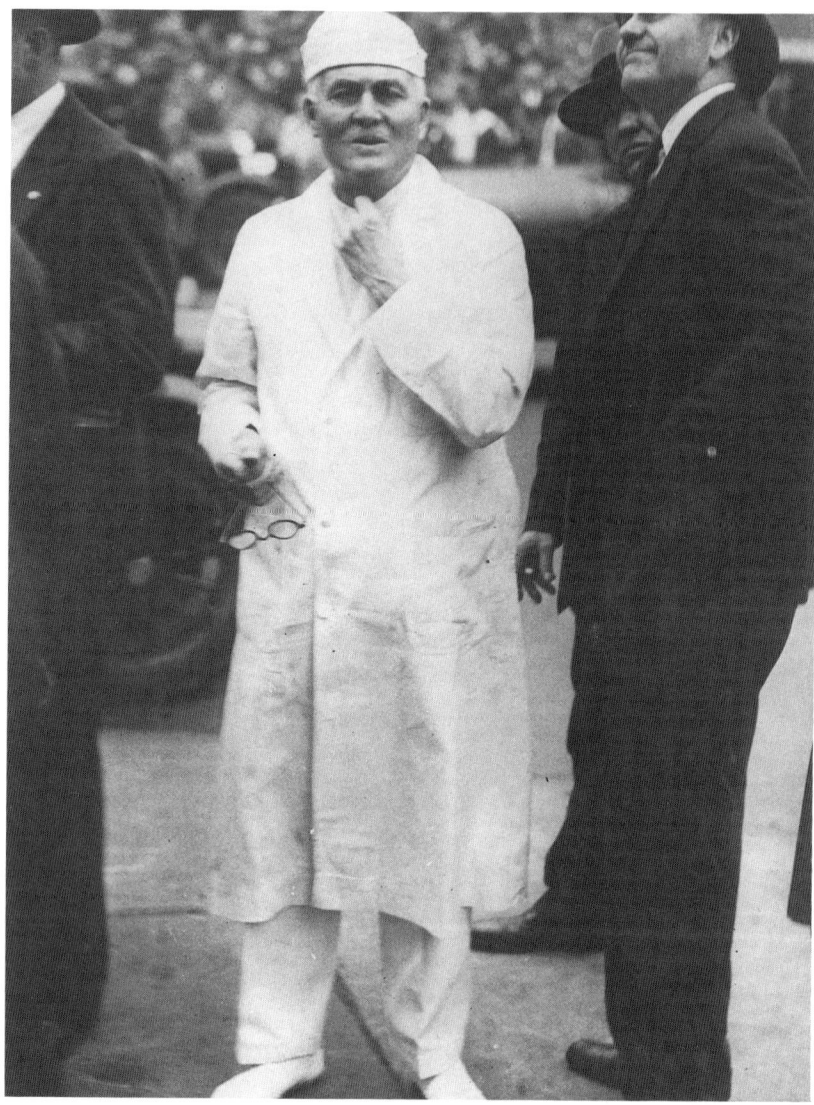

The Clinic disaster, May 1929. In shock, Dr. George Crile, Sr., and his son-in-law Hiram Garretson stand on Euclid Avenue witnessing people jumping from the Clinic's third and fourth floors into rescue nets.

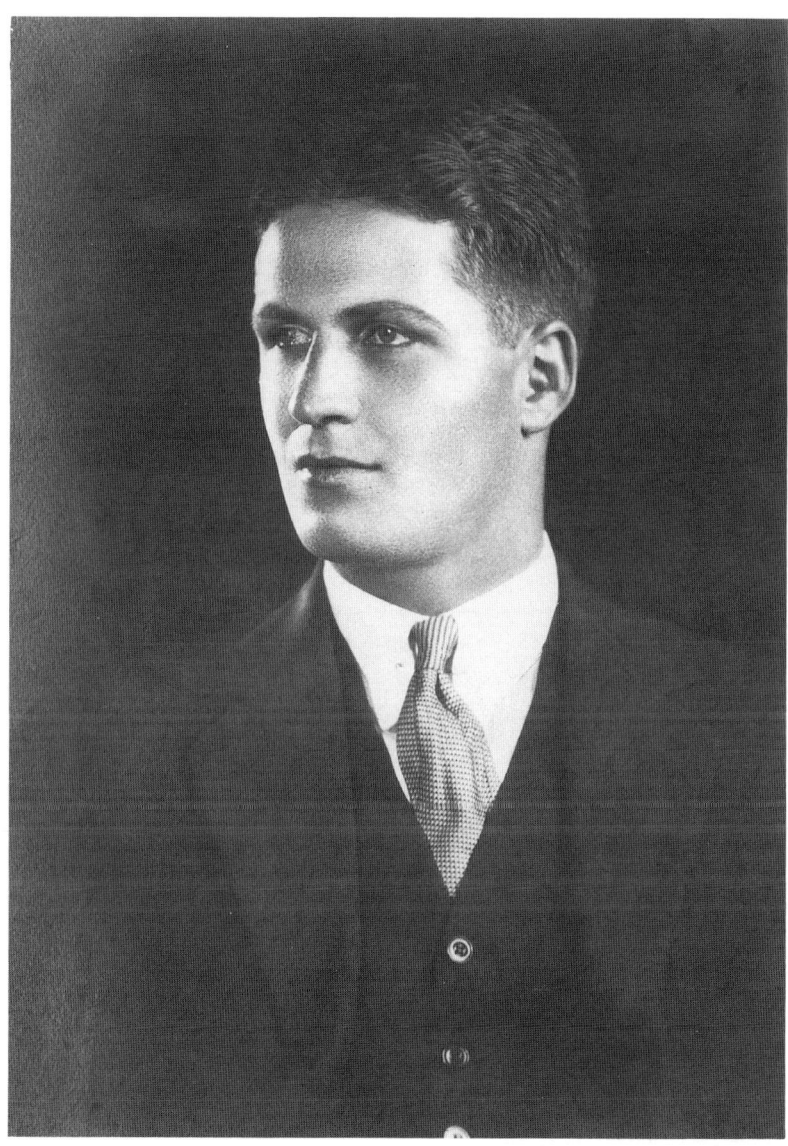
Barney Crile in September 1930, at the start of his second year at Harvard Medical School.

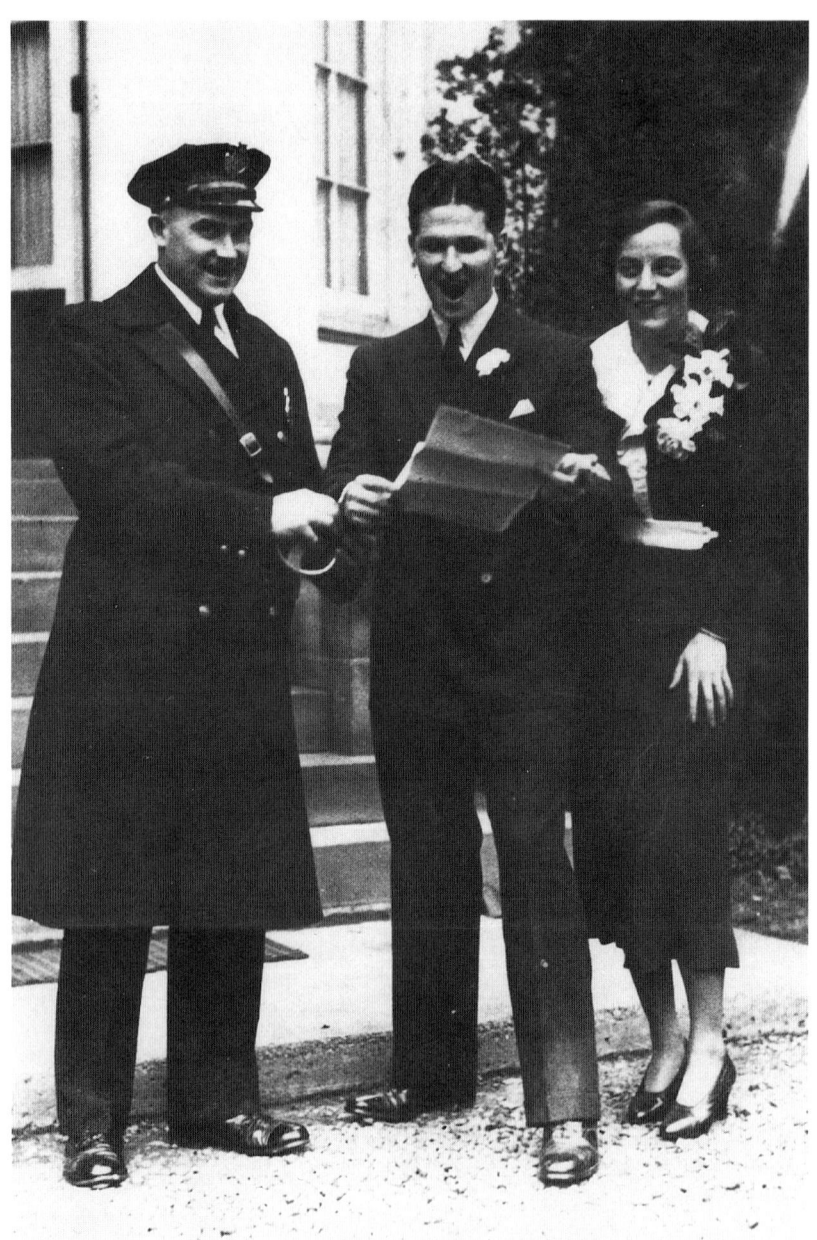

On their wedding day, December 5, 1934, Barney and Jane were handcuffed and served with a warrant—a prank concocted by friends Boots Britton and Ted Williams.

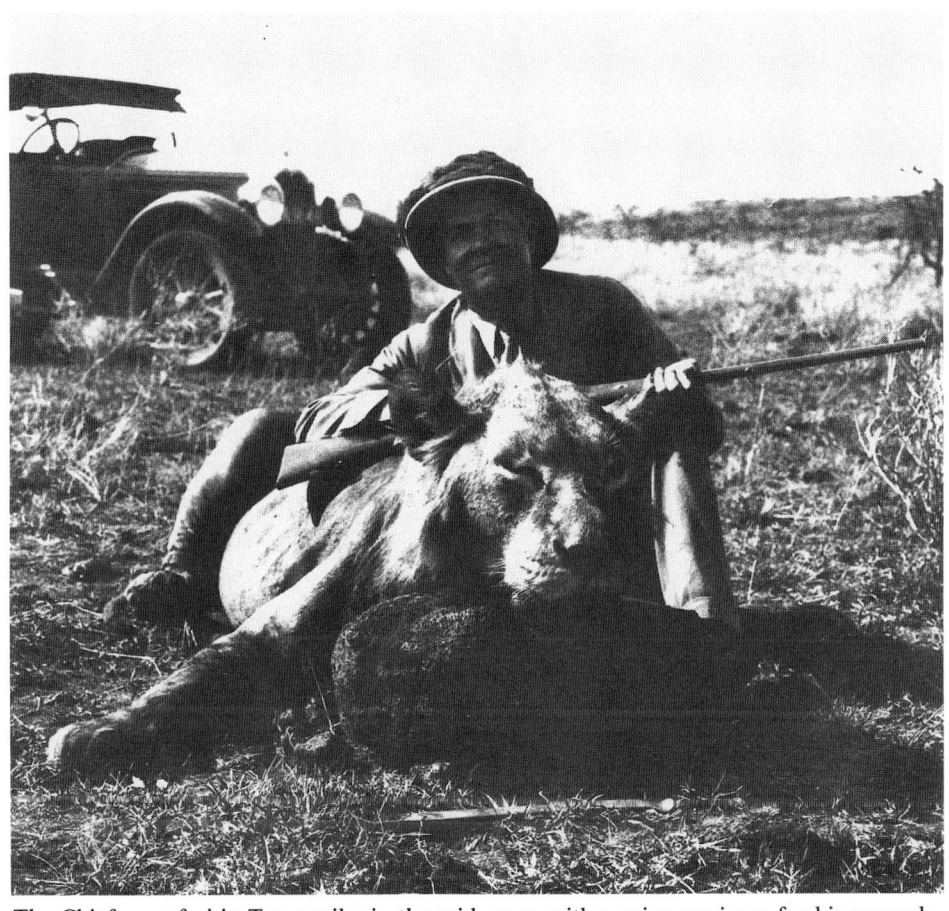
The Chief on safari in Tanganyika in the mid-1930s, with a prize specimen for his research.

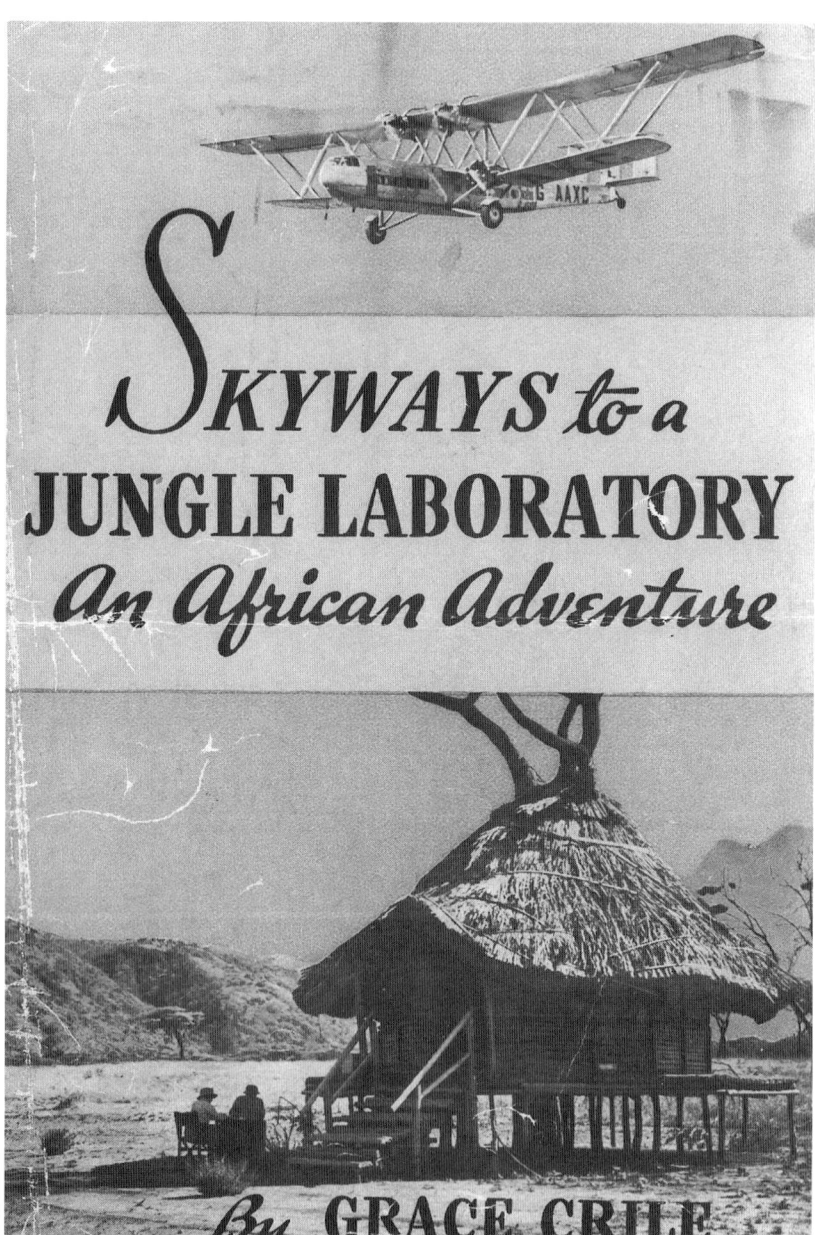

Grace Crile's meticulously kept journal of the Criles' African trip was the basis for her book *Skyways to a Jungle Laboratory,* published in 1936.

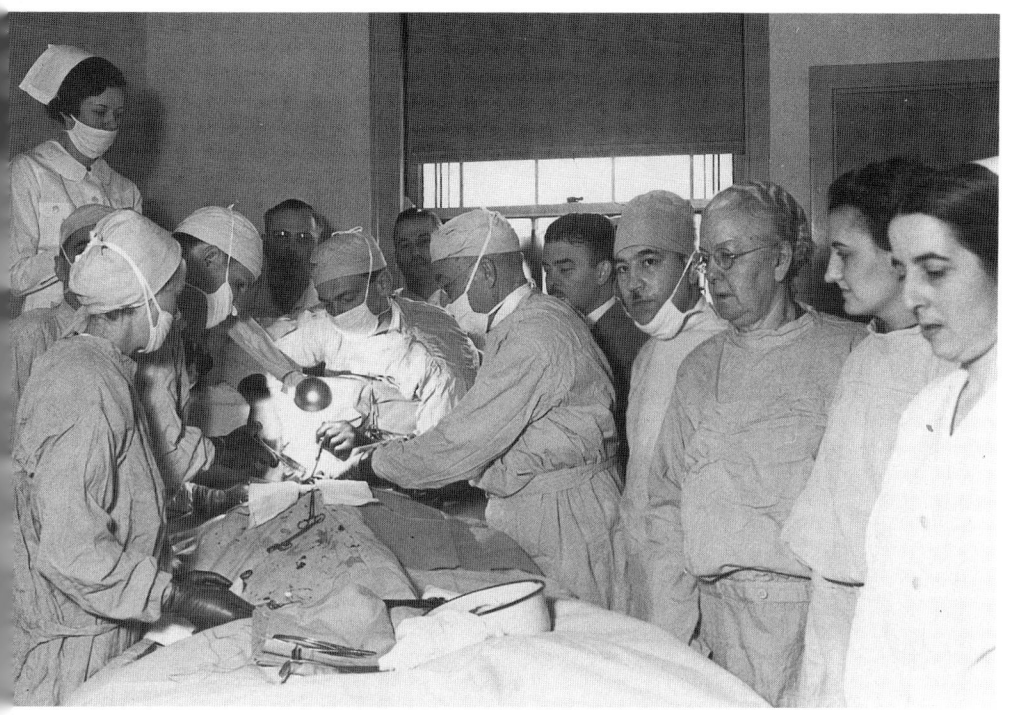

On the occasion of Dr. George Crile, Sr.'s twenty-five thousandth thyroidectomy (June 3, 1936), thirteen people crowded around the patient—some without masks or gowns. Barney is the fourth from left; his father is across from him. Third from right is the Chief's longtime secretary, Amy Rowland.

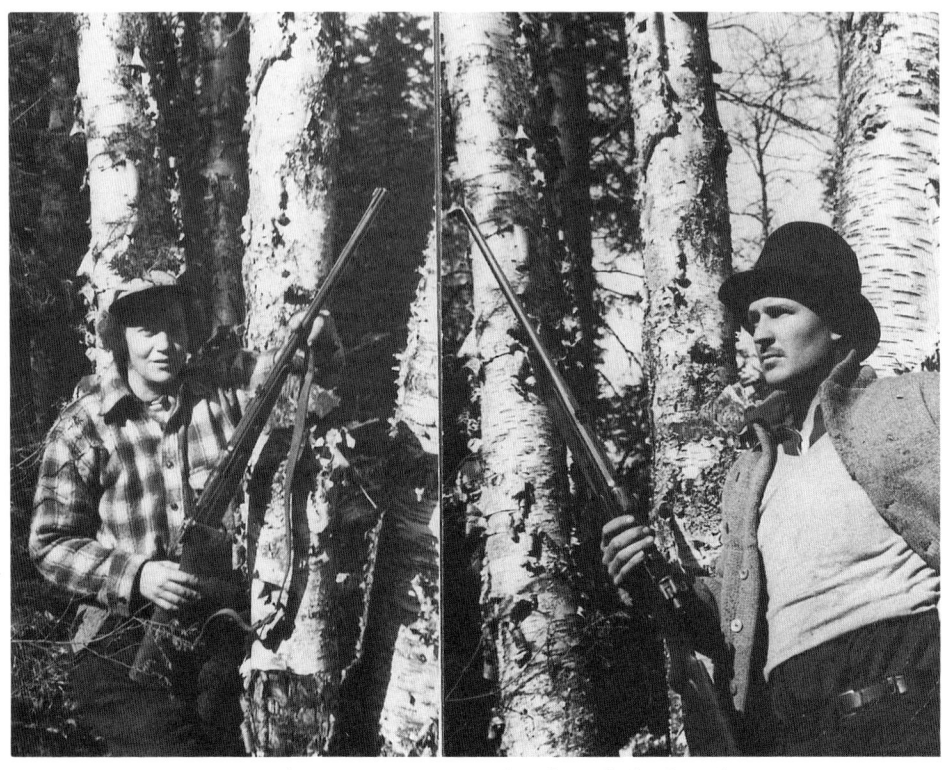
Jane and Barney on a moose hunting trip in Canada.

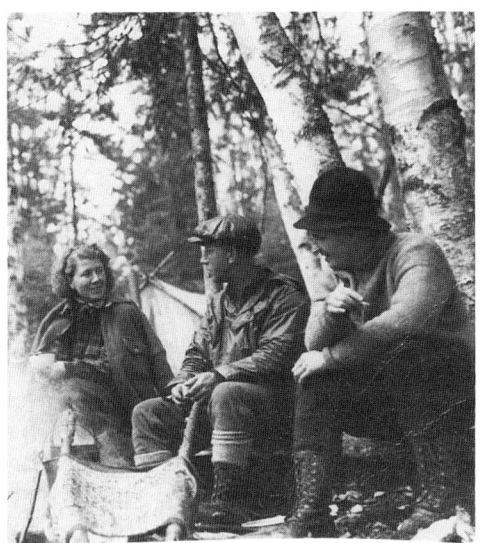

At camp in Canada. Their hunting guide, Tom Bell, is between Peg and Barney.

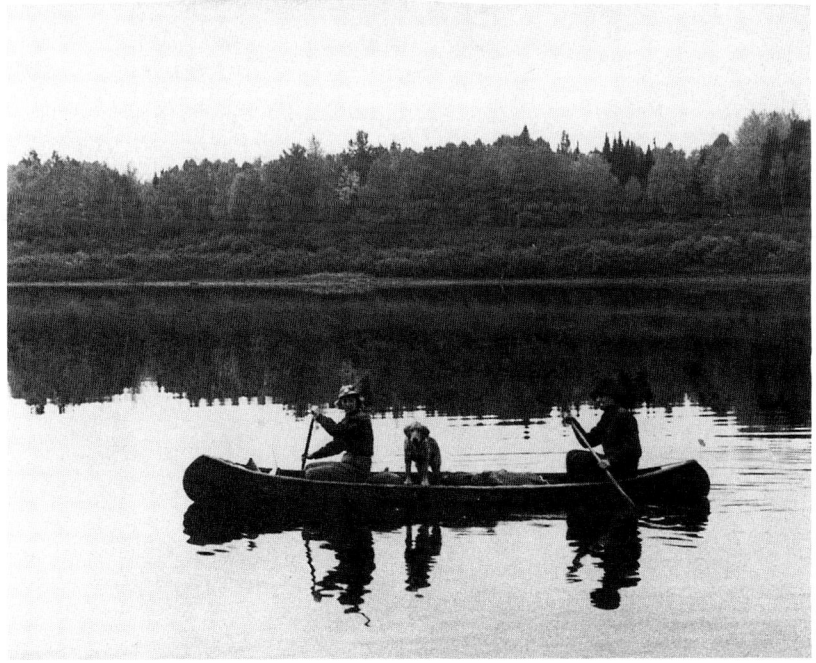

Jane and Barney loved the beauty of the Canadian wilderness during their hunting and fishing trips.

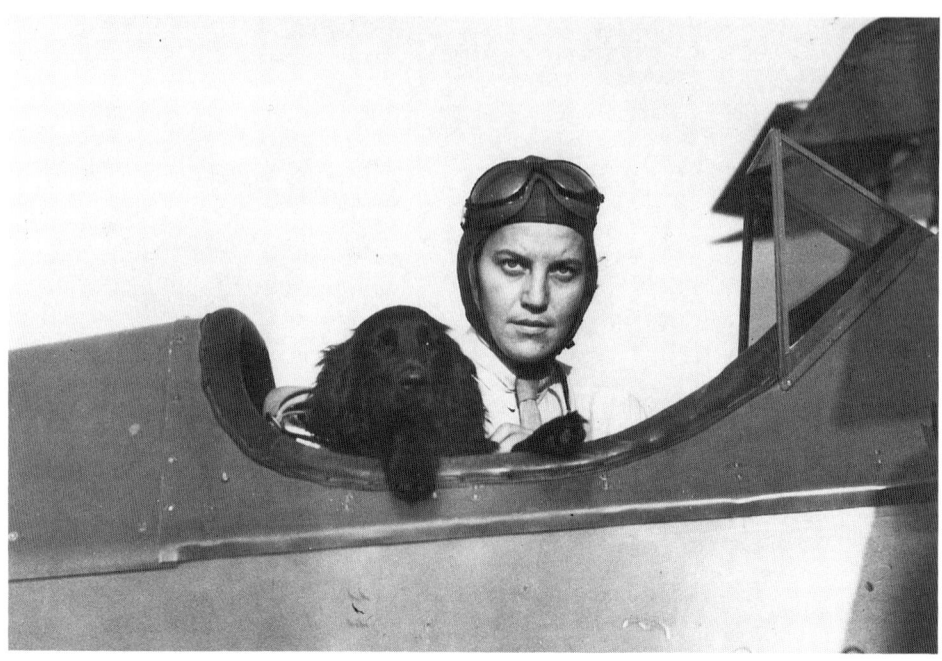

Jane shared an interest in flying with her father, Sam Halle. Here she also shares the cockpit for a photo taken in 1937.

Those were pleasant years, at the end of the 1930s. Everything was conventional—the surgery, the society, the pack trips, the hunting, and the fishing. I did everything just as my grandfather and father had done—fly fishing and duck shooting. Soon the time would come when my ideas about both vacations and work would change. But for now the children were growing and were fun to have with us on holidays. Only one event marred the happiness of those years. Jane's third pregnancy ended in the birth of a baby with a typical Down's syndrome—a "Mongolian idiot," the victim was then called.

The first time I saw Jane with the baby, she said, "What's wrong with her? She doesn't eat." I was no pediatrician, but I suspected the worst. Our pediatrician said everyone knew it. When the obstetrician had come in the afternoon of the day of delivery he had seen the baby in the ward and asked who that mongol belonged to. I talked with Jane. The baby steadfastly refused the breast, didn't react, didn't cry. The very expert and most understanding pediatrician told me, "Why don't you take Jane home? We'll take care of the baby. It's not going to survive anyway." So I did.

Those were unhappy days for Jane. Once or twice she wept, "I can't help thinking that she is hungry." To get her mind off the baby, I took her duck hunting in the marsh. We were wading in knee-deep water when suddenly Jane hit a bog and down she went, way over her boots and waist-deep in that frigid mud. She just stood there and cried. It wasn't the usual postpartum therapy. But before long, we were sitting in front of the fire and with a sip of rum, the world seemed better again. I was very proud of the way that Jane handled that tragic occurrence. I shudder to think what would have happened if there had been available and mandatory all the life-sustaining devices that prolong the lives of some of the children that are born today with severe manifestations of Down's syndrome.

In 1941, my father and mother were returning from a collection trip in the Florida Keys where they had captured and dissected a sea cow (manatee), when their airplane hit the center of a tornado and was dropped straight into the muddy water of the Florida Everglades. Miraculously no one aboard was killed, but my father's pelvis was fractured, and Mother broke two ribs and her sternum (chest bone), and cracked a vertebra. The plane seemed to have had little forward headway. It just dropped into the swamp and the seats, with the people in them, went straight on down through the floor with the result that all the people in them were up to their waists in water. They sat there in stunned silence. My father was the first to recover his voice, if not his senses. "Grace," he is reported to have said, "Grace, would you mind turning on the hot water?" No one laughed at the time, but Dr. Quiring, who was with them, remembered and related the story.

Jane and I along with my sister Peg and the rest of the family from all over flew down to try to help, but we found that all was going well and there wasn't much to be done. So we contented ourselves with staying at Vero Beach, exploring the Everglades, hunting and fishing and having a good time for a few days. Mother and Dad made slow but perfect recoveries. Impelled by this experience, in which for the first time he had experienced the effect on the circulation of sudden changes in gravitation, and stimulated by his knowledge of the role of aviation in the upcoming World War II, my father started out to redesign the old inflatable rubber suit that he once had used to prevent shock by squeezing the blood out of the abdomen and lower extremities and back into the essential brain-lung circulation. This development was indeed used by flyers in the war and later by brain surgeons when they wanted to have their patients sitting up for their operations.

The war was imminent now, and a Cleveland Clinic Naval Medical Unit had been projected. Jane and I viewed the war as almost inevitable and were determined to make the most of what might be our last months with our families. We moved out to the country for a month, living in "the Stables" of the Halle farm where there were good quarters for the family of the long-ago stable master and groom. I commuted, and was not too enthusiastic. I had, as usual, an old Ford and the forty-five-minute drive was not luxurious.

We traveled a little, taking a week with our friends, the Brittons, on their plantation in Thomasville, where everyone was devoted entirely to hunting quail and wild turkeys. It was a great place, built and operated in the tradition of *Gone With the Wind*. All of our best friends kept coming in and out.

Back in Cleveland, on one long weekend we drove over to Cook's Forest—a national park in Western Pennsylvania, where there are famous ski slopes, but I had never learned to ski well and I still, as had been the case in medical school, preferred to linger with Jane by the fireside instead of burying my awkward body in the snow.

One day at home, we decided that the ancient wooden garage behind our house needed updating, so we invited in all our friends, got a demolition permit, and one Saturday afternoon, with a keg of beer to encourage us, demolished the structure amidst shouts and screams and songs that were so loud that the police came and wouldn't go away until we showed them our permit. There were about forty of us there temporarily threatened with jail. Bob Little, a budding architect just out of school, had married Jane's sister Ann, and it was to him that we gave his first commission—to build for us a new and more appropriately located garage, suitable for cars rather than for the horses for which our old one had been built.

By this time, Jane was deep in photography. She had recovered from the loss of the last baby and wanted another, and in the meantime turned her talents to photography. She had even outfitted a darkroom in our basement and was beginning to enter some of her pictures in competitions.

My father's birthday was on November 11. He dressed up in his World War I uniform with general's stars and formally gave me a sword which he advised me to carry in case I went to war, so that if all did not go as we hoped, I would be able to express my desire to surrender and survive. I accepted it, and I would carry it all through the coming war without ever having to use or abuse it.

December 7, 1941, was a Sunday, and I was sitting in our sun porch reading and listening to the radio when the program was interrupted. Pearl Harbor had been bombed.

Our unit had been organized and was ready to go. We knew it was just a matter of time. We made our preparations. Among mine was a decision to write a paper on the treatment of hyperthyroidism, on which I felt myself an authority, because I had had a large practice in it and I thought I had developed some ways of making the operation safer. This paper I set aside so that after the war it would be there for me to send in as an announcement of my return and availability. But wasn't it my father who had said the average life of a scientific fact is seven years? If the life of a fact is seven years, the life of a favorite treatment is half of that, and in this case, by the time I would return, the need for the treatment would have vanished. The control of hyperthyroidism by thiouracil would have come into use and radioactive iodine would have been discovered.

There was, however, one last mistake I was privileged to make before we were called. It was made in the report of a new type of thyroid cancer—papillary cancer of the thyroid—which suddenly began to occur in children and young adults. The tumor metastasized widely throughout the lymph nodes of the neck, but rarely to distant organs and rarely was it fatal. This was so unlike the behavior of all other tumors—almost all of which, when there is extensive nodal involvement, metastasize to distant organs and are fatal—that I (along with most of other surgeons) took up the myth that the tumor in the lymph nodes was not metastatic cancer, but a strange, heretofore unrecognized, type of congenital anomaly. We thought it was a flaw of development in which there were deposits of thyroid tissue, known as lateral (side of the neck) aberrant (wandering) thyroids. There was no mention as to why, for the first time in history, these strange anomalies were being reported in increasing numbers.

My first papers, "Tumors of Lateral Aberrant Thyroid Origin" and "Papillary Thyroid Tumors," had been published in *Surgery, Gynecology & Obstetrics* and in the *Journal of the American Medical Association* in 1939. They reported twenty cases of papillary carcinoma of the thyroid and thirteen cases of papillary tumors arising in lateral aberrant thyroid tissue. I noted that in nearly half of the cases of lateral aberrant thyroid disease, the lobe of the thyroid on the affected side contained the same type of tumor. I also noted that only five of the twenty patients with papillary carcinoma of the thyroid died of the disease, a finding quite different from that in earlier cases where most papillary cancers proved fatal. In spite of my inability to realize that we were looking at a different type of papillary tumor occurring in people a generation younger and provoked by entirely different causes, I did comment, "It is often difficult to distinguish between lateral aberrant thyroid tumors and metastatic papillary carcinoma in lymph nodes." I continued, "Tumors arising in lateral aberrant thyroid tissue are essentially benign. Only two of the 45 patients classified in the literature as having malignant tumors of lateral aberrant thyroid origin have been reported to have died as a result of recurrence of the tumor following operation. None of the 13 patients in this series has died."

It would be eight years before increasing experience would confirm my observations about the relatively benign nature of the disease, and show that in almost every case a primary tumor could be found in the lobe of the thyroid on the affected side. Now, of course, we know that "aberrant thyroids" are metastases from what was then a new type of cancer that in a few years would be proven to be the result of radiating the necks of infants and children in the treatment of relatively harmless benign diseases. As an interesting sidelight on the way medical fads wax and wane, in the 1920s and 1930s radiation treatment of benign conditions of the neck and chest became so popular that at one time there was a bill before the New York legislature that would have made it mandatory for every baby at birth to have its thymic gland (in the neck and upper chest) irradiated in order to prevent "crib death" from supposedly enlarged thymic glands blocking the airways. These "enlarged" thymuses that the pathologists were reporting in babies dying suddenly were normal glands. When children are sick, the thymuses shrink. Therefore, it was the thymuses of long-ill children that were weighed and used as a standard instead of the thymuses of healthy children who had sudden deaths.

Although by 1947 I would make up my mind about the treatment of papillary carcinoma, many of the head and neck surgeons would continue, for the next twenty-five years, to treat it by radical and seriously deforming operations. During that period my chief and most gratifying occupation would be trying to disprove the theories and contentions of the cancer-specialized surgeons.

In the last few months before the war, I was busy working on my first book which, in 1934, when my father had suggested it, I had promised to write. It was practically finished when I had to leave, and the last touches would be added by its coauthor, my former resident Frank Shively, who took my place when I went away. *Hospital Care of The Surgical Patient,* with an introduction by my old chief, Evarts A. Graham, would be published by Charles C. Thomas and go through two editions. The four sections covered "Physiological Principles Related to the Care of the Surgical Patient," "Management of Surgical Complications," "Technic of Common Hospital Procedures," and "Relationships of the House Officer." The last contained a warning that I had found was a wise principle: "The house officer should realize from the first that his relationship with nurses while on duty should be entirely professional, especially in the presence of a patient." The book was dedicated to Dr. George Crile, Sr., thus fulfilling the prophecy of my chief in St. Louis who had written to my father, saying that soon he thought that he would have to so designate himself.

I still have a clear memory of Pearl Harbor Day. When the Japanese attack was announced, I knew that in a few weeks our unit would be mobilized and on its way. That was the end of surgery for a while and the beginning of a very exciting, educational, and thoroughly worthwhile experience. The only trouble was that I couldn't bear to leave Jane.

9

The War Years

NEW ZEALAND

A S SOON as war was declared my father, who held the rank of general, went to Washington to talk to some of his friends in the military. He took me along, and we interviewed the plan-makers. It was decided that our naval unit would go to New Zealand to prepare for what was not then mentioned, but which would turn out to be the Battle of Guadalcanal. When we returned to the Clinic with what we thought was great news, we were met by resentment and stony silence. Dr. Haden, the outspoken head of the Medical Department, told me what was on his mind: "We had been trying to arrange for you to get duty here in the States so you could do some teaching in naval hospitals and could come back to the Clinic from time to time." That may have been Dr. Haden's idea of war duty, but it wasn't my father's or mine, and it didn't come to pass.

It would be a while before the unit was mobilized, and we made the most of our time. Jane and I drove my mother and father west to what had been the Castalia Trout Club, which Mother's uncle, Lee McBride, had founded and where her father and my father had for so many years had such pleasure in fishing. After the trip, Mother wrote Jane and me,

> The Chief said it gave him an out-and-out thrill to feel the play of a light rod again. Over and over again he expressed the "kick" he got out of the day, his interest in seeing the old club again, his utterly satisfying visit with you, his talkfest with Jane, his delight in seeing you and Jane in action with your children, includ-

ing of course Cynnie [our dog]. Beside the joy of his being with you, the day to me recalled so many early memories of Father. You and your rods reminded me of how he used to bundle Mother and all five of us into a three-seated buckboard—fishing rods, lunch baskets, always a dog, sometimes a bicycle, and we too were off with worms, to fish small streams or in Shaker Lake, then seemingly miles away.

Mother, now with complete change of heart towards Jane, went on to compliment us on our "adaptable mechanisms and philosophies."

I remember the last night before our unit left. We went to Mother's house for dinner and afterwards sat in the living room and talked. I felt that this would be the last time I would see my father. His eyesight was nearly gone. A few days before he had had a bad tumble down a flight of stairs. He was seventy-eight. Perhaps he too felt that it was good-bye when we embraced. When Jane and I went home there were tears in my eyes.

The unit met in New York where every day, on the huge dock, we took an indoctrination course in naval etiquette, manners, and medicine. It was incredibly boring. But it lasted only a little over half of the day and then we were free. Jane and I had found a nice apartment in Brooklyn, with a king-sized double bed. We had never slept in one, for in those days they were considered to be faintly sensuous and immoral. We loved it and enjoyed New York, about which both of us, from college days, had many happy memories. Bud Yandell, who also was in the unit, found "La Cigne" piano bar, where we could drink beer and where everyone enjoyed listening to him play. This lasted eight weeks and then we were off to San Francisco to meet our boat.

On the way out Jane and I, incurable fish fanciers that we were, went first to Oregon and, by boat and ashore, wove our way down the Rogue River, fishing for trout all the way but catching only a few. It was a good last vacation together, and then we joined the rest of the unit in San Francisco, another new adventure for us, because it was our first trip to the West Coast.

San Francisco, with the Golden Gate Bridge, Chinatown, the nearby seal rookeries, cable cars, and the view of the harbor from the "Top of the Mark," was a memorable experience. We had a couple of weeks there, with nothing much to do except see the sights and think sad thoughts. Then sailing time was announced. Jane flew home to our children, and Bud Yandell and I boarded the ship, and with the rest of our unit and thousands of Marines waited for it to take us to The War.

We lived aboard the harbor-bound ship, and I wrote Jane about the delicious and classily served meals. "So far, we all agree, this is a great war and we are all enjoying it immensely. Just save your sympathy for yourself, because there is no question but that the only tough job is the one at home. It is odd how quickly one can adjust to new surroundings—including a very narrow, although comfortable, berth in place of the sumptuous double bed and the warmth of a little round body. [Jane was pregnant.] I guess I'll miss that more as time goes on. All my love, Barney."

Our ship was a 28,000-ton luxury liner that had been converted to a troop transport. The quarters for the officers were comfortable enough—but those for the men were cramped, with bunks four or five tiers high. There were seven thousand Marines on board. Sailing with us was another large converted liner, (the *Matsonia*), two Navy transports, a cruiser (the *Boise* with six-inch guns and two seaplanes), and one indeterminate sort of medium-sized vessel, probably a transport. As we sailed out through the Golden Gate, scanning the sea for submarines, a huge black shape rose through the water and a hundred feet to the port broke the surface. It spouted, waved its enormous flukes and sounded again. Outside the harbor, a destroyer joined the convoy and planes droned overhead.

Clear of land and a few days at sea, we lost all of our escorts except a single cruiser to guard the five troop transports and three freighters. The voyage was to take between twenty-one and twenty-five days. We were somewhere far west of Panama and about ten days out when I wrote in my journal,

> Last night after a long movie in the jammed and stinking-hot ward room we came on deck and looked out at the convoy moving along in ghostly procession in the light of a nearly full moon. The sea, sky and ships were a thrilling spectacle in the vast expanse of the universe. The foam made weird and changing patterns in the moonlight at the side of the ship. Not a sound, not a light, just grey forms stealing through the water. Three of us were leaning on the rail thinking these thoughts when someone suggested that if a man went overboard the ship would never stop. Another wondered how strong the rail was. We all stepped back, in step.

Other journal entries recount life aboard ship:

> *Sunday, July 5.* Last night I was sitting on the top deck watching the stars come out and thinking about submarines, when

suddenly the ships all blew great blasts of their whistles, shot up green rockets and made a sharp 40° turn. Practicing, I presume, but for a moment it made us all sit up and take notice.

Friday, July 10. We had a tremendous poker game on Wednesday and never left the table until Friday A.M. That, however, took into account the fact that we skipped Thursday by crossing the equator. This morning it is clear, fairly warm, a smooth sea, and in the distance is the land. We caught the first glimpse of it under the arc of a huge rainbow, the right side of which was anchored to the escorting cruiser. All we can see is the outline of rugged mountains, snow-capped and huge, in the distance. I am sure that the rainbow over the cruiser is a good omen.

Our mail is censored, and we are not supposed to tell anyone where we are. One of the Marine soldiers wrote a note saying, "We went under the Golden Gate, crossed the equator, lost a day, and are going to a large island noted for sheep-raising which is near a country noted for kangaroos. I can't tell you where it is, however."

I too wrote a letter from the ship, but I did not include any material that the censor might strike out.

Dearest Jane,

When we sailed we were all keyed up a bit and there was of course much joking and talking about submarines. A rumor went about that a tanker had been sunk 14 miles outside the harbor the night before.

Nick, Bill Engel, Saint, Red and I are at a table together and have a lot of fun. Bill is always entertaining and has plenty of tall tales. The food has been very good. Rare roast beef at least twice a week, steaks of the best order at least once a week, chicken or turkey once or twice a week, and all of the food well prepared and of fine quality. There is much more of it than we can eat, especially when it is hot. Celery and olives, salads, iced tea, everything one could wish for, and served on a white table cloth, with one steward to a table, and nice silver. It is really first-class cabin service.

The men have had a number of amateur shows with a band, piano players, guitar players, singers, story tellers, clowns, etc. They are quite amazing and serve to pass the time away. The only trouble is that there is little or no room for the spectators.

Our officers lounge was taken over by the men and so we have no place to sit. That, however, is our only hardship.

The water has held out well. We have a salt shower in our bathroom and have had enough fresh water for sponge baths all along. In the tropics, however, it was no use bathing as you sweat so much that you are soaked again by the time you get your clothes on again.

The morale of the men has been extraordinarily high, in spite of the fact that their quarters during a large part of the trip were nearly unbearable. Many of them slept on deck during this period. Our room got pretty hot, but actually little worse than many an August night in Cleveland.

The first day out was rough and many of the men were seasick. Fortunately, none of the officers of our group succumbed. The rest of the trip has been quite smooth. The men's quarters were a mess that first night!

Periodically come the damnedest epidemics of rumors. Submarines sighted, course changed, Captain having a nervous breakdown, engines broken, meeting up with other ships, ships leaving us, all of these and many more go the rounds, starting no one knows when and based on no foundation of fact. Still it keeps one interested and makes conversation. Most of the time one forgets all about danger and can scarcely remember to hang on to the life preserver. The best rumor of all was that there were a lot of girls (nurses) aboard another ship and that they would pull alongside one night and have a dance. Next that the girls had hung out their laundry and that a marine officer with glasses had counted 200 brassieres. Everyone with glasses rushed topside to look, but was not rewarded with any satisfaction.

If you have never crossed the equator on a transport you have missed an experience. The initiation into Neptune's realm is a real one that no one going through it will soon forget. They start the build-up several days in advance by broadcasting on the loud speakers and posting notices—remarks, such as

"All pollywogs—all pollywogs (those to be initiated), you are betrayed. Father Neptune knows your sins. Repent. The day is at hand." (This will be repeated from 2 to 5 times.)

"Attention all sharks, whales, and barracuda and monsters of the deep. There is plenty of fresh meat. Pollywogs!"

"All shellbacks (those who have crossed the equator), Attention. Corpses should be well weighted before being thrown over."

"Attention all pollywogs. Are you too hot? Are you sick of the chow? Are you seasick? Do you wish you were dead? Wait until the day. Ha Ha Ha." (Ghastly laugh).

They built a large butcher stand and a dunking pool on the aft deck. When the day came we found that they had not exaggerated the difficulties of entering King Neptune's kingdom. Davy Jones, in red shirt, black breeches and a patch over an eye, came aboard at 7:00 P.M. Tuesday, was received by the band and the guard of honor and gave his message to the captain. The guard of honor wore evening dresses, grass skirts, pirates' clothes, battle equipment, skyvvies (underwear) and one "lady" was adorned with two half grapefruit with an olive stuck on the front of each with a toothpick. They paraded the deck, the band leader using a broom for a baton.

The next morning the shellbacks drilled the pollywogs in full equipment and overcoats in the equatorial sun. At 9:15 King Neptune came aboard with his retinue of judges, executioner, hangman, etc. Those receiving charges of mutiny, plotting, spying, etc., were brought up first. There was a mutiny among the pollywogs who turned a fire hose on the shellbacks. But this was controlled and they started them through the line, crawling on hands and knees while a line of 100 paddled them with barrel staves. And they really paddled too.

When they got through the line they were tried, brought up to the King, put their hand on an electrically charged bible, were shoved and ducked into the dunking pool. Nearly drowned by repeated dunkings, shocked with an electric pitchfork, and down the line on the other side, running through another 100 paddles. All the officers and most of the men were eventually put through. My tail was black and blue for a week. There were several minor fractures and a concussion during the course of the day. We are now the proud possessor of cards announcing that we are members of the ancient order of The Deep. We are now very comfortable and quite well adjusted to life aboard, although the days seem to go more slowly than at first. We are eagerly anticipating seeing Jim and the Captain and finding out what we are to do next. So far it has been a great war! Aren't you glad you aren't with us?

Love,
Barney

We disembarked in Wellington and spent a couple of days there before going north to Auckland, where our hospital would be built. The New Zealanders were almost overly hospitable. We were invited to parties. They gave us meals and drinks and found young women for us. Of the latter, there was no scarcity for twenty-six thousand New Zealanders were on duty overseas, and there wasn't left in the country an able-bodied man between the ages of eighteen and forty.

The New Zealand women were amazingly versatile. "When a girl walks you have to canter to keep up with her," I wrote in a letter to Jane. They had a special accent—not like that of the New Zealand men and not at all like that of Australians. New Zealand women of all classes spoke like girls from the Boston colleges and "finishing schools." The accent was exaggeratedly refined, and unlike many Australians that I have met, the New Zealanders refrained from using the four-letter language of the United States Marines.

Wellington was a dry town. We searched without being able to find anything but a glass or two of native wine. "The Marines have drunk us dry," they told us, for thousands of them had been stationed there, preparing for the Battle of Guadalcanal. Moreover, the New Zealanders were honest and law-abiding citizens and did not use or even tolerate bootleggers.

Along with four officers and thirty men, I boarded the *Lipscomb Lykes*, a 6,500-ton freighter loaded with our medical gear and bound for Auckland in the North Island. The captain of the ship welcomed us aboard with drinks from a large bottle of Scotch and we were given comfortable staterooms that contrasted sharply with the accommodations on the transport. We played poker with the crew and had a good time except for an interlude shortly before landing, in which a great storm blew up, the compass broke, and we were lost in an area said to be haunted by submarines and set with a myriad of Japanese mines. There was wind as well as fog, and my diary says, "The ship would come up out of the water, crash down on a wave, pitch her propellers out of water, vibrate and shake and then do it all over again." Finally we reached the harbor and landed. The details are contained in a letter to Jane:

The Captain and Donahue went about getting the field (on which the hospital would be built) surveyed and arrangements made with the local authorities for help. Zup [Dr. Zupanic, a general surgeon] took charge of the storage warehouse, Ken [Dr. Kennedy, Clinic ophthalmologist] took charge of the building supplies at the field and I took charge of the unloading. (All of us, of course, were surgeons and had no idea of how to do what we were doing.) Each of us was on 24-hour duty, and had under us a detail of seamen who worked in shifts. For three or four days we didn't get over four or five hours of sleep a day.

My job on the wharf was terrific as we had to correlate the efforts of all the stevedores (whose only idea was to do nothing at all if they could find an excuse to do so), the Navy (whose idea was to get the ship unloaded and back to work as soon as possible), and the local Army (whose trucks we were using to haul the material and whose chief object was to throw everything into a truck and haul it away to anywhere, no matter where). Our chief motive was to get the stuff (building material and supplies for a 300-bed field hospital) sorted out so that our perishable supplies would not stand outside and get wet and so our building materials would all get out to the field. I had to cajole and threaten and practically bribe all persons concerned in order to accomplish these ends. I learned more about stevedores and stevedore bosses and the Army and the Navy in a matter of 24 hours than I ever hope to again in the rest of my life. We finally developed a system in which each piece was marked "F" for field or "S" for storage and educated the stevedores to load the marked material into appropriate trucks. But I can tell you that when they began to unload the unsorted cargo from several ketches at once and pile it all up on the dock it was the damndest state of confusion you have ever seen—nursing supplies, mattresses and bedding being stacked out at the field in the rain!

At the field, Ken did a wonderful job of unloading the stuff and keeping it all together in stacks. He worked like hell day and night for four days in the cold rain up to his knees in mud and Zup did an equally good job arranging the store houses which were nothing but a lot of black, dirty old cellars and garages. Our men and ourselves were all exhausted by the time the rest arrived, and we were given a night off.

I next described how we went out to see the town and ended up at a spot named "Orange Hall" which was famous for its dancing. The great ballroom was filled with people, some in couples, some as women dancing together, all very formal, joining hands in marches, and parades, and after each episode each person returning to his or her appointed seats.

THE WAY IT WAS

If anyone sat in anyone else's place there was hell to pay. This is the most orderly and arranged country I have ever seen or heard of.

At last Bill and I picked out a couple of girls and gave it a try. Both of us got so battered and bruised when we missed the first reverse that we had to give it up. You might as well step in front of a herd of stampeding buffaloes as try to go against the grain in one of those dances.

The next morning we started building. [The buildings would be one-story, tin-roofed wards each holding about forty beds.] Since then I have been on the night shift. We work from 8:00 P.M. until 8:00 A.M., get breakfast and sleep from 9:00 until 5:00, go for a walk, supper at 6:30, and off to work again at 7:30. There hasn't been time for anything but work.

Digging the footings is a hell of a job in the rain and mud at night. The ground is hard as a rock and we have to chip it out at the bottom as best we can. It is tiring work, and if you just stand around and watch the men you feel so lazy and mean that you are miserable, and if you dig yourself, you get so tired that you are more miserable. So I compromise and dig about half the time and appear to be busy supervising or go to get something somewhere the rest of the time.

The officers are living at the Royal Hotel—the most rundown and notorious house of ill repute in Auckland. The lounge is constantly filled with harlots and there appears to be plenty going on upstairs.

When I wrote the above I hadn't learned that there are absolutely no harlots in New Zealand. If there ever had been any the war-induced scarcity of men and the avidity of the nonprofessionals would have put them out of business.

But the food is wonderful—steak for breakfast, lunch—about six courses, and dinner starts with fruit juice, then soup, then fish, the entree if desired, then roast beef, steak or mutton, next chicken or duck and then dessert and ice cream. Often after a day's work I don't miss a single course. [Later I mention that in restaurants you can buy the finest steak you ever tasted for the equivalent of thirty cents.]

The beds are broken down and the sheets are dirty, mouldy and full of holes. We have all been badly bitten by some kind of bed bug or flea, but we are so tired when we go to bed that we don't notice it at all. In the A.M. the chamber maid wakes us up

230

with a pot of tea in bed. There is no toilet in the room, but the sink is handy. The shower has no head on it—just a broken-off pipe at the end of the hall. But it is too cold to use anyway. The whole damn thing is rather like a moose hunting trip, and I don't know when I have had more fun.

I went on to say that my brother's best friend, Charley Neff, suddenly appeared in civilian clothes, for he was connected with some aviation project. Charley had everything under control, as usual, for he had "found a way to buy whiskey by the case and had heard of a woman who distributes dates to lonely Americans." Before Charley left, he would do me a great favor. He would introduce me to his favorite Auckland girl.

My first letter from Auckland closed, "We have had invaluable experience learning to handle men and organize work. I wouldn't have missed this for anything. We have been too busy to think or be homesick. Only in the little interlude after the work is over and before sleep do I feel the emptiness which your being away brings."

We were working on construction twelve hours a day seven days a week. I was best when it came to laying down the wooden floors, for then my manual training course at University School all came back to me. I found I could lay the boards and pound the nails just as fast as any of the corpsmen and at the same time organize and provide the necessary materials. I enjoyed it.

Later in the period of construction, when the buildings were almost completed, I stopped in at headquarters and said I was going to go out for about an hour and gave a number where I could be reached. It was the number of my friend Dr. James Fitzsimmons, who had visited me in Cleveland and stayed at our house. He lived just a few blocks away, but no sooner had I arrived than the phone rang and I was told to return at once to the construction. Mrs. Fitzsimmons ran me back and I was met by a furious skipper. "You have deserted your duty. That is a court martial offense," and he went on without mercy. Although I had at that time nothing at all to do in the construction and although I was only minutes away and had left my number, I had no real excuse. I apologized. The next day the skipper was all smiles and he never again mentioned the episode. That was the last time that I ever bent any of the rules of naval behavior.

The hospital ward buildings were completed on schedule, and so were those for the officers and men. Our quarters consisted of a building the same size as the wards but divided into rooms just big enough to hold a bed, a small table, and a chair. Some of the rooms had a single bed, some had an upper and a lower berth. There was a pleasant veranda outside with chairs enough for those who wanted them, and a croquet court. All of this was set in a grove of ancient greenery surrounded by a wall, for this had once been the site of the exclusive Remuera Golf, Tennis and Cricket Club. A small portion of it was still extant, providing a lawn for bowling on the green. At the far end of the building that housed the officers' bedrooms there was a single "head" (the naval word for toilet) with showers and all necessary facilities. An adjacent building housed the officers' mess, with living space, a dining table for the officers, and the kitchen in which the officers' mess was prepared. Everything was highly organized by our experienced and intelligent, regular-Navy-Captain Robbins. He put Dr. Nichols, the dentist, in charge of the officers' mess. There was a liquor ration, derived from naval supplies and available in limited amounts for about a dollar a bottle, and there was excellent food.

My base pay as a lieutenant was $200 a month, all of which was allotted to Jane. But I was paid a $20 bonus for sea duty plus a $90 allowance for rent and a $43 subsistence allowance, a total of $153. Out of this I had fixed expenses of $21 for food, $7.50 for insurance and $10 for laundry and pressing. That left me $114.50 a month, so that, with steak at thirty cents a serving, I could afford to go out to dinner whenever I wanted to.

The most expensive thing in New Zealand was transportation because there was severe gas rationing. There were few taxis and those of our local friends who had cars weren't able to get gasoline. A group of us got together and rented a car, at a shilling a mile, pretty expensive, but a ration of gasoline went with the rental and occasionally we could supplement that by borrowing a little from the gas-operated drilling machine in the dental office. Nevertheless, a weekend in the car would cost us about $30, which we'd split, usually coming to about $10 apiece. That was the only way that we could see the great beaches and parks and catch the trout that had made the country famous, and hunt the deer that lived in the hills, and visit the geysers and hot water springs of the sulfurous volcanic resort of Rota Rua.

At first we were mystified by the New Zealand women. There were many of them around—Red Cross workers, volunteers working at the hospital, girls that we'd meet by accident or that friends would introduce us to. They all seemed so refined and well mannered, and they really were. The only thing that we didn't at first understand was that they were eager. This, of course, was because they had for so long been without the company of men.

Thirty-year-old wives, eighteen-year-old girls—all of them were charming and available. It took most of us a month or so to find this out, but some of the smarter members of the unit made the observation when we first moved into the hotel and the chamber maids brought tea to them in bed. Bud Yandell and I were among the more retarded members. I remember a long drive that we were taken on one evening by a couple of ladies whose husbands were overseas. I have often thought that those two must have thought that we were two of the world's most innocent dummies. But we began to watch the skipper and to notice that there was a motherly looking lady who seemed to be with him almost every evening, and we saw that most of the enlisted men seemed to be pairing up. Finally, we got the word. My brother's friend, Charley Neff, was my teacher. He introduced me to a lovely twenty-one-year-old girl, Jean Milson, who was engaged to a flight officer now overseas in the air force. Jean and I became fast friends and although there were no pledges of fidelity and each of us went out with whomever we chose, we did have an understanding that I would take her each Saturday night to the weekly Officers-Mess party.

When the construction of the officers' quarters and mess were completed, the skipper called a meeting. "We assumed he was going to give us hell, because he looked very stern," I wrote to Jane. "He started by stating that there were two rules that could not be broken by the officers living in our one-story bungalow quarters. The first was that no women were to be allowed on the second floor, and the second was that the ladies had to be out of the officers' rooms by 8:00 A.M. The skipper then opened up the mess hall, which he had secretly furnished and in which he had all of his private stock of liquor. He gave us a big cocktail party. There was singing and Bud at the piano, and it wound up very happily. Nichols, the mess officer, began planning a big party for Saturday night." The skipper was one of the greatest and most inspirational leaders that I had ever known. Everyone was behind him all the way, and in New Zealand he never made what I could call a mistake.

On September 3, I wrote to Jane in answer to some of the questions she had asked me about life in New Zealand:

> The whole situation here is almost exactly like college all over again. We might just as well be living in a fraternity—a damn good bunch of fellows—congenial. No scraps or feuds anymore —busy enough to keep us out of trouble, but not too busy to have a lot of fun. Work is over at five o'clock and there is plenty

to do in the evenings. The local people have been wonderful to us, and we have gone out a lot to parties etc. When I say it is like college I mean in every way. This life without women brings about strange reactions in a group of married men, and makes them all think and talk about such business much more than ordinarily. The usual masculine wit and vulgarity is ever present and as delightful as ever. Philosophical discussions and crude humor are blended into an entertaining melange. It is just like college in that although you may talk a lot you do little. Remember I was a virgin throughout college. I don't think I could persuade you, even if I tried, that my thoughts don't occasionally stray, but so far I have been able to keep them in handcuffs.

In the same letter I went on to speak of the corpsmen who assisted us in the operating room and took care of the patients on the wards:

They are just as good as nurses in most ways, and better in some. For a ward full of men they are definitely superior. And our operating room lads are as good as any scrub nurse I have ever worked with. Tomorrow we have seven cases scheduled, the biggest day so far. I am keeping the work equally divided between the four general surgeons. Most of it is really minor surgery, but some of it is quite interesting and there has been a scattering of very good cases to do. The general surgery department has had the best break so far, as the specialty departments haven't had much to do and time hangs heavy on their hands. Censorship forbids any details.

The dance halls are quite amazing. It is worth the price of admission to go and see the sailors do the Jive. They really have taught the local girls how to hoof it. The colored mess attendants tell their girls that they are full-blooded American Indians and they are the toast of the town. There is no drinking allowed in any dance place, and they are really very respectable. Bud and I are thinking of taking up dancing.

A little later on, in a letter to Jane, I expressed some bewilderment by the situation, "At times it seems entirely wrong to be having a good time in times like this. I wonder if we're not just a lot of old damn fools trying to be kids again, but there is no other choice because there isn't anything else to do."

Sometimes there was a different type of reversion, this to the outdoor sporting life instead of to the sporting life with women. On October 12, I wrote of a fishing trip that we took and of the country we passed through:

This weekend I really did miss you every second of the day and night. I started missing you the night before we left when I began to pack up the fishing gear and thought of all of the places and streams we had visited and the fun we had had with that equipment. And, as usual, when you aren't around, all of my things were lost and dirty, and I couldn't find anything that I wanted. So at last I just rolled up a big ball of equipment and shoved it into a sea bag along with Bud's and Charley B's, and we were off. Joe R. [Root, a radiologist] came along too—not to fish, but to go on a sightseeing tour with a friend of his who lived in the village we were headed for.

It was a perfectly beautiful Spring day, and the four of us, with our gear strapped onto the fenders, piled into a little bug of a car about the size of a sewing machine, and with Bud at the wheel, we drove away. There was over a hundred miles of beautiful rolling country, and each hill was as green and smooth as a golf course fairway and dotted with sheep and cattle. If you could imagine a golf course 100 miles long, that is the way it was. We followed a river valley all the way up, with mountains on each side and the pastures' rough hillsides covered only with tree ferns, scrub palms, and gorse. The tree ferns are huge things with leaves just like a fern but thirty or more feet high with big trunks six or eight inches in diameter. Every bit of the land between the mountain ranges is fenced and filled with cattle or sheep, and each half mile or so there would be a cute little house, neat as a pin, surrounded with green grass and such a brilliant display of flowers as you have never dreamed of. Rhododendrons grow taller than two-story houses and the individual blossoms are as big as your head. Camellia trees, covered with the most gorgeous waxy pink, white, or red flowers, stand thirty feet high and are a blaze of color. Each farmhouse has its flower garden neatly laid out and perfectly tended, and the humblest of these would win a first prize in any garden show in America.

Through the valley ran a great river, about the size of Cook's Forest's, with clear water, big pools, and rapids that made your mouth water for a canoe. We saw dozens of hares and rabbits feeding with the sheep on the hillsides, and alongside the road covey after covey of California quail scuttled into the underbrush. We saw several of the biggest pheasants we have ever seen and twice, as we passed lakes or marshes, we saw wild duck swimming on the water or setting their wings to come in.

After a drive of 100 miles we came to the Hotel, a typical tourist type of resort, badly in need of renovation, but clean and nice enough. It was located in the center of a golf course. Around it were scattered tennis courts, and through the backyard wound a lovely clear trout stream.

Joe detached himself from the party at this point and looked up his friend with whom he was planning to drive farther on to visit a famous national park the next day, and Bud, Charley and I set up our rods and employed the services of a small boy, "Barry," age seven, and his dog "Chum," age seventeen and black. They were to act as guides for us.

We dashed down to the stream and tried one fly after another with no observable effect. But, fortunately, with my customary foresight, and in spite of the glowing accounts of the fishing that all the natives had regaled us with, I had made provisions against just such a contingency. At midnight the night before I had gone quietly out into the garden with my flashlight and had picked up a big can full of night crawlers.

In this land of British sportsmanship, fishing with worms is a penitentiary offense, prohibited by law. So I had carefully concealed them in the flaps of my fishing jacket. Barry, Chum, and I proceeded to detach ourselves from the eager fly fishermen who were still ardently slapping the water with useless flies, and went downstream where I heard a waterfall. The stream wound down through precipitous banks much like that roaring stream we found in the gorge at Glacier Park—through impenetrable damp green forests of ferns into a rocky cleft and then over a waterfall into a giant punch bowl. It looked like Dawn Mist Falls.

I climbed out over slippery rocks onto a ledge where there was a natural seat, and proceeded to break out my can of worms and relax. The little boy kept asking me what I had in the can. I kept telling him it was fly oil. The dog said nothing but sniffed and looked wise.

I let the worm drift down with the current and soon enough began to drag out what seemed to me to be exceptionally fine fish—twelve to sixteen inches long—beautiful rainbows. I had five of them when the crowd began to gather. First came three civilians, all of whom looked like the game warden; then a group of girls; then four boys about fourteen or fifteen years old, and finally a group of twenty native soldiers. Everyone sat down comfortably and watched me fish. I had a big old snelled hook on my line and two big dew worms on my hook. The Army officers kept yelling, "What are you using for bait?" I pretended I could not hear because of the waterfall. Finally, one of them came across to me and yelled in my ear, "What fly are you using?" I thought of saying, "No speakee English," but thought I might be judged as a spy. So I said I was using an American fly. He went back across the stream and reported to the crowd that I was using an American fly. Just then I got a strike and gave a big yank so that the line flew out of the water and the hook and worm landed right in the middle of the crowd. At that we all had a good laugh and I was much relieved that the game keeper was not numbered among those present.

That night, as usual, Yandell and I took over the hotel, bought drinks for everyone in sight, got the manager drunk, ran the telephone exchange, and found a wonderful blond woman who sang Irish songs all night. Bud was of course at the piano, and the affair was a small edition of our night at the Beaverkill.

The next day we got our small boy and dog and started out to fish. The boy said that his school teacher's husband knew a good place to fish, so we stopped by their house. He was out, but she was willing, and we drove up to pick up her friend who lived on a farm five miles away and the two girl guides, the boy guide, and the three fishermen set off.

We drove to the end of the road, then opened a gate and started off across country, scattering sheep, rabbits and quail in every direction, over mountains, down valleys, through dry stream-beds. For miles, it seemed, we drove, and finally came to the lost valley. Surrounded with hills brown with gorse and palmetto and scrub, the valley with its winding stream was incredibly smooth and green. Sheep were everywhere, but no sign of human habitation. No trees, no shrubs, just the crystal-clear stream meandering through the fields. Big pools, rapids, ripples, high banks, low scrub for cover, and all in all the most beautiful stream I have ever seen for fishing. Bingham chased the farmer's wife up a mountainside, but kept in plain view of us all the time and apparently behaved himself. Bud was dressed in Worder's bathing trunks, identification disc and officer's cap. The sun was bright and warm and the sky as blue as the grass was green—an incredible sight and experience in these days when nothing should look right. But we fished and fished and saw nothing.

Finally Charley tried to lure a frog into taking his fly but with no results.

We then went back to the farmer's wife's house and helped her put her cows in the paddock. We were wonderful at it.

The farmers here are amazing. She was a young woman of twenty-four or twenty-five and as well educated and well dressed as any one in the country. They had a *modern* home of stucco or some such thing, immaculately clean, with a lovely lawn and flower garden. Inside, they had a piano, telephone, radio, frigidaire, electric range, and modern sink and toilet. The cow barns and milking station were as clean as a kitchen, and everything was exactly in its place. They had 95 cows on 105 acres of land. The standard of living of the small farmer here is remarkably high and the people who are farming are perfectly happy in the life that they lead. That part of this country is like a little Utopia.

We drove back that afternoon, arriving home about eight, and we all had a fish fry in the officers' mess hall. It was a great weekend and gave us a real insight into the workings of the rural part of this country.

Love,
Barney

A little later in October, I was invited by Dr. Hercus, the dean of the Medical School in the North Island, to visit the school and lecture. Dr. Hercus was a thyroidologist and knew of my work and of course of my father's. He even arranged for me to do a thyroidectomy while I was visiting them. I stayed with the Hercuses. They were a charming family, and did everything for me.

About this time my birthday came along (November 3) and I wrote Jane about the party that Yandell gave for me—cake, thirty-five candles and all—at the Royal Hotel with all of our best friends and a bevy of local beauties, including my special friend, Jean Milson, who by now had made a little dress for my new daughter Susie and had written Jane a letter. Bud, of course, played the piano, and somewhere, during the evening, one of the New Zealanders caught a hedgehog "which," I told Jane, "is like a porcupine, but more so, and had rolled itself into a ball of quills. He threw it to Jean who caught it, like a damn fool, and filled her arms with quills and dropped it on her legs. We then gave it a drink of beer and the animal, which was no bigger than a baby's head, proceeded to piss the biggest puddle you have ever seen right in the middle of the floor. For a half-pint animal it has a two-gallon bladder."

The letter continues, "If I am busy and active and don't hear from you, I can fit myself back into the more or less aimless unsatisfied way of life that I led before I was married. There was lots of fun, a certain amount of humor, but no deep real satisfaction." And I went on to tell of my admiration for her letters and "the most perfect gift of self-expression and mail-order love making that I ever dreamed of."

By this time, I had more or less settled down with Jean as my Saturday night companion, but would go out on any other night with whomsoever came by. I told Jane about this when she asked me to tell her about our life here and whether I approved of her going out at home:

Those are hard questions to answer because different people react differently to the same situation, and I am sure that no one should censure another's behavior. Each individual, confronted with a situation, does what he or she thinks right for himself or herself, and if it turns out that it wasn't right he will change his ways if he has any sense. Almost anyone will make mistakes on one side or the other, and these shouldn't be held up as examples of what that individual's true behavior is. When such a fundamental thing as a person's married life is broken up by separation there are very difficult adjustments that have to be made, and few people will arrive at once at the solution that is really the best for them. Some attempt to live by some theoretical, child-taught idealism. Others go to the opposite extreme of utter abandon. Somewhere in between, I believe, lies the proper solution for the majority of people, but that balance is hard to hit at first.

Then I went on to tell about the plight of the manless New Zealand women and about the behavior of the members of the unit, all but one of whom ultimately settled down into some sort of relationship with one or more of the many women who were available.

And then at last came action—the Battle of Guadalcanal. We were to receive the casualties. None of them were fresh, for there was no air transport and by boat the island was several days away. I wrote about it to Jane:

November 27, 1942
This has been a hell of a week. Not only is the hospital in the greatest state of confusion, being full to overflowing and at one point having 30 more patients than there were beds, but all of the

239

surgical patients are on medical wards and vice versa. Now it is gradually getting okay again.

Then I sneaked off downtown one afternoon and went to the cable office to send Bob a cable. Every so often one forgets that a war is on. And it is especially funny because I was on the censor board out here that week. Anyway, I cabled Bob the following message, "Deliver Jane December fifth two bottles French champagne, can Russian caviar, Spring onion, three Belmont gardenias, and all my love. Money order for $25.00 follows." Needless to say, I had no sooner returned to the hospital than Naval Intelligence phoned and said the cable could not be sent. It naturally sounded like some kind of a code. It would probably indicate that the French would attack the Russians on December 5th and eat onions in the Spring. Anyway, I found out that nothing but the most routine messages passed censorship on the cables and hence could not make the necessary arrangements. I could not even cable flowers. It has to go by mail. But if you did not have any remembrance from me on December 5th it was not because I was not thinking of you or did not try well in advance to get something through. I would have done it by air mail a bit earlier except that I thought you would rather have the cable, and by the time I found out it was impossible, it was too late. I am probably now on the list of suspects and all other cables will be censored!

Then your cable about Dad came. Naturally I was deeply concerned and distressed. It sounds terribly serious at his age. The more I think of him and his unique personality and philosophy, the more tragic it seems that he has to get old. Lord, but I hope he gets well again so that he can impress his memory on the children. We have been most fortunate to have our wonderful memories of him—memories of his operating in the days when he was at his peak, of his humor, his vitality and his handling of people. He is a rare and universal type of genius. I hope nothing happens to him. You will keep me frankly in touch, won't you?

This was the beginning of my father's final illness. He had bacterial endocarditis—universally fatal in those days before antibiotics. He was beginning to have embolisms that lodged in the vessels of the brain.

In the same month I wrote my friend Dr. Tom Jones, head of Surgery at the Clinic,

Perhaps you were never in a base hospital during the last excursion. If not, you can't really imagine how confusing life can be. There is always some ignorant buzzard who outranks everyone else and the chief concern of all concerned is to politely maneuver the political wires in such a way that he is kicked upstairs out of everyone's way. I was assigned control of "plastic surgery." My ability to visualize the fine points and artistry of plastic surgery is about on a par with my appreciation of other artistic things. Fortunately there have been few cases requiring anything on the face.

There was one plastic problem that I remember vividly. A man had been shot in the mouth and his whole lower lip was gone. He couldn't hold food or fluids in his mouth or suck a straw. By sliding tissue flaps I closed the defect. Of course its appearance was a disaster, but the man could eat. I was very proud of the result until a year later, when I would be in San Diego and the plastic surgeons would present the case at a meeting as an example of what disasters the front line people perpetrated when they tried to repair tissue defects.

All of our life in Auckland didn't revolve around the hospital. We took weekend trips when it was our turn to be off duty—fishing, hunting in season, sightseeing. The beaches were of black volcanic sand and were spectacular with the white surf breaking and the sparkling blue beyond. There were great fishing trips. One I remember well, to Rota Rua, New Zealand's famous lake, surrounded by mountains. The skipper headed the party, so one of the corpsmen drove us up in a transport vehicle which we left by the side of a stream while we went out on the lake in boats provided by friends. When we returned with three or four small fish we were astonished—and our law-abiding sportsmen New Zealand friends were horrified—to see the corpsman standing by the stream with a baseball bat and with a waist-high pile of salmon-sized rainbow trout beside him. They were running up the river to spawn and to the corpsman, who knew we were on a fishing trip, they looked like fair game!

It was mid-November, which in New Zealand is like May. "It is the most beautiful spring day," I told Jane.

The sky here, when it is not raining, is the brightest clearest blue that you have ever seen. There is no smoke and no dirt and everything looks green and freshly washed. Best of all, the air always has the invigorating tingle of an autumn day at home. One has a constant feeling of exhilaration. It feels like the rare days of autumn in New England when everyone is gay and the sun is bright and you pack up to go to a football game. Perhaps it is the air, perhaps it is just that we get plenty of rest and exercise and have little worry or responsibility compared to the life at home, but I just feel wonderful all the time. I am getting to be a pretty hot tennis player, by the way. I am just wondering if this would be a good afternoon to go rabbit shooting.

A few days later, I wrote her another letter about the hardships of our war:

Spring is really here, or rather summer—because for the first time it has been really pleasantly warm. Spring was in the air, so I promptly commandeered a Red Cross driver—a 31-year-old Irish, born-in-England gal who has traveled all over the world. We packed up the blankets and bottles, and went out to a beautiful point overlooking the harbor and established ourselves on the rocks. It was just like the opening of the blanket season in Northampton—except actually I had never seen this girl before and as Engel, who later came along and caught us sitting on the rocks, can testify, it was all very up and up. We had glasses and cigarettes and it was moonlight and ghostly, with the waves washing in on the rocks and huge white cliffs behind us and the shadowy outline of the islands in the bay—very mellow—as Yandell would have said—It is the most beautiful place to drink that I have ever seen. Later on a fisherman came by with a 40-pound eel.

Yesterday I got miserably defeated in tennis by a little 19-year-old blonde who lives in the neighborhood. It really is interesting to see the approach that we have to any girl we meet. We grade them in accordance with whether they have:

    1 – Coal-burning car—A, priority, as there is no problem about gasoline
    2 – Regular car with some source of gas
    3 – Tennis court
    4 – Piano
    5 – Country place
    6 – Husband away at war

It is very interesting to see the officers try to get all this information. The last item—husband away—is the least important because for some strange reason even those whose husbands are right here seem to take great delight in chasing after us. Poor old Bingham and Bud have been violently (and unsuccessfully) pursued. We are quite elusive.

I have been seeing an occasional interesting civilian case in consultation with some of the local M.D.'s, and that, coupled with a slightly increased activity here, has served to keep up the interest. For the greater part, however, the work has been pretty routine—appendices, hernias, pilonidal sinuses, hemorrhoids, and the usual run of casualties. I have an interesting case on hand now with an external carotid, severed about ¼ inch above the common carotid, loose in an infected neck and will probably ligate the common carotid tomorrow. We have pretty good equipment now and the operating room personnel are fine. We hear that perhaps sometime we are going to be given some Navy nurses. We do not know whether that is a good thing or a bad one.

We are becoming very proficient at our drilling. That is to say we do not all fall down any more when we make a right turn. Sinclair, when he drills, looks as if he is doing a modification of the shag. Joe Root is, of course, most professionally military and as a matter of fact is a darn good drill master. We will be all right Sunday when we march to church if the turn is to the left, but we will have to walk around the block if it is a right turn because we have not mastered that yet.

We have badminton and baseball and football each night in our back yard. From 4:30 to 6:00 we exercise there or sit and drink beer on our porch or in steamer chairs and watch. What a life!

Great interest in the radio these days. We just heard the news of the Solomons' naval victory. That, coupled with the good news from Africa, and the stalemate in Russia, is almost too good to be true.

In the next letter I told her about another friend of mine, Beth Dove, who was a Red Cross transport driver assigned to our hospital. On several afternoons we drove out into the country in search of a proper Christmas tree and Christmas decorations for the Officers' Mess, for I was in charge of this detail:

Beth is a nice little girl, but only about 20, and the night before I had taken her mother, also very charming, to a dance at the Fitzsimmons. The women were all about 40 and couldn't dance at all. [Coming from me that was a truly derogatory remark, for I had always been known as one of the world's worst dancers.]

We had an interesting letter from a friend of ours—a medical officer on Guadalcanal—and apparently he is enjoying his experience there but not really doing very much in the way of surgery. Actually there isn't much surgery associated with the casualties. The trend is towards conservation in the treatment of wounds and extensive debridement and excision and primary wound closure are considered inadvisable. We do a lot of skin grafting and secondary closures here. And that's about all except for hernias, appendices and hemorrhoids. I just got a glimpse of one of our ten new (female) nurses. Have to stop now!

Love always,
Barney

How Jane tolerated such a letter is beyond my comprehension.

After Guadalcanal everything settled down again and there wasn't much to do except play golf and tennis and go hunting and fishing and take the girls out at night. But I wasn't happy.

> I would in many respects rather be aboard ship or up in the islands than here, because I would at least feel that I was making some sort of sacrifice for the cause and that what I was doing was worth while. I realize that it would be even less interesting from the professional standpoint, but it would be a welcome change and it would make me feel worth while again. If you can't be home with your family and the things that really interest you, it would be better to go the whole hog and see what it's like in the field.
>
> This is idle talk and I am not contemplating applying for a change of station. But it would make a nice change for a couple of months.

At home Jane was taking it all remarkably well. We were perfectly frank with one another, and I think that was what saved us. On December 28, 1942, Jane wrote:

Dearest Barney—

Christmas is over—

The funny thing about me is this—that instead of being jealous of you, Barney, I am envious. I really have a terrific sense of sex. No man has ever appealed to me at all, really, since I have been married to you. But now that you are away the old game would be fun again. Some people can be most attractive. I am *envious* of you because you can play the game and I honestly can't. At least I think I can't. Don't forget what propinquity does—

Never think you made a mistake in writing me anything. To me this just makes you close to me. If I can't know something of your feelings and emotions you will have shut away a part of yourself from me and that I couldn't ever bear for a minute—Oh H. What I mean is that damn it I love you and want you and want to be with you. Loving you—and I don't want anyone else loving you when I can do it better than anyone else.—

In going through the files of World War II, I happened to come upon a misplaced letter from World War I, in which my mother told my father, using her nickname for him, how she felt when he was away in France. Following it is a letter to me in which a quarter of a century later, Jane expresses similar feelings.

Love Letters
from
Two Wars

May 22, 1918

Jerry Dear,
   Your wonderful letter from Paris has just come and I'm overwhelmed with a longing which seems impossible to again curb. These days of inhibition are simply stifling. As I look back I wonder how I have ever endured it and if I allow myself for one moment to more than live today I feel as if a flood, a torrent of something would burst its bonds and rend something asunder.
   "Packing up troubles in a kit bag" doesn't express it at all. It is simply a proud, grim carrying on—an endeavor to unsex oneself in the midst of a world drunk with the radiance of spring and when everything about one reeks with the great urge for Life—is mad with the mere joy of possessing his mate.
   Yesterday morning Elo called me to her room and there, on her very window sill, as if to taunt one, was a pair of doves. The children were elated. Poor unawakened things! I was cast into a tempest of unrest.

The letter ended, "With all I have—as you know, Grace."

Sunday, December 20, 1942

Darling Barney,
   It's the Sunday before Christmas. Ann and Joan have been little bright comets all morning. [Her letter went on for six pages telling of the children, our friends and the preparations for the day.]
   When I think of that period in our life, Barney—those fun days in Brooklyn, Oregon, San Francisco—it's like a dream. The thought of that big double bed and you close to me is like dreaming of heaven. And I knew it was heaven then, too. One thing I have never taken for granted was you. I have always thought and

felt at the time—this is the life—"Here is my heaven and now." Sometimes it makes me mad that you are so wonderful and that I love you so deeply because you make all other men seem rarely vivid. What I wouldn't give to run my hands through that woolly head of yours, and feel those strong shoulders against mine. That warm muscular weight of you—There is something so intrinsically powerful and masculine about you, Barney, that I can't resist you even in thought.

Oh Barney. Come home soon—
Barney—
Barney—
Jane

In contrast to the tender sentiments expressed by my mother and my wife are the cruder, but still strong feelings that I wrote of.

Dearest Jane,

This is Saturday. Last night was the big Army-Navy dance. Most of us took nurses—I had the one from my ward. She bears a superficial resemblance to a horse, but is a lot of fun. This party was a dandy. Our Mob 4 orchestra "The Robinettes" (Our skipper is Captain Robins) is excellent. I can hardly wait to get home and dance with you. I have gotten so that I really enjoy it now. . . .

I love you and miss you and love you more

Barney

The nurse that was assigned to my ward and whom I took to the dance was a marvelous nurse, a philosopher, and a good companion. But the winds of change were beginning to blow. I wrote to my mother:

New Zealand
January 5, 1943

Dearest Mother,

I feel so sorry for you, Mother dear, with the load that you are carrying these days and I know that my being away makes it that much harder. I just received your V mail letters through December 15th. This brings us through the time that you decided to take Dad home from the hospital.

I am completely in accord with that decision. If chemotherapy is not promptly effective, it is a waste of time to continue it. And it does make one feel so miserable when taking all of that stuff. If he can rest comfortably at home and have visitors and be happy, that is all that can be done.

And now, looking at the thing from another point of view, hasn't he had a marvelous life? He is nearly eighty; he has accomplished everything he ever set out to do; he has attained an unrivaled position in American surgery; he has satisfactorily completed and published his theories and his story of the life-long quest; he has had you, and he has seen his children grow up healthy and happy, and has seen four families of grandchildren come along. His life has been very full and complete. And the time was coming when, in the natural course of events, even if he had not had this illness, he would have had to give up more and more of his interests because of his physical disabilities and the handicap of his vision. I think that in some ways we can be grateful that his illness is not one such as cancer or angina pectoris, in which the end must come with pain.

And one bit of philosophy, Mother dear, that every doctor, and you too I believe know. When a person is really sick he is perfectly happy. People with strokes and paralysis do not suffer mentally or physically because of their inability to do the things they once did. People who are a little bit confused mentally, live in a dream world of their own—merging indistinguishably into delirium—and these patients remember nothing afterwards and are in a twilight sleep. Dad once said, "Old age is its own analgesia." So is severe illness. You need not worry over the outcome because these things take care of themselves. There will be no pain; and for that we may be grateful. And Dad is so wonderful as a patient and so sweet even when disoriented that I feel perfectly sure that he will be happy and content to be at home with you in the familiarity of his room.

The hardest thing about going away last June was saying good-bye to Dad. You and Jane and the rest of the family were young and strong and independent and I knew that no matter what happened you could all get along and that you would be waiting for me when I returned. I felt, and Dad felt, that we two would not meet again. We both were emotional and I have felt so since over the memories of that moment. I think that you know, in spite of our differences of opinion about certain things, that Dad and I have had a wonderful time together and that he has been my guiding star. His loyalty to me on certain occasions when I badly needed it, his idealism, and his ever present humor and virility have been the bastions of my career.

Your Christmas presents—more of them—cards and a chess game—came yesterday, Mother dear, and thank you again.

Love,
Barney

At about this time I heard from Frank Shively that our book on hospital care was coming out and wrote to thank him for all the work he had done editing and preparing the index. "As to the royalties, I always assumed we would share them 50–50. Don't be surprised at unfavorable criticism because the critics will probably all be from schools and their theories may not coincide with our rather practical attitude towards many things. I think the book will be OK for the average intern." This was my first written statement about what would become a more or less lifelong battle against the medical school establishment.

January 11, 1943

Dearest Jane,

The news of Dad's death reached me Saturday, following fast on the heel of Charley Hartsock's telegram telling of the hemiplegia—in fact when I left home I knew that in all probability I would never see him again. So in a sense it was a relief to know that he had been spared a long period of chronic invalidism and pain. Nevertheless, it is hard to think of home without The Chief—hard to think of making important decisions without talking them over with him—hard to realize that he won't be there when I return. But that will probably be only one of many profound changes in our own home life and in that of all Americans in the post-war period. We read this morning of a $100 billion budget for 1943! Things are bound to be different.

Perhaps things would be different at home, but in New Zealand they seemed to be about the same. In my next letter I said:

Practically no work to do—and we are still occupying our time with golf, tennis etc. Last Sunday Red Williams, Charley and I went fishing to a valley about 35 miles away. It was a beautiful drive through the Bush Country—wild and desolate. Huge banks of tree ferns, precipitous mountains and lovely valleys. The one we fished was about 15 miles long—access via a one-track road which ended blindly. There were only six farms in the whole valley and a lovely little stream about the size of the ones we fish in Pennsylvania, clear with rapids and pools running through it. The trout were all in the pools and we didn't even see one.

We broiled pork chops over a fire and watched a unique phenomenon—a Blue Moon—rise over the mountains. The moon was as blue as azure. I have never seen anything like it. None of us had ever seen such a thing. Once in a blue moon.

Time was hanging heavy on our hands. Some of our officers were being reassigned to hospitals up in the islands, closer to the front. An application was sent out for surgeons who were interested in taking a course in plastic surgery. There was a shortage of people competent to do the final repairs. I applied.

There were still enough patients with tropical diseases and convalescents requiring rehabilitation to keep the hospital fairly full, but there were very few who required surgery, and the life of the surgeons became progressively more boring. Even the skipper, Old Sea Hawk that he was, seemed to be undergoing a regressive sort of change. He built a private kitchen and dining room next to his quarters, and more or less withdrew from the rest of us.

For our depression, we had no psychiatrist to turn to and the Church had little to offer. About our religious officer I wrote, "He is the most narrow, intolerant, uneducated excuse for a prelate that the witch doctors of the Papuan Jungle could imagine. I am going to spend the rest of my life in the dedicated purpose of destroying the Catholic Church. That old bastard tried to make out that he is God's right hand man and the blood brother of Jesus Christ." In addition, we thought that the prelate's behavior in respect to both the use of liquor and women was something short of exemplary.

Jane, this is a hell of an existence. We are happy and gay and kid ourselves into no end of fun, and when it is over the whole world is empty and dead and futile, and you feel as if you were living in the upper reaches of the stratosphere where everything is either non-existent or the beginning of things to come or the end of things past. Atoms torn from life and carrying nothing but a faint perfume of the realities we once knew. Jane, do you know how empty a single bed can be?

In addition to the depression that came from having nothing to do there was the episodic sadness of having one after another of our good friends detached from the unit and sent away to sea duty on destroyers or up to the islands. There was one episode, however, that livened up this last part of my stay in New Zealand.

The most dramatic incident of the past week was the return of Jean's fiancé (the sole survivor of the nine New Zealand flyers who went to England). Russ Blood and I were down at the Milsons for Sunday night tea, and were going to take the girls (Jean and her sister) out to Artie Shaw's concert, leaving at 7:50. At 7:45 the phone rang and Ray (Jean's fiancé) announced that he was at the foot of the street and on his way out. The scene that ensued was comparable only to the evacuation of Dunkirk.

Blood, who is naturally very excitable, became panic-stricken, grabbed my hat and started running down the street. I stood my ground firmly, as the rear echelon, and began running around the house hiding all the American cigarettes, bottles and magazines in sight. Jean, her eyes as big as saucers and laughing and crying at once, tried to get Margaret, her mother, and herself all dressed at once. Poor old Auntie had gone out to church and was expected back any moment, and no one knew how she would be kept from making some kind of a break when she observed the sudden change of personnel. We all scurried out of the house like rats from a sinking ship. It was funny as hell, but apparently everything went along smoothly, as the two characters are very happy.

In September my orders came and I was delighted to find that, after a couple of weeks of leave in which I was free to go to Cleveland, I was assigned to study plastic surgery at the Mayo Clinic. I had faint hope of succeeding in these studies, but I was as happy as I could be to have the opportunity of spending a few months at Mayo.

In the last few weeks that we were in New Zealand, Bud Yandell wrote the music and I the words to a song called "Piha Bay" that expressed our feelings about the country and its people, some of the last lines going:

> The skies of New Zealand
> Will call us back to you
> With clouds on the hill tops
> Against the rain-washed blue
> We'll stand on the mountain
> To watch the Tasman Sea
> And dream for a moment
> Of the days that used to be

At the last Saturday night dance, our rendition of "Piha Bay" brought tears to the eyes of those of us who were leaving and a standing ovation from our New Zealand companions. Jean, by the way, with her fiancé's permission, was my companion at that last dance.

The trip home was uneventful. There was no further need to be tortured when the equator was passed. Jane met me in Chicago. To be with her again seemed to me to be perfectly unreal. She hadn't changed at all. I was head over heels in love with her, but I wasn't used to saying it or proving it. We went back to the hotel. After the long trip I felt dirty and wanted to take a bath. "Not yet," Jane whispered, and so the bath was slightly delayed.

It was incredibly good to be home, and then to see the children, one of whom I had not met before—Susie, rosy and chubby and sweet. Even Cynnie our dog, with whom we often had been moose hunting and duck hunting, welcomed me back. It was a glorious ten days. Then I left for Rochester, to be followed, as soon as I could make the arrangements, by Jane and the children, and our new helper, Barbara Thaine, an elderly Scotch lady who had supplanted Mary Margaret and would be with us for the rest of her days, an expert in the care of children.

10

The War Years

MAYO CLINIC

I HAD BEEN assigned to spend three months learning plastic surgery at the Mayo Clinic. Through friends in Rochester, we were able to rent an apartment big enough to take care of the six of us, including Barbara. Our stay in Rochester was like a second honeymoon. It was autumn and the ducks were flying. The pheasants were in the fields, the leaves were beginning to turn. We stayed in a simple apartment just a few blocks from the Clinic and spent our extra time out-of-doors.

We had many friends. There was Alice Mayo, wife of Chuck Mayo, the son of the founder. We had known Chuck and Alice through the Surgeons' Club. The Priestleys and the Grays also were in the Mayo Clinic and the Surgeons' Club. All the men were away at war, but their wives took us in like members of their families. Dr. Balfour was there—one of the senior members of the staff, for whom I had great admiration and who had been a great friend of my father. There was Dr. James Clagett, a general surgeon about my age, who was the best upper abdominal surgeon I'd ever seen. For a long time I thought he was just lucky because he never had a case that presented any difficulties. Finally, I discovered that Jim just made everything look easy.

One of my best friends, and Jane's and my favorite hunting companion, was Malcolm Dockerty, a young pathologist and a true master of that art. He not only had skill and learning but also a vast amount of originality and common sense. He had one of the world's greatest senses of humor and that made him the perfect companion on those autumn weekends in the fields and in the marshes. Autumn in Minnesota is a hunter's dream. Jane wrote her parents describing it:

> Mayo Clinic
> Rochester, Minnesota
> October 21, 1943
>
> Dearest Mother and Father,
>
> You will never know how wonderful this is for all of us to be together again. Everything is working out well here. The children are very happy and Barbara seems contented.
>
> Barney and I went pheasant and duck hunting for the weekend with two doctors. It was back at our old activities again. It makes the past year soon slip away into oblivion with all its emptiness and loneliness. We had a perfect time.
>
> We hunted on the nicest farmer's land you have ever seen. The farms out here are a beautiful sight to see. They are prosperous, well kept up, and with good equipment. This farmer had 6 or 700 acres—mostly corn—lots of pigs—cows—chickens and ducks. He was a philosopher, as all good farmers are, and interesting to hear. They certainly all feel that the Farm Problems aren't being solved by farmers. They invited us to spend the night and gave us their best sheets and beds, a wonderful breakfast and insisted on our coming back to lunch.
>
> We got up at 3:30 AM, then walked thru the corn fields and swamps until 6:15 PM at sundown. I am really a hunter at heart, because I am never ready to go home. We got our limits which is three cocks and a hen (pheasants) out here. Barney and I did a little duck shooting too in farmers' swamps and eked out 3 or 4 ducks—which we ate tonight with the children.

And that was the way it was as Jane and I suffered out the war in Minnesota.

There was also fishing, not too far away, in the shallow upper tributaries of the Mississippi. If there were parts of my life that I would like to relive, one of them would be that autumn with Jane and Dockerty and the ducks and the pheasants in the countryside of Rochester.

At the Mayo Clinic it soon became apparent to everyone that I would never be a plastic surgeon. After considerable consultation, and without a guilty conscience, I transferred my activities to watching, following, and learning from Claggett and Dockerty. I spent a full day five days a week doing this and I went to the staff meetings and I learned many lessons in almost every field except the one I came for. I learned, among other things, to marvel at the organization, the morale, and the all-around excellence of the Mayo Clinic.

This Clinic was the pattern on which the Cleveland Clinic was based, but it was at least three times as large and at that time it was much more highly specialized. It was in my three months there that I decided that if we, at the Cleveland Clinic, were going to be able to compete with the technical excellence of the Mayo, we would have to introduce many specialized surgical departments including plastic surgery, gynecology, thoracic surgery, vascular surgery, and colorectal surgery.

The organization of the Mayo Clinic was a thing beyond belief. Most of the patients were examined in the huge, relatively new Clinic building, and some in the older areas. The hospitals were scattered all around. How the surgeons managed to see new patients, follow them to their hospitals, operate on them, and give them postoperative care is still a mystery to me. Besides my memories of the superb organization and of the skills of the doctors, I remember also my visit to the history-filled board room and meeting halls where the pictures of the Mayo brothers were displayed along with many historical documents and instruments that brought back to me many memories of my father.

Long before I met Chuck Mayo, I had known the senior Mayos, because one of their daughters, Edith, had been a classmate of my sister Peg at Cleveland's Laurel School, and her father had visited her. I had also seen and heard the Mayos at meetings. Both were dominant personalities. Will seemed more reserved and intellectual—Charles was more tangible and humorous. They were a magnificent pair. They were models for what both brothers and founders of institutions should be.

Soon the three months were over and the hunting season too. Jane and I were ready to move on. As I boarded the plane I felt grateful to the surgeon general, to the Navy, and to the United States of America for granting me a three months' education leave at the Mayo Clinic.

11

The War Years

BONITA AND SAN DIEGO

A FTER TWO WEEKS' leave in Cleveland, I went to the United States Naval Hospital, San Diego. Jane and the children would follow, as soon as I could find a place for us to live. I had been assigned to the Plastic Surgery Department, headed by the famous Dr. Kirkham. Fortunately for everyone concerned, the department was fully staffed with well-qualified experts. The chief of the Surgical Division, Captain Pugh, who was a well trained and highly qualified general surgeon, knew of the Cleveland Clinic, recognized my name, and realized that I didn't belong in Plastic Surgery. He put me in charge of the seventy-five-bed acute surgical ward where all injuries, and acute abdominal diseases such as appendicitis, were treated. Every day six or more patients with acute abdominal pain were admitted to the hospital, and on the average three a day were operated on for acute appendicitis. Occasionally also there would be a perforated ulcer, intestinal obstruction, or an acutely inflamed gallbladder.

In San Diego there was plenty of work to keep a surgeon busy and interested. It wasn't at all like New Zealand. The Naval Hospital was built on 250 acres of land, much of it in adjacent Balboa Park. There were six units with 213 buildings, 11,000 beds and a staff of 3,500. An additional 3,000 corpsmen were in training. A new annex was under construction to furnish eight new wards for patients and barracks for the corpsmen. It took five butchers and six power saws to prepare the 100,000 pounds of meat that the population of the hospital ate every week.

Every type of activity was available on the compound from religious services to athletic events. There was organized basketball, boxing, baseball, bowling, golf, swimming, touch football, and beach parties. The hospital cared not only for the thousands of casualties transported from the war fronts in the Pacific, but also for the sick and injured from the huge Naval and Marine bases and camps in the San Diego area.

The commanding officer was Captain (soon to be Admiral) Willcuts—a dominant and decisive personality, who ruled the huge hospital with a wise head and an iron hand. His executive officer was Captain Jacobs, whose function it was to see that the skipper's orders were obeyed. Captain Willcutts was in command of what was then the world's largest hospital, but he had read of a hospital in some previous war that was a little larger. That was why most of our patients who had had any training as carpenters, plumbers, electricians, or masons were kept on the sick list and never were discharged to duty. They just lived on in the barracks in luxury (compared to sea duty) and worked away at enlarging the hospital. This growth was a sort of self-fulfilling prophecy, for the more patients the hospital treated, the more builders it was able to add to the staff that was constructing the additions.

By the time I arrived in San Diego, my book, *Hospital Care of the Surgical Patient*, had been favorably reviewed in the *Journal of the American Medical Association*, and was headed for its second edition. In addition, in March 1943, my article, written in New Zealand on Solomon Island casualties, had appeared in the *United States Naval Medical Bulletin*. It advocated conservative treatment of wounds with the use of antibiotics instead of extensive debridement and showed that there need be no hurry about removing bullets or shell fragments and that many of the smaller ones didn't need to be removed at all. Later I would publish a similar article in the April 1944 issue of *Archives of Surgery*. All of these publications on subjects that I really knew very little about, made me seem like such an authority that Captain Pugh, in spite of the fact that I was only a lieutenant, made me assistant to the chief of Surgery, a position that in some ways put me in charge of many surgeons who were commanders or lieutenant commanders.

When I first arrived in San Diego, I had been put up in the El Cortez Hotel with a roommate, whom I described, in a letter to Jane, as "having the build of Man Mountain Dean. He is the Standard Oil contact man for the west coast, has a trunk full of whiskey, an address book full of telephone numbers, a head full of ideas and an utter disregard of the laws of nature in respect to sleep. He weighs 250 pounds and takes vitamin pills for his arthritis which he has suffered from for 20 years—ever since his first case of gonorrhea." This relationship lasted for only two weeks, until I could find a place to live and arrange with Jane to move out.

Exactly how it happened I can't remember—probably just seeing an ad in the paper—but fortune was smiling the day that I drove south to Bonita, a tiny settlement about thirty minutes drive from the Naval Hospital and about seven miles from the Mexican border. Here lived Judge Robert Burch and his wife Bea. Next door to their house was an empty one that they would rent. All of this was in an orange grove at the foot of the mountains, and the houses were surrounded with olive and lemon and eucalyptus trees. In addition there was a barn and a pasture, and Judge Burch had gone to Yale and was my brother in Skull and Bones. The rent was a bit higher than we had anticipated, but the location was ideal for the family. The post office and general store were only a couple of hundred yards away, a neighbor with children of the same ages as ours lived about the same distance, there were no other houses in sight, and the school was only two miles away. I signed the papers and rejoiced. The whole family was elated when they saw where we would live. By this time Ann and Joan were of school age and Susie was two and talking. We became much attached to our neighbors, the Burches, and Bea was so fond of Jane that she kept a diary about her.

During the first few months, the hospital was very busy and my ward was full. We worked every day, all day, Monday through Friday, until three o'clock on Saturday, and on every third weekend I had "the duty." Jane wrote my mother that "our 'weekends in Mexico' have consisted of three three-hour trips to the beach over the border, which is seven miles from where we live. Barney has not got one hour off from the hospital since he came here." But there was no reason to go to the beach or anywhere. Our home was a complete change and a delight. There was rationing of meat and we had three hungry children to feed plus a pregnant-again mother and Barbara, who looked after the children. Jane and I became cordon bleu chefs.

In view of the meat shortage, and with our pasture and the barn, we decided to raise goats, sheep, and pigs. Jane had had some experience with animals on her family's country place, and I had had the Knob and a summer on my uncle's farm. Moreover, butchering came easily to a surgeon. We also raised ducks and geese and chickens, and the children gathered the eggs. When I would come home with a few people for dinner, it alarmed no one. We just wrung the necks of a couple more ducks and put them on the fire, for we cooked outside.

There were plenty of fresh vegetables in the market at the corner, and the grove was laden with oranges and avocadoes. All we needed was a cow, but Jane had never learned to milk. Instead we bought a little burro that we used as a pet and to carry milk and groceries from the market.

When autumn came, there was hunting. Work was through before five and there were quail in the fields and ducks in the ponds. Best of all, we were near the ocean, for as time went on and the hospital had more medical officers and not as many acutely ill patients, I could get away for weekends in Tijuana and on the beaches of Mexico. By then Jane and I, and the older girls too, had a new obsession. We had become skin divers and were learning to live on the octopi, lobsters, and fish that we speared.

It was no accident that we again took up diving. A little to the north was the Marine camp where Dr. Rupert Turnbull was on duty as a medical officer. I went up there to give a lecture, met Turnbull, learned of his interest in skin diving and told him of Jane's and my diving hood. Rupe introduced us to the face plates and rubber flippers that the West Coast divers had learned about from the Japanese pearl divers and which were widely used in Southern California and on the coast of Mexico's Baja Sur. We outfitted ourselves and were ready to go. At the time we never dreamed that this was the beginning of what would turn out to be almost a new career. It was one of the turning points of my life, because through my experience in writing about diving, I was to learn about writing books and articles for nonmedical readers. For this it is chiefly Dr. Turnbull who must take the blame.

Rupe was about thirty, a few years younger than I. He was tall, strikingly handsome, and married to a lovely lady, "Dougie," who once had been a Canadian and a nurse. Rupert was a Californian, born of a successful father whose hobby was the ocean and who owned and operated an enormous yacht. Rupe had been raised to the sea and to speedboat racing, and lately he had taken up diving.

The beaches of California were rocky and it was tricky to get through the surf and into the water. The water was cold, too—even in summer—but once in, if you had a face plate that allowed you to see, the bottom waved to you with sea fans and billowing kelp and there were schools of fish, big and little, to say nothing of the lobsters that wiggled their antennae at you and the abalones that clung so firmly to the rocks. That part of the Pacific was a cold but beautiful place to dive.

Both Jane and I were good swimmers, so it took little time to master the underwater techniques. Nevertheless Jane was once frightened by being swept by a surge into a dark and airless tunnel from which she had no way to escape except to wait for the returning surge to take her back. Ann and Joan soon learned to dive with us, and at low tide the family went octopus hunting on the rocks, feeling for their bodies with long bamboo wands. When the creatures were located, we would squirt a syringe-full of Clorox in the hole. The octopus, irritated by the chemical, would jet propel itself from the hole and we could spear it or net it before it could escape. Our fridge was soon filled with octopus, speared fish, abalones that we dived down for and pried off the rocks with tire irons, and lobsters that we collected by tickling their antennae until they came out of their holes far enough for us to spear them. It was a great adventure and it gave a rewarding menu.

We became lifelong friends with the Turnbulls and after the war Rupe would come to the Clinic for training in colorectal surgery and become one of the country's leading surgeons in that field. I always claimed that it was his technique of prying the abalones off the rocks that made him such a master of getting the cancers out of the pelvis.

We had many friends on the staff of the hospital and many others who came through San Diego and looked us up. Bud Yandell was one of these, and we nearly lost him when we took him abalone diving. He had never done any diving and was extremely thin. As a Texan, he was unused to cold water. He got so chilled that he became disoriented and started rowing his dinghy out to sea. We managed to get him ashore and up the cliffs and into a hot bath, where he made a speedy and complete recovery.

We had some marvelous trips to the Coronado Islands that lie off the coast of San Diego and Mexico. At that time, the Navy controlled the islands and forbade them to fishermen—except those of the Navy. From time to time, we would get one of the regular Navy officers to come with us for a fishing trip and in a Navy boat we would go out to "inspect" the islands. We "inspected" them under water too, and on one occasion I came home with an eleven-pound lobster as long as my arm. There were also many sea lions that we were swimming with and some of the world's most beautiful kelp groves replete with foot-long scarlet Garibaldi perch. The rocks were literally covered with eight- to ten-inch abalones, their shells like rainbows spun in silk. There were many octopi there too, and once we arrived home with a dozen for a feast.

As autumn came, we got to know the country around San Diego. South of the border, we found many places where duck hunting was good. With the supply of shotgun shells that we had brought from home and the box that we were eligible to buy every three months, for we were now ranchers, we kept ourselves well supplied with meat as well as seafood. Our life outside of work hours was a continuous holiday, and our meals, which we shared with many friends and cooked over charcoal in the patio, were a series of feasts.

To provide an adequate amount of the necessities, we purchased a pregnant pig named Bonita Houdini Crile—Bonita for the town, Houdini because she was an escape artist, and Crile because she was a member of the family. About six months before Jane herself was due, she wrote her parents about the delivery of the sow and an interesting local annual event:

> Box 184
> Bonita, California
> August 15, 1944

Dearest Mother and Father,

Many great events have taken place since I have written to you at length about us all. The greatest, of course, is the fact that we got so fascinated in the whole problem of reproduction that we became pretty involved in it ourselves.

The next and perhaps even, at that, the greatest was the arrival of ten baby pigs by our lovely Bonita Houdini Crile. She went into labor at five one evening and you have never heard such excitement in all your lives as then ensued. Ann and Joan were besides themselves. They could not possibly have seen a better delivery for their first. As I told you they come catapulting out like a Christmas package all wrapped up in cellophane. The old sow just would give a grunt and a push and out would fly another one. Even Susie stood by the fence with her curly head hanging over watching in complete absorption yelling; "See babies! See babies!" Ann and Joan brought their suppers out on a tray and ate while Bonita delivered! Neighboring children wandered over, other children were sent to bring them home for supper but they would get so interested they would stay too. We should have sold tickets. We will next time. If times get bad Barney thinks he will open up a night club and instead of a floor show he is going to have a sow deliver each night. There will be betting on the sex, the color, interval between births, and whether it will be a breach or a head first delivery. The children stayed on into the dark and even watched her eat her placenta by flash light. I must tell you what Ann said after that, "Mummie, did Gangie [Jane's mother] eat *her* placenta?" Nothing like a farm to learn the facts of life!

Another great sport we have indulged in is grunyion fishing. Did you ever do it, Father? The first time we went we had been at a dance at the Naval Hospital. We stopped by afterwards to have a drink with a doctor when someone said that the grunyion were running, at midnight. Until we actually got on the beach I thought it was some kind of a snipe hunt. When we got to the beach there were hundreds of fires with people all milling around them. At the stroke of twelve everyone moved en masse into the ocean in a sort of mass hysteria. Being swept along with the current we all went in too, and in varying and in an odd assortment of clothing. Barney had his blues on so he just took off his pants and went right in with his coat and hat still on. I just took off my best dress and went in in my slip. There were two Navy Captains along who left on their hats with all the gold braid. It was quite a sight. It seems that the grunyion, which are a fish resembling a smelt and somewhat larger than a sardine, come in on the seventh wave of the seventh high tide when the moon is in a certain phase and mate on the beach. They are protected to the extent that no one is allowed to use any net or tool to catch them. You grab for them by the light of a flash light when they swoop up on a high wave. It is very slippery and difficult, everyone dives for the same fish, and there is great excitement. Barney and I devised a new way to catch them. We jumped up and down as fast as we could and grabbed them between our toes when they swam up under our feet! It worked so well that we had every one along the beach jumping up and down like mad creatures.

My work at the hospital was interesting from several angles. I found myself assisting Captain Pugh when he had special operations to do and I grew to know and like him well. He was fully aware of his limitations in technical surgery and when a special problem turned up, he always turned it over to someone who was competent to deal with it. When distinguished visitors came to the hospital and were in need of recreation, they often were sent to Mexico or to the islands on hunting or fishing trips under my guidance and with Navy transport.

In addition to my increasing "social responsibilities," I was deeply involved in the study of acute appendicitis, which before this I had seen little of but which now came in at the rate of as much as ten cases a day. Moreover we were beginning to hear of patients being operated on for acute appendicitis when they were at sea, on small boats, with inadequate operating room facilities. There was even an example of a corpsman who tried to do an appendectomy in a submarine with no medical officer present.

Penicillin had just become available and was being used in small amounts—doses of 30,000 units every three or four hours. This worked miracles in the control of hemolytic streptococcal infections, but seemed little better than the sulfonamides in controlling the peritonitis that often came from appendicitis. I began to experiment with larger doses and found that 100,000 units given every two hours for two days usually had a dramatic effect in controlling the mixed infections of appendiceal peritonitis. Usually it subsided without forming an abscess or requiring emergency surgery. From the standpoint of the patients on naval vessels, where good facilities were not available, conservative treatment with massive doses of penicillin would be a great advance. I discussed it with Captain J. R. Fulton, who had just replaced Captain Pugh and whom I found to be just as intelligent and cooperative as the former chief. We decided that we would try treating patients who had appendicitis more than forty-eight hours with large doses of penicillin. It worked. The infection was always controlled. We were able to report in the *United States Naval Medical Bulletin* (September 1945) that more than 1,500 appendectomies had been done on enlisted personnel at the United States Naval Hospital, San Diego, with only one death, and that that one was not from peritonitis, but from an infected hematoma arising from the appendiceal artery. There were also a number of patients who were not seen until they had what appeared to be extensive peritonitis as a result of appendicitis and these were not operated on, but treated with massive doses of penicillin. Only one of these died, and that one died not of peritonitis but of a thrombosis of the mesenteric vein.

We concluded that the inflammation caused so much swelling of the appendiceal stump and surrounding cecum, that the swelling completely plugged the lumen of the appendix at the site of its attachment to the cecum. This resulted in a buildup of pressure in the pus that filled the lumen of the appendix, and that, in turn, resulted in the rupture of the appendix. The pus then escaped into and contaminated the peritoneal cavity, but the resulting peritonitis was bacterial, and hence controllable by antibiotics, for it was not the result of intestinal contents escaping into the cavity. "The question is raised whether in view of the efficacy of treatment with large doses of penicillin, the risk of appendectomy at sea on small ships is not greater than that of conservative therapy."

This message was repeated in a publication in *Archives of Surgery* and later in America's most distinguished surgical journal, *Surgery,*

Gynecology and Obstetrics. In the latter, fifty cases of peritonitis of appendiceal origin (so proven by appendectomy done after recovery) were reported. No such treatment or results had ever before been reported, but the surgical profession did not shout out its acclaim. For surgeons, appendectomy for acute appendicitis was almost a religious principle.

I had been reared in strong surgical traditions, at home, at Harvard, and at Barnes Hospital, and it was astonishing to me to discover that a policy as universally accepted as the necessity of appendectomy in the treatment of appendicitis might be wrong. I began to look about for other chinks in our profession's armor. One that I very soon found, had to do with pilonidal disease. Pilonidal means hair nest and these nests occur betwen the buttocks of hairy people, just above the coccyx. Sometimes they appear as cysts filled with pus and hair and sometimes as hair-and-pus-filled draining sinuses.

Long ago in England, pathologists had reported that these cysts and sinuses contained no hair follicles and that the hair that was found in them and that acted as a foreign body causing infection and irritation was the result of the ingrowth of normal hairs. These sought out and grew through the little dimple that many people have over the base of the spine where in the development of the fetus the epithelium curves in to make the nervous system. I wasn't aware of this at the time because my teachers and associates had mixed up in their minds the common pilonidal sinuses, resulting from ingrown hairs, with the rare congenital dermoid cysts that sometimes occur in the same area and contain hair, skin, hair follicles, and even teeth. (These are so rare that one is lucky to see one of them in a lifetime.) But almost all surgeons firmly believed, or at least operated as if they firmly believed, that the hair came from follicles in the cyst or sinus and that the lesion had to be widely excised like a cancer. As a result we had a whole ward full of patients who had been there for months with huge unhealed wounds that had resulted from the unnecessary radical treatment of pilonidal disease. Some of them had been in the hospital as long as a year, and they didn't seem unhappy about it because life in the San Diego Naval Hospital was a lot safer and more pleasant than in the islands of the South Pacific.

The strange thing about the unhealed pilonidals was that no one did anything about them. The pilonidal was caused by ingrown hairs and in order to get one you had to be hairy. This hair was shaved off at the time of the operation, but after that, no one bothered about shaving it or using a depilatory to keep it from growing back. These men had scraggly hair growing from their buttocks and rubbing the sores when they walked, thus destroying any newly formed skin. My attention was riveted to this problem when I encountered a Wave who had had three operations for persistent pilonidal disease and refused a fourth. I thought I'd try something so I put a mushroom catheter in her cyst, cut it off and secured it from falling in by putting a little safety pin through it. The patient had no discomfort and went about her work for a couple of months. The cavity filled in and the sides of the tract epithelized. When I removed the catheter, the tract simply closed over and was healed. "Why not do this always?" I wondered.

I asked the pathologists if they ever found hair follicles in the pilonidal tracts and they said rarely, if ever. I went to the literature and found the British account of the true nature of pilonidal disease. So I began to operate on the cysts by inserting a catheter (and I later used the same technique successfully in the treatment of abscesses of Bartholin's vaginal cysts). The pilonidal sinuses I treated by shaving the buttocks and painstakingly removing the hair with a crochet hook, which fitted nicely into the sinus and easily caught the hairs. Most of the sinuses could be cured in this way, if one kept the external hair shaven. The rest, too complicated for us to be able to reach all the hairs, were treated by simply opening them up, curetting them, and then allowing the skin to fall back in place. Nothing but the hairs was removed. If the hair was kept shaven the wounds healed promptly.

This experience, in which I found that the surgical profession had for so long done such absurdly large operations for simple ingrown hairs, combined with my knowledge that the profession had had no idea of the lack of significance of the rupture of an appendix, but had viewed it as being as dangerous as a perforation of the bowel, led me to have a profound distrust of any accepted surgical principle.

I would spend the rest of my career taking unpopular public positions, in which I consistently stood against many of the things that most surgeons believed. I was through with accepting as gospel what American surgeons taught, and I was ready to explore other branches of science that might be of use in my practice. I also wanted to see in other countries what other surgeons had discovered. I no longer felt that American surgeons, whether at Harvard Medical School or the Cleveland Clinic, had the answers to all questions. When I returned to Cleveland I would start on a different type of career.

The conservative treatment of appendicitis never did gain favor among surgeons, but in the May 1987 issue of the journal *Surgery* there would be an article by a Danish gastroenterologist that reported the successful "nonoperative management of the ultrasonically evaluated appendiceal mass." In his series there were no deaths.

While I was in San Diego, I published a paper in the *Journal of the American Medical Association* that described the forerunner of the modern ileostomy bags that in patients with intestinal openings protect the skin and collect the intestinal contents. The type of cement that binds rubber or plastic to the skin had become available, and we were using it to fix a protective covering over the skin of patients who had ileostomies. Before leaving the service, I also wrote and later published in the *United States Naval Medical Bulletin* a brief note entitled "Injection of Iodized Oil as an Aid to Closure of Draining Sinuses" (1946). This called attention to the fact that the oil used to visualize the sinus so that its extent could be seen on an X-ray often resulted in the permanent closure of that sinus.

The Naval Hospital was a great place in which to work. The morale was high, everyone cooperated, the leadership was superb. After Captain Fulton moved on, Howard Gray of the Mayo Clinic became chief of Surgery. No more able and amiable a chief could be imagined. "Howdy" was not only a superb general surgeon, but he was also a man of flawless character who was married to an equally able and attractive woman, Wint. We were old friends, dating from my initiation into the Surgeons' Club, so that to be together in San Diego was like a reunion. There was only one fault that I could find in Howdy Gray. He was just too honest. As chief of Surgery he had to turn in fitness reports on all those under him. If he allowed our friendship to alter his report, I probably would have been advanced to the rank of commander. Instead, when it came to the section on neatness and orderliness and whether or not the uniform was appropriate and well pressed, he gave me a less than perfect mark! Tragically soon after the end of the war, and when he was at the peak of his career, Howdy would be drowned in a boating accident.

As the war came to a close, there were fewer casualties, and by refusing to take my accumulated leave I was able to take weekends off to dive and hunt and explore the hinterlands of Mexico. Usually we took the older girls with us and left Susie with Barbara. It was a relaxed and happy life. The surgery was interesting. We had organized meetings, in which the doctors gave reports. One officer who was assigned to the sick officers quarters—a special unit where officers were hospitalized—read a paper in which he concluded that operations for gallbladder disease were more dangerous than the disease and shouldn't be done. He based this on the results in the last two years of a couple of dozen cholecystectomies that had been done on officers (mainly retired) and in which there had been several postoperative deaths and severe complications. This of course was not the fault of the operation, but of the surgeons who were performing it, because compared with the main hospital there was little surgery to be done on the officers and consequently the most competent surgeons were usually assigned to the areas in which most of the surgery was done.

On the other side of the ledger, it was at the Navy Hospital that I witnessed the very beginnings of vascular surgery. One of the surgeons had begun to repair injured blood vessels. By today's standards the technique was crude, but it was an exciting beginning.

One frightening incident occurred. A sailor had been hospitalized because of a hernia. Whether because of religious convictions or because he wanted an excuse to avoid being sent to sea duty, the sailor refused operation. This infuriated Captain Pugh, and he ordered that with or without consent the hernia was to be repaired. A group of sturdy Marines grabbed the struggling sailor and held him down while the anaesthetic was given. Captain Pugh then ordered me to have him operated on. I ordered my next in line to do so, and so on down to the most junior one, who had no choice. The command of the commanding officer must be executed and it was. But I am still glad that it wasn't I who had to do that operation.

It was the autumn of 1944 and my mother came from Cleveland and stayed with us for a few weeks. She of course had been reared to shoot ducks and ride horses, and there used to be cows on her father's pasture right in the middle of what is now the east side of Cleveland, so she felt perfectly at home and loved it. She wrote to Jane's mother about Christmas.

Dear Blanche,

It's Christmas Eve. The stockings are hung by the chimney with care in the hopes that St. Nicholas soon will be here. The children are tucked on the sofas in the living room. Nine stockings—lovely, decorated, red ones hang from the mantel. Why nine? Well they include Barbara and me and Jake, the dog, and White-foot, the cat, as well as the family. A glass of milk and two bananas are on the mantel for St. Nick.

I still remember how it happened that there was a glass of milk on the mantel. We had been talking about Santa Claus and we had asked Joan, who was seven, whether she believed in Santa Claus. "No," she replied, "I don't believe in him, but don't you think that just in case he is hungry we ought to leave him a glass of milk?"

Mother went on to tell how she had gone shooting with Jane and me, and how I had gone into the swamp up to my armpits to pick up a fallen duck. The letter ended, "There is something that gives one real confidence in life, even today, when problems bear everyone down, in the close companionship and understanding that Jane and Barney possess. One knows it will surmount everything and always be constructive."

Again, in another letter to Mrs. Halle, Mother said:

Here I am in Bonita, out under the olive trees, sitting on Jane's pretty brown furniture with the cushions, reminding me of the log-cabin patio at Halle Farm, and right ahead are the orange trees, quite golden with fruit, the big palms, the roses, the poinsettias, the beautiful symmetrical monkey tree. The skies are blue—not a cloud to be seen. The far away mountains are clearly outlined. The grass—in fact the whole world is green and refreshed from the short rains. Two dogs at my feet, three cats wander about. I can see the turkey strutting and hear the pig, the ducks and the chickens. Although they tell me that neighbors are tucked away in among the shadows of this hill, one is unconscious of them. It is as if all the world belonged to this House of Crile.

Later in a letter to my mother, Jane would tell of a party in our Bonita home:

There was a magnificent moon that arose behind San Miguel Mountains into a cloud-streaked sky. It was cold, but the fire was warm and Barney's drinks stimulating. After we had opened the last of the oysters and tossed away the last chicken bone, we went in for coffee and a long evening of the piano and singing. Both Rupe Turnbull and Dr. Young play the piano well and the singing was lusty. Even Susie awoke and said, "Daddy singing, Susie want to go down right now."

It was during the pleasant days at the Naval Hospital that George Crile III was born on March 5, 1944. "So far he looks as though he takes after Barney's musical and poetic side rather than his primitive and predatory side," Jane wrote her parents and enclosed a clip of the baby's hair. "A boy at last!" Needless to say, everyone was delighted.

After the baby came, there was much discussion about naming him. Everyone of course wanted to honor the departed George Crile, but I had experienced such confusion between George W. and George H. that I had had to go to Junior. I thought III might be confusing. Jane and I settled on Jerry, which was my mother's nickname for my father, but Mother said no—he should have a dignified name. So finally it was George III. That has been all right so far, except that George would in time become the Columbia Broadcasting System producer responsible for the Westmoreland documentary and the multimillion dollar lawsuit that followed, and by then he would have dropped the III. I, of course, would remain George Crile, Jr., obviously George Crile's son. When George would become famous and win the suit, I would be proud to have him as my father.

To celebrate the final naming of George III, Mother sent him a pin that long before my father had given her. With it was a note:

> Barney dear,
> It seems a long time ago that the Chief and I floated among fleur-de-lis at Winous dreaming dreams that have yielded many a milestone along the way, but none of them more important than you.

Mother went on to explain that the three petals of the fleur-de-lis represented the three Georges. She enclosed the letter that my father had written to her when he gave her the pin.

> Dearest Grace,
> I have always been proud of all of your accomplishments and deeply appreciative of what you have made these years mean to me, but greater than all else—earthly—our babies. To remind you in future of these golden days I have made from a design, which you will recognize as my own, a pin which I want to see you wearing during many many happy years. Always with fondest love
>
> George

The letter was dated November 3, 1907, the day I was born.

In that spring of 1945, the work at the hospital had fallen off a lot and many of the officers were being sent overseas to be closer to the activity. My orders came. However, the commanding officer was aware of my ongoing studies on penicillin in the treatment of appendicitis, for I had presented them at a staff meeting and he called Washington and had my orders changed. I stayed on as a lieutenant commander in charge of acute surgery and was surrounded by commanders and captains. We were overjoyed to be able to remain in San Diego, for the summer season of diving was coming up. The warm weather was marred by only one incident. Susie, who frequently supplemented her diet from the ground, was found to have worms— easily treated and cured of course, but nevertheless quite dramatic for a few days.

In August the war was over. Then that autumn, shortly before we would be returning to Cleveland, one of the brush fires, for which California is noted, started about a mile away from us. Swept our way by a strong wind, it burned everything in its path until it came almost to the pine grove on that side of our house. If it had hit the pines, the wooden house would have been gone too. We all stood by the road with shovels and what water we could carry and succeeded in keeping the fire from crossing. Why the Californians don't clear the areas around their houses of inflammable brush and trees, I have never understood.

Life was so pleasant in San Diego and Jane and I and the children enjoyed it so much that I was sorely tempted to go into private practice and not return to the Cleveland Clinic. However, my experiences in the treatment of appendicitis and pilonidal disease made me aware that there still were frontiers in surgery to be crossed and new territories to discover. I knew that I needed to be a part of a large institution, where I would be able to see many patients with the kind of problems I was interested in. At about this time I reread a letter written soon after my father's death, from Dr. Lower, cofounder of the Cleveland Clinic. Dr. Lower was my father's cousin, and I had always called him Uncle Ed. I realized, when I reread his letter, that I had no choice. My future, my opportunities to explore the fields that interested me, lay in Cleveland. In private practice I could never find the opportunities that the Clinic could give:

Dear Barney:

Your Dad and I discussed, up to the last time we had an interview, the question of the future of the Clinic and as we have felt for some years that it was time for us to withdraw from the executive side of the work, this was done and on January 1, 1943, Mr. Daoust took over as President of the Cleveland Clinic Foundation and Chief Executive Officer. He now has his office here and puts in full time. Mr. Grill has gone into the Army as a hospital administrator.

There is an Administrative Committee, composed of five Staff members, and they function as far as every care of the patient is concerned, while the financial and business side of the organization is in charge of an Executive Committee of the lay Board of Trustees, and your Uncle Hal Sherman is Chairman of the Board.

The Clinic is in good condition and when your father and I turned it over, it was free of debt and in good financial condition with the pension plan functioning and certain reserves for contingencies. We are extremely busy and very short of help. Today, on Monday, February 1, with a snowy, wintry day, we had between 140 and 150 registrations, 62% from out of town. It isn't necessary to put up any argument that the Clinic now is widely recognized, well equipped to help solve the problems of the sick and has gained the confidence of the public at large as at no other time in its history. We still believe that the end of its possibilities is far from being reached. However, we also recognize that we are going to go through a social and economic revolution after this war and just how it will influence the practice of medicine or the practice of anything, nobody knows. We have never tried to sell the Clinic to any of our professional staff (and I mean sell it figuratively) but we still believe it has great possibilities and opportunities.

We feel that the members of your Unit, with their age and energy and perspective, if they so desire, can play an important part in the future of this organization. Whether they will elect to come back and carry on the tradition is entirely up to them. Neither your Dad nor I felt that because of our relationship in this organization, it must necessarily follow that any of our family must carry on here if other places look better. On the contrary, I feel that with the new setup, the Clinic should run fairly and smoothly for all concerned, offering them wide opportunity for research and practice, and when their active career is ended perhaps place the Clinic on a higher pedestal than *we* were able to do. We cannot promise anything, as we never have, except the opportunity which it affords.

I have asked the members of the Surgical Divisions to be tolerant with me as it is the only place in which I have great interest and just how long I shall be hanging around here, I don't know. I want to help in every way I can and am working harder than I have for years, but only operating such cases as I feel sure I can do satisfactorily. The curtain is closing down on the Founders but going up for the new actors. Talk it over with Bill [Engle] and Ernstene [Carl, a cardiologist] and let me hear from you.

As ever,
W. E. Lower

12

The Postwar Years

THE CLEVELAND CLINIC

I T WAS GOOD to come back to Cleveland and to move back into our Kent Road house which, while we were in San Diego, we had rented. Everything was the same there, but at the Clinic there had been changes. Dr. Shively had stayed on and so had a couple of residents who were on the assistant staff in the General Surgery Department. Soon these departed and once again it was Dr. Jones, Dr. Dinsmore, and myself, with plenty of work for all of us. But times were changing.

During my stay at the Mayo Clinic and in San Diego, I had observed and been impressed with what specialization does to increase the technical excellence of surgery. At the time of my return the only surgical departments at the Clinic were General Surgery, Orthopedics, Neurological Surgery, Ear, Nose and Throat, and Ophthalmology. In addition our great pathologist, Dr. Graham, had retired. Through my contacts at Harvard, I was able to reach Dr. Beach Hazard, a young Harvard-trained pathologist who had not yet settled down after the war. We persuaded him to come to Cleveland, and he would turn out to be one of the greatest assets the Surgical Division ever had. He would coauthor, with me alone, at least a dozen papers, some of them highly original, like the one which gave the first clinicopathological description of medullary carcinoma, a rare but highly malignant cancer of the thyroid. Beach would stay with us until his retirement, and earn for himself the affection and respect of his colleagues.

At the end of the war, anaesthesiology was in a state of transition. In my father's days, specially trained nurses had given the anaesthetics.

Gradually physicians began to enter the field. At the same time, there were technical advances that made it more difficult to give anaesthetics. Reluctantly, we admitted that we needed physician anaesthetists and fortunately I had met some during the war. One was Dr. Donald Hale, who became the Clinic's first physician anaesthesiologist and began a training program for residents. By 1987, the Department of Anaesthesiology would have more physicians than any department in the Clinic and run smoothly. But there would be some exciting years during the period of transition, when the physicians were in charge without enough well trained ones to do the job properly. I know of at least one tragic accident that occurred in that period, as a result of residents, still in training, taking the place of skilled nurse anaesthetists.

Next Dr. Rupert Turnbull, the abalone diver from San Diego, came to us to take a general surgical residency. Dougie and Rupe and their small children would live in a house that Jane and I found for them not far from our country place at the Knob. It was marvelous to have our California friends in Cleveland. Turnbull was a brilliant resident. He was liked by all and then, when he had just been appointed to the assistant staff, it happened that Dr. Tom Jones, dressing for surgery, leaned over to tie his shoelace and fell forward, dead. He had ruptured an aneurysm of the heart's right ventricle. Rupert stayed on, was promoted to the staff, inherited Dr. Jones's colorectal patients, and in his first year, the small proportion of patients who died in the hospital after his operations was almost identical to that which had been attained by the departed master. Turnbull was a genius and would remain so until his retirement—back to California—at the age of sixty-five. Under his direction, colorectal surgery grew to what it is now—a four-man department—one of the first in the country and one of the best.

In 1955, in conjunction with Dr. E. R. Fisher, of our Pathology Department, Turnbull would demonstrate for the first time the presence of cancer cells in the blood draining from cancers. Their publication of this observation would not be the world's first, but their work would precede the other report and consist not of a case report but of a large series. Based on this, Turnbull would write several articles urging that surgeons refrain from handling the cancers they were removing until the blood vessels to the cancer had been tied—"The No-Touch Technique," he called it.

In 1950, I persuaded my colleagues that we needed to make gynecology a specialty department, and we found Dr. James Krieger in Ann Arbor at the University of Michigan. Krieger started the department, built it up skillfully, and led it until his retirement at the age of sixty-five. In spite of the national tendency to do more and more hysterectomies for any excuse, Krieger remained conservative and refused to remove all of the uterus just because the cervix had a little dysplasia or a localized carcinoma in situ that had not invaded the underlying tissues. Krieger only removed a cone of the cervical tissue. This was just as effective as hysterectomy, and now, in different forms, using cryosurgery to freeze the cervix or lasers to remove the cone, most gynecologists are following the lead of Drs. Tom Jones and Jim Krieger and are controlling the disease by local treatment.

In the same year, through friends of mine who had known him at Harvard and in Columbus, we located Dr. Stanley Hoerr and persuaded him to join us in general surgery. Dr. Hoerr had a special interest in surgery of the stomach, and would begin to lecture and write about gastric cancer and about the treatment of peptic ulcer. Dr. Hoerr was not only a competent clinician and a surgeon with flawless judgment, but he also was a person of complete integrity, a combination that resulted in his being elected, in the course of time, to be the head of the Division of Surgery. And while Stan would be elected to many offices in the local and national surgical societies, these were positions I was never considered for, perhaps because I always seemed to be in the minority in my views about controversial treatments.

It was becoming obvious that the Clinic needed a plastic surgeon. Dr. Dinsmore, who used to operate on harelips and do some plastic repairs, had now departed. I turned to my old friend Dr. Bill Byars, who was still on the plastic service at Barnes Hospital, and he recommended one of his residents, Dr. Robin Anderson. It couldn't have worked out better. Anderson was not only well trained but superbly skillful, sensible, and very attractive. Needless to say, his practice and the department grew rapidly and Andy obtained national recognition.

By 1955, the first publications on the results of vascular surgery were beginning to appear. I happened to be in England, where I had been invited to lecture before the Royal College of Surgeons, when I watched one of the English pioneers in vascular surgery use an artery from a bank of frozen arteries to splice into a badly damaged and almost occluded femoral artery. They had just begun this work and had no long-range follow-up. I thought it looked good and when I returned, I was able to persuade Dr. Dinsmore to send Dr. Al Humphries, a young orthopedic surgeon, to England to learn the art of grafting vessels. The reason I selected Humphries was that he was an orthopedist and if the graft failed he would be able to amputate the leg! Fortunately, my caution was ill conceived, for rarely was amputation necessary. Dr. Humphries was an innovator, who devised and carried out many complex vascular operations. He also was the first person I'd ever heard of who suggested the use of vein grafts to bridge the defects in the coronary arteries to the heart. This suggestion, which was made in writing at least five years before the first bypass graft was done, was contained in a letter to the Board of Governors, who disregarded it. When he retired, Al left a splendid three-man vascular surgery department.

The only other contribution that I made in bringing competent surgeons to the Clinic was in the case of Rene Favaloro, the cardiac surgeon who would do the world's first coronary bypass operation. Unfortunately, it was not done in 1962 when Dr. Al Humphries first suggested it, but six years later, prompted by a necessity that arose during an operation. The only credit I can take for Dr. Favaloro's success is that it was I, on a visit to Argentina, who met Rene and discussed with him the possibility of his coming to the Clinic for training in thoracic surgery. His request was turned down by the military-type physician who at that time was in charge of the Clinic's Department of Education and who had much to do with appointments to the residency program. However, I had been favorably impressed with Dr. Favaloro and recommended that he be accepted. Fortunately, my advice prevailed, and a few years later when Rene was on the staff he did his Historic First.

13

The Postwar Years

THE LIGHTER SIDE

A FTER THE WAR, things were a little different at home. It was 1945 and there were four children now, the two older ones eight and ten. Barbara Thaine had become a member of the family, caring for the younger ones. There was a cook too, who prepared everything and then went home for supper. We subdivided one of four big bedrooms to make a place for George III. We closed in a porch and made a playroom out of what had been the living room, a living room out of what had been the dining room and, with a little addition to the kitchen, we put in a dining space. Here there was a round table that seated up to twelve, with a lazy Susan in the center. All of this was ideal for conversation and discussion.

The Knob had changed a lot. Jack and Mary Bell, the Scotch couple who had cooked for my father and cared for the place, had long since left. The groom and the horses were gone. Jane and I had bought the house and stable and two hundred central acres of my bankrupt father's estate shortly after his death and while I was still in New Zealand. In the little house that the groom and his family had lived in, there was a new family—the Konicks—strong, ethnic people with several children and more to come. They stayed on the place free of charge and saw to it that vandals did not destroy the property.

Saturdays weren't true holidays because until noon there were meetings and teaching programs at the Clinic. We would go to the Knob every Saturday afternoon and come back Sunday. We didn't keep horses of our own, but close by there was a women's college with a riding program and dozens of horses. In exchange for the privilege of riding our trails, we were allowed, on weekends when the horses weren't being used, to ride them. That and the walks in the woods and through the caves of Little Mountain, with the children big and little leading or tagging along, made the weekends active and good fun. We had electricity at the Knob now, and a telephone. What more could we want?

There were many parties out there on Saturday nights. In California we had learned to cook over an open fire, and now there was no longer meat rationing and we would barbecue goats and sheep along with anything else, such as coons or groundhogs that we had caught, or even beef ribs—prosaic as that may sound. There was a keg of beer and plenty of songs, for in those days television hadn't yet robbed us of our ability to remember the words.

At least once every summer, Jane and I gave a huge party for all the general surgery-related specialties, including colorectal, gynecology, plastic, thoracic, and vascular. All the surgeons and their wives and all the residents and their wives would be there, and some of the older children too. In the afternoon we played baseball in the pasture, then we would go for a swim in the pond and all the while, the goats were roasting and someone was tending the fire. We did it all ourselves, without caterers. We had learned the art in California, and our Goat Roasts would become legend.

There were also parties held at the top of the Knob, that the Clinic gave for the entire staff—usually stag parties, for in those days there were no women doctors. These were clambakes and we'd have chicken and lobster, and as the Italian caterer used to say, "Plenty Clam. Plenty Clam!" Again it would end in unprintable stories and songs. In spite of the drinking and the problem of driving home afterwards, there were no bad accidents. One dark night, at the top, one of the guests stepped down or tumbled down the first drop, just before the thirty-foot-high cliff that overlooks distant Lake Erie, and was heard to say, "That's a big step." His next step was over the cliff and into a bushy treetop that broke his fall. On another occasion, one of the guests missed a bridge on a narrow road, and drove into a creek. Fortunately, he was driving slowly and was not injured. Gradually, it seemed wise not to hold these big beer parties because thruways had been built and it was too dangerous to drink and then drive on them. Moreover with the advent of television and the departure of Dr. Jones and some of our best singers and performers, and with the advent of women as members of the staff, the stag parties were replaced by such trivia as banquets and dances.

In 1947, two years after the end of the war and five after my father's death, Mother finished her book called *George Crile, an Autobiography,* with the subtitle, *Edited, with Sidelights by Grace Crile*. She put it together by using his papers, public and private, and adding her own opinions and observations. There was a foreword by her, a list of the twenty-four books he had written, copious wonderful photographs, and a sixteen-page index. Lippincott published it in a handsome, boxed, two-volume edition.

Mother managed to survive the surprise publication party, for which the family from all over the country had assembled. My sister Elo and her husband, Gus, and their children had flown in from Memphis, my father's brother Austin had come from Texas, my brother Bob and his wife Sally from Virginia. The party was complete with full evening dress and the American Beauty roses that had symbolized my parents' romance. There were speeches and of course, when it came to poems, I had to have my say.

For Gay—November 11, 1947

The threads of life are intertwined
And woven in its loom;
Some spring from our environment
And some stem from the womb.

Now Grace was born her Father's child,
A rugged hunter, he;
He killed three hundred ducks a day
And ate them all at tea.

The poem went on for a total of fifteen biographical verses including:

In heart of darkest Africa
She stands amidst the gorse
And aims her gun with steady eye
At a rhinoceros.

It was not long after the celebration of her book's publication that Mother died. She was seventy-two, and although she had had a dissecting aneurysm of the aorta (her brother died of a ruptured aneurysm) she had remained as sharp mentally as ever. Her death came as a result of Rocky Mountain spotted fever, contracted from an insect bite when she was visiting my brother Bob in Virginia. She had had a marvelous career for, in addition to working with my father and editing most of his books and innumerable scientific papers, she herself was the author of two books. My mother was one of the best organizers and most industrious and efficient women I have ever known.

14

The Search for Sunken Treasure

THOSE POSTWAR years were satisfying ones, not only because I was happy in my work, but also because Jane and the four children made it a delight to be home. We had the Knob for weekends and there was bass fishing in the local lakes and trout fishing in the Castalia stream and in the autumns we continued to go duck hunting. Often we took the older girls with us on those hunting trips west to the marshes near Port Clinton. Jane had become an excellent shot and even Ann and Joan were beginning, although not very effectively, to shoot clay pigeons. The children were developing well and doing well in school. We could have gone on forever like this, but then something happened that completely changed Jane's and my life. As a result she would start a new career and I would take on an additional one.

In 1948, we were vacationing in the Florida Keys, and there, on the Delta Shoal near Sombrero Light, we discovered the Ivory Wreck. It was filled with elephant tusks, coins and artifacts that dated from the seventeenth century. Overnight we became treasure-divers, underwater photographers, and writers.

The story had its beginnings on the West Coast when Rupe Turnbull taught us how to use face plates and flippers. The next year, we revisited San Diego with the older girls and tried to take some underwater motion pictures in the kelp beds, using a disastrously leaky plastic covering for the camera. The camera was destroyed, but the film of the scarlet Garibaldi and opal-eyed perch swimming through the waving fronds of kelp made us realize that there could be a future to this adventure.

Back in Cleveland, I came home from the Clinic one day, waving a rubber bag. It was a rebreather bag taken from an anesthetic machine. "This is what we've been looking for," I told Jane. We cut the end off it and put the camera inside. I had had a device made to close the open end and clamp it shut, and we mounted a glass window into the other end of the bag. The lens of the 16-mm Eastman Cine Kodak movie camera fitted it perfectly. We could wind the camera through the rubber, and with a 9.5-mm super-wide angle lens set at infinity, everything would be in focus within the thirty-foot range of underwater visibility. To smooth out the action, the camera would be set on slow motion, and we would be careful always to photograph with the surge of the waves so that motion would not make the background rush past, first one way and then the other. We measured the light by putting a standard light meter in a mason jar. The alternative to our pocketable device would have been to buy an awkward, one hundred-pound, five thousand dollar camera and tripod that we couldn't carry with us as we explored the reefs but had to set up in a fixed spot.

Our device worked perfectly. All we needed now was something to take a picture of and in the meantime, the children needed training in diving, and we needed to perfect our photographic techniques. One evening, we had a telephone call from a young man who introduced himself as Davie Dyche. He had heard that we were interested in underwater photography. Dave was a professional diver, and he wondered if we could get together sometime and talk. Our first conversation was recorded by Jane:

"How deep do you dive?" we asked him.

"Not very deep," he replied, "Never over two hundred and twenty feet."

This stopped the conversation dead in its tracks. We looked at Dave with awe and a little skepticism. Barney changed the subject to octopuses and, foot by foot, he stretched the diameter of our La Jolla octopuses to six or seven feet.

"Do you ever see any big octopuses down there?" I asked Dave.

"No," he replied, "No really big ones. I've never seen one over twenty or twenty-five feet."

Again Dave had the last word, but we were in the trap and had to go through with it.

"What do you do when you run into one of those?" we asked.

"There's nothing to it," he replied, "We have our heavy dress on, you know, and the octopus just wraps his arms four or five times around you and then he unwraps and goes away because he doesn't like the taste of the canvas."

We became fast friends and soon Davie was our diving companion. He had cruised the pirate haunts of the Caribbean with actor Errol Flynn, had dived on some ancient wrecks in the West Indies, and knew of the famous Spanish treasure fleet of thirteen galleons that in 1715 had gone down on the reefs near Florida's Key Largo and left sixty-five million dollars' worth of gold and silver on the bottom of the sea. Our next vacation would be as soon as we could arrange it, down in Florida. There Davie and Jane and I rented a boat at Key Largo. Enrico, the captain and owner, was the navigator. Davie had his Jackie Brown Diving Gear (a face plate with a rubber tube leading to an air compressor) and we had our homemade underwater camera gear. We were prepared to photograph the salvage of the gold and silver ingots.

In the water, we became absorbed in photographing the beauties of the reef and later, when we should have been heading back to Key Largo, we were examining and photographing an enormous anchor—ten feet long, corroded and nearly rusted away. Its hauser-end pointed seaward, so it was seaward that we swam—straight away from the setting sun, to search for the wreck. In 1945, no sensible person would ever have gone swimming on the Florida reefs where everyone knew the sharks and barracuda lay in wait. But in San Diego, we had learned that they do not molest a swimmer who minds his business and carries no fish.

Back on the boat, Enrico had been so intrigued with the novel diving apparatus and camera equipment and with the fact that these fools were swimming that he had forgotten about time. Suddenly he wailed, "Look, it's seven o'clock. Tavernier is the only harbor and it's thirty miles south. We can never get home!" Enrico was deadly serious, for he had just bought the boat, was not a navigator and had never been out at night. He sobbed in gratitude, when he found that Davie could read the maps and get us back. We could anchor for the night in Angel Fish Creek.

On the way there, Enrico turned the tiller over to Davie, while secretly he became a swiller on a bottle of rum. Once anchored, all of us went to sleep, Jane and I in the forward cabin. About midnight we were awakened by a shout, "Mama mia!"

Jane stepped out of the lower berth and found herself waist-deep in water. We were sinking by the bow. Captain Davie Dyche, as might be expected, took charge. "Bail," he commanded and threw us a couple of buckets. However, the water was coming in as fast as we could throw it out.

"Get me a potato," Davie called to Jane. Disbelievingly, she obeyed. Davie leaned over the stern and jammed the potato into the exhaust pipe, a connection of which had broken and allowed the water to pour into the boat. Later, when the story would be told as we became writers, the title of one chapter would be "Saved by a Potato."

Jane and I remained so obsessed with the beauties and excitement of the world beneath the sea that on our next vacation we decided to take the three girls with us to the Dry Tortugas, which we had visited before the war. Susie had just turned six and was a good swimmer. In Key West we rented a little boat, with a competent captain who brought us past the Marquesas Keys and Rebecca Shoals and to the southwestern tip of the Keys where the great Civil War fortress stands. We lived there for a week in the dungeons where Dr. Mudd, who treated the assassin of Lincoln, had been confined. The girls learned to dive among the branching corals and sea fans and to spear the groupers that inhabited the caves. Susie even rode on one of the great sea turtles that the shrimp fishermen caught and kept in the moat.

Then we returned to Key West and rented a car and drove down the overseas highway, built on the trestles of the now extinct railroad that Jane and I had taken to our honeymoon hotel in Marathon. That hotel was gone, but there was a new motel run by Bill Thompson. He was something of an adventurer and in his pleasure boat he often explored the reefs searching for wrecks. He said that once, on a reef near the Sombrero Lighthouse, he had found and raised an ancient cannon. It sounded promising to us, so we rented a boat and set off for the reef with Captain Parkhurst (Parky) at the wheel.

Bill Thompson, in his own boat, guided us to the area. On the way I had spotted a magnificent shallow coral bed I had wanted to photograph, but Bill didn't have time to wait. So on we went, until we came to the area on the outer reef where he had found the cannon. Bill left us then and we stayed on with Parky to search for the wreck. All five of us were in the water, floating with the tide on our life preservers or on air bags. We all were dressed in long black tights and long-sleeved, yellow cotton turtlenecks to protect us from coral scratches. On the rear end of our pants were sewn strips of white cloth made to look like malevolent faces that we hoped would frighten away the sharks and barracuda.

We swam for an hour over the deep, dull reef, while I kept thinking of the bright shallow coral bed we had passed on the way. It had seemed so promising for photography that we decided to return there, while the sun was high, and to continue our search for both treasure and beauty. We went overboard at the new location, known as Delta Shoal, and spread out, ten yards apart, to scan the bottom for wreckage or artifacts. As we were drifting with the tide there was, below us, a majestic vista. In the coral there was a canyon that led out to the open sea. A school of silver tarpon, almost invisible behind the mirror of their scales, drifted around us and then dissolved into the far blue reaches of the reef.

I was following and photographing a purple parrot fish when suddenly, as I dived down, I saw on the bottom of the white-sand channel, the straight line of a log or of a manmade object. Then I saw the telltale knob at the end of it. It was a cannon! My diary reads, "When Lord Carnarvon, digging in a valley of sand, found the sealed door to Tutankhamen's Tomb, he could have had no greater feeling of promise than did we as we looked down on the cannon, with its golden sea fan waving in the tide."

We set a buoy over the cannon and went back to Marathon for equipment to help us in digging and diving. There things were happening fast. A week before, a man named Halley Hamlin had raised a cannon just like ours from the same area. Also, Art McKee, famous for his retrieval of ingots of silver and for his Museum of Sunken Treasure, had just arrived in town. What we didn't know, but we were pretty sure of, was that he was after our wreck.

We made a deal with Hamlin that if he would take us to the wreck in his diving and salvage barge, we would split any salvage with him. And then, in order to beat McKee to the wreck, we had Parky hurry us back out there. I had no sooner jumped overboard than I saw something peculiar on the summit of the reef. Lying in water only about ten feet deep was an elephant's tusk, all overgrown with coral! I dived down and brought it up. It was three feet long, with a little square hole in the butt end.

No sooner had we brought up the tusk than Hamlin's barge arrived, and in it was Art McKee and his diving helmet and pump and a young man. Art was willing to work with us, Hamlin said, so he brought him along. We showed McKee the elephant tusk. "That makes two of them," Art said, and his young companion held up a similar one that a couple of weeks before he had found on the same reef. The coincidence that the two tusks had lain there for three hundred years and then had been discovered, each independently in the same week, was astonishing.

We decided to work together and share the spoils, so down went McKee and began to dig in the sand and to pick up objects from the bottom. There were musket barrels, bits of wood from the hull, riddled with worm holes. Some of them had live sea worms as big as snakes sticking out of them and wriggling. He uncovered brass cooking kettles, pewter cups and plates, brass pans, a clay pipe, and more elephant tusks—twelve of them. The tusks that were buried deep in the sand were the best preserved. The ship must have been carrying slaves and ivory from Africa, we decided, and we worked all day diving and bringing up relics. We photographed Susie coming up with a "scrivello," a baby's tusk.

For three days we dug through the remains of the Ivory Wreck, McKee sometimes staying down as long as seven-and-a-half hours at a time. Susie was our greatest worry. She had no fear of anything, least of all fish. The fifty-pound barracuda, larger than herself, which lurked below our boat made no impression on this little girl who, at the Tortugas, had swum with a three hundred-pound Jewfish and ridden a huge sea turtle.

We found bar shot, cannonballs, lead musket balls, and pewter spoons. There were samples of everything that the ship had borne— everything except the gold, silver, and jewels we were looking for. All was photographed with our now waterproof and efficient moving-picture camera. There was a winch on Hamlin's barge, so we were able to raise the cannon that had called our attention to the wreck. It was a Saker, seven and a half feet long and named for a ferocious variety of hawk. Although it was engraved with a provocative JN and the number 170 1/11 24, we were never able to identify the ship. Historically, it is recorded that the Africans who were taken to this country as slaves were forced to carry the ivory from the jungle to the ship, and then all were brought to America. Naturally, the finding of the wreck with its ivory and cannon and artifacts attracted much attention from the press, which gathered to report the salvage.

By now, Jane and I were confirmed treasure hunters. As soon as we could get away again, we organized an expedition and returned with better equipment and with our expert diver, Davie Dyche, to search for more wrecks. Bill Thompson, who had guided us to the area of the Ivory Wreck, said he knew of a cannon at Looe Key, which once was an island but now was just a shallow reef. Jim Rand, the inventor, and his wife Mary had come along with us from Cleveland. We were all scanning the bottom in the area that Thompson had indicated when Jim called from the shoreward side of the reef, "Look below you!" We swam to him and saw that the bottom was covered with oblong bars— heaps and piles of them tumbled and strewn as far as we could see. The channel also was filled with cannons and there was a huge anchor, half of it overgrown by the coral. We tried to move the bars but couldn't budge them.

Davie came up from a tour of the bottom. "Look what I found," he shouted and showed us a handful of coins and metal buttons. "I just scooped them up from the sand—right out of a drowned sailor's pocket." One of the coins looked like gold and was dated 1720. We turned our attention to the metal ingots. The bars were so heavy that we couldn't lift them. If they were made of gold or silver, they were worth a king's ransom. We tried to chip or saw off a piece, but they were covered with chips of flint, probably part of the cargo, and the chips were bound together by coral. "We've got to go home," Thompson said. "It's getting dark, and the wind is rising." Reluctantly we obeyed.

The next day was Friday, the thirteenth. We left for the wreck early, before the weather reports. By the time we reached Looe Key there were ominous clouds over the sea. It was windy, and the waves were breaking high over the reef. On my first dive at the site, I found a circular copper ring that was a barrel hoop. "Perhaps the barrel was filled with gold coins," I thought. Then as I started to swim back to the barge, I noticed that it had slipped anchor and was adrift. Hamlin had been in the engine room, repairing the motor. We yelled to him and he came up, saw what had happened and threw out a reserve anchor. The rope of the other anchor had been sawed in two by the coral.

Hamlin had an hour of repair work to do before the engine could be started. In the meantime, the wind and waves were rising. It was the start of the 1950 hurricane that would do millions of dollars' worth of damage to Miami. In the distance there was a speck on the horizon. It was Bill Thompson who, after hearing the weather prediction, had come to warn us of the approaching hurricane. He stood by until the motor was repaired. Then we all returned, Thompson's Chris Craft nearly swamping in the mammoth waves. That was the end of that year's adventure.

The next season, with a huge band of friends who had become fascinated with the moving pictures of our previous expeditions, we went to the Keys again. This time Ed and Marion Link joined the expedition. They had been sailing the Keys in their sporty sailboat and had heard about us from Bill Thompson. Ed was the inventor of the Link Trainer for airplane pilots and was a daring adventurer on land, air, and sea. Marion was a writer, and a suitable shipmate for Ed. They became Jane's and my lifelong friends both above and below the water.

To shorten a long tale, we raised one of the Looe Key ingots and found it was made of iron. We also raised and identified a cannon. It was from the HMS *Looe*, from which the Key had gotten its name, which had been wrecked off Florida in 1744. Mendel Peterson, naval curator of the Smithsonian, was with us, and this time the salvage, cleansing, and organization of the artifacts was done in a more scientific manner. We found hundreds and many are still on display at the Smithsonian, but no more coins and no gold. It looked as if we would have to find some indirect way of prospering from our treasure hunts.

15

From Sea to Screen

OUR NEXT undersea adventure was with Ed and Marion Link, who as a result of their experience with us on the Ivory Wreck had switched their interest from sailing to treasure diving. Ed bought a ninety-foot shrimp boat and converted it, so that it had comfortable staterooms. All of its shrimp-lifting equipment was now available to haul up what gold or silver we might find. Link, who of course was a superb aviator, navigator, and seaman, needed no professional sailor to run his boat. He did all that himself—the mechanical genius who had invented the Link Trainer needed no help in the engine room. Marion, too, was better in the kitchen than any professional chef. The crew consisted of Vidal, their French Canadian guide who had never before been at sea, and Kemp, a Bahamian who couldn't start a motor but could read the bottom through fifty feet of water.

Jane and I met the Links in Cap Hatien, where before setting off for treasure-laden Silver Shoals, we climbed to the top of the ruins of King Christophe's mile-high citadel and looked out across the mountains to the blue stretches of the Caribbean. Then we set sail across the oily reaches of the weed-strewn Sargasso Sea. We were searching for the wreck of the *Golden Lion*, a Spanish galleon that had sunk centuries ago and in 1686 had been partially salvaged by William Phipps, who recovered 170 of her 300 tons of silver. The rest of her treasure still remained on the bottom. The silver had come from Peru's Petosi mines, a vein 300 feet long and thirteen broad "with a great outcrop above the ground, the height of a lance—half silver and in part all silver with flukes projecting out from the level of the hill."

The sea was smooth, the wind was hushed as we sailed out to the reef where the ship was said to lie. We were out of sight of land, and the flat and quiet sea looked lovely—too lovely—perhaps ominously lovely. From the crow's nest in the mast, I spotted spouts of white water, like those made by whales. Then we could see the coral of Silver Shoals—flat-topped towers of it rising from what our fathometer said was the ninety-feet-deep channel, right up to the surface. When the ocean swells encountered these walls of coral, they produced the spouts I had seen and that Phipps had called "The Boilers." Some of them, even on this calm day, sprayed water up twenty feet high. I asked Kemp what Silver Shoals would be like in a storm. "We'd better not be here," he replied.

At the periphery of the shoals the water fell off to the unfathomable depths of the ocean where there was no bottom to anchor to. We had to set our anchor in the channel and hold the vessel with an anchor at the stern too. This we did, and within a hundred yards of a piece of coral that was protruding three or four feet from the water. Phipps had described a similar protrusion and had called it "the dry rock." We all went overboard into the clearest water we had ever seen. Visibility was up to two hundred feet. Near the surface, the craggy vertical walls of the coral banks mushroomed out in response to light and edible plankton. We hung onto the overhanging edges and looked down, dazzled by the sunlight on the purple and gold coral and by the myriad of tiny fish which were as bright as the corals. Over the bank a six-foot barracuda hung like a torpedo, ready to strike.

Below us we began to see the coral-encrusted granite stones that had been the ballast of the ship. Then Link found a huge anchor and, scattered in the ballast, a few silver coins, now changed to black masses of silver salts. There were musket barrels and broken bottles, but no pattern of a shipwreck and no bars of silver or gold. We found what we thought might be "ye bellie of ye ship" and Link set a dynamite charge in it. We got out of the water and set off the charge. There was a bump and a cloud of yellowish smoke and then a few fish floating belly up. We had blown a six-foot hole in the reef and that led into a cave, but it was empty—no artifacts—no treasure.

We spent seven days on Silver Shoals—and seven black, mysterious nights, as the reefs groaned and threw up their threatening "boilers." Every night it blew a gale that threatened to break loose our anchorage. Every day we searched and found nothing but a few coral-coated artifacts. We were uneasy and we were out of reach of the radioed weather reports.

Jane and I remembered the time, in another trip in the Caribbean, when we had been on the Great Bahama Banks with the Links looking for wrecks. They had left Jane and me in a dinghy with an outboard to explore the endless expanse of coral. There was no land within a hundred miles of us and yet no water more than eight feet deep. As we had searched the banks suddenly we had found a cannon, then a dozen of them. We had gone overboard to examine our find. Jane had thought I had hold of the rope to the boat, and I had thought she did. We had been so fascinated that we didn't look up. When we did, the boat was almost on the horizon. Although Ed had known where we were, two heads floating on a life preserver in the vast expanse of ocean would have been hard to find. Luckily, the drift of the boat had been from the current, and we were able to use the same current to catch it. If the drift had been from the wind, we never could have swum it down.

After seven days all of us had had enough of Silver Shoals. None of us mentioned it aloud, but finally Jane and Marion got together and each found that the other was nervous. Then Ed and I talked it over and with the crew too, and found that every one of us was afraid. "We are in a hurricane nest," Kemp said. "Let's get out of here," Vidal suggested. And we were on our way back.

The pictures that Jane and I took in the crystal clear water of Silver Shoals were magnificent and coupled with the movies that we had made on the summit of the Citadel, where the cannons of King Christophe still lay rusting, we had some marvelous sequences. We also were able to fit in scenes from the Ivory Wreck and elsewhere and make a ninety-minute documentary, so good that in 1953 the National Geographic would ask us to show it at one of their public meetings in Washington. Jane narrated the first reel and I the second. The house was filled and we were happy. At about that same time, we had been in contact with John Craig, a California producer who bought rights to several of our films and later would show them on the national television program "Kingdom of the Sea."

When we were first beginning to put together our films, I had had a patient who was a film producer from Hollywood. I had asked him to dinner and to look at our films. "Cut them," he had said, "cut them. When you've said it, you've said it. Don't repeat." It is a temptation, when you have a good, steady clear shot of something, to show it, even if it's all been shown before. We corrected our ways, and our films improved. At that time, both Jane and I could hold our breath for nearly a minute, and at slow motion this meant a minute and a half of showing time. We could catch plenty of action by diving freely with our hand-held camera—much more than could those who had to set up a tripod and wait for something to happen.

Bill Finn ran a travel agency and a lecture program at the Masonic Hall in downtown Cleveland. The auditorium was huge—holding perhaps two thousand people, and Bill had had such noted travelers as Lowell Thomas, Sr. and Jr., and many others who lectured and put on slides or movies there. We became one of these, and with the aid of friendly critics and a helpful press, we sold the place out, the proceeds going to the Museum of Natural History of which I was a trustee. This was long before competition from television destroyed the travelogue business, and it was before Cousteau had begun to show his professional pictures made on the bottom of the sea.

Jane and I had great fun making and narrating our films. Together we cut and spliced them. She was more dextrous at the splices and I was more brave with the scissors. We would time each segment and then write the script so that there was a perfectly timed narrative that either Jane or I could read. I was at the peak of my surgical career and turned most of the lecture business over to Jane. She did it splendidly, in her strong contralto voice, and you can be sure that she held her audience.

Our movies were becoming famous, even internationally, and the exclusive English surgeons' organization, the Hunterian Society, asked me to show the film. We did so, and it was well received. On the same trip, I gave the Moynihan Lecture at a meeting of the Royal College of Surgeons, which included my friends Reginald Murley and Arthur Porritt, both of whom had been among the first in England to reject radical mastectomy. Arthur by now had been knighted and became Sir Arthur and soon would be president of the Royal College. Later Reggie, too, would hold that office.

We had a good week in London, visited the various clinics and learned a lot about surgery, for the British surgeons were not only highly trained and experienced, but also very specialized. My trip to London was well worthwhile, particularly in seeing novel approaches to the treatment of cancers of the stomach and of vascular disease of the extremities, and for the first time to see other surgeons who thought that it was not an immoral act to treat cancer of the breast by anything less than a radical mastectomy.

In England, we met producers of motion pictures and were overjoyed when one of them contracted with us to make a regular 35-mm film out of our 16-mm and pay us royalties on the receipts. We were so happy that we went out and spent much money on a banquet to celebrate with all of our friends. The next day the movie man called and apologized, saying he had not been fully authorized to make the deal, but they did want to use the pictures on the British Broadcasting Company's show. That deal went through, and I'm glad to say that we got back the money that we'd spent on the banquet and a little more.

Jane continued to be a hit in the world of entertainment, and we continued to travel and dive and make movies both above and below the water. On the advice of Phillipe Diole, the French archaeologist, explorer, and author, we took all four children on a kayak trip down southern France's River Tarn. "It is fourmillant de rapides," Diole had said.

Our trip down the Tarn was for travel what my mother and father had said about their relationship with their children. "This is the peak of our life with the children," Mother had written in describing an evening spent in reading aloud before the fire. Similarly, for Jane and me, the trip down the white water of the Tarn represented the peak of our travels with the family. George was then seven. Ann was seventeen, Joan fifteen and Susie ten. We were all together and not yet torn apart by budding adolescence.

We bought our kayaks in Lyons, the chief city of South Central France, and we prepared to go southwest towards the sea. The canvas kayaks were feather-light and equipped with long double-bladed paddles with which we could paddle alternately on either side. It was early summer, the floods were just over, the water was clear, the air was warm, we all were happy. We had a rented car in which we kept our baggage and then, after each day, when we had stopped for the night, I would take the bus back and pick up the car. By the time the rest were settled, I would be back with the baggage.

It was lucky that we left our baggage in the car, because the stream was about twenty yards across and sometimes quite deep. It was white water almost all of the ninety miles of our descent. The children, who were inexperienced in rapids except for a very short adventure on a Canadian river near Lake Timagami, capsized two or three times. All were expert swimmers by now, so we had no worries on that score. It was a great experience to whiz down that river, as the beautiful countryside of southern France passed by. My memory is of cattle, fat pigs, orchards and vineyards, stone houses, men in boats that were filled with ripe red cherries, and towering cliffs, with miniwaterfalls gushing from springs in their sides. These were the gorges of the Tarn. Further downstream the land was flat and there were plowed fields with the green shoots of starting grain. Trout scooted away from our kayaks as we traversed the pools, and now and then there was a fisherman on the bank.

There were three kayaks for the six of us and Joan's friend Peggy French. Each of the older Crile girls had a kayak, and Susie and George were with Ann. But they kept getting into so much trouble that we made Ann's kayak lighter by switching George to ours. By this time we'd twice had to patch the bottom of Ann's.

One night we spent in a walled castle, with moat and drawbridge, which now was an inn. We were the only guests. The landlord told us that it had been built by a noble to protect the virtue of his seven beautiful daughters, known as the "Seven Nymphs of the Tarn." In spite of the baron's efforts, nature prevailed and all seven of the daughters ultimately were borne off by lovers. After supper that night, we all sang the French song that the landlord taught us, called "Chevaliers de la Table Ronde":

> *Chevaliers de la table ronde,*
> *Goutons voir si le vin est bon,*
> *Goutons voir, oui, oui, oui,*
> *Goutons voir, non, non, non!*

I was grateful to my parents for their foresight, when I was six years old, in having Madame Klein spend that time speaking French with me.

There were many villages along the banks of the Tarn and we had no problem finding lodgings. Most of our lunches we would take along with us, picnic style, sometimes making a fire and cooking baby goat or trout before paddling on down the stream. All of this we kept photographing on our 16-mm color film, including a Saints' Day Parade in the Village of la Malene, complete with crosses and costumes, and later a series of famous rapids that had been given the names of "The Pass of the Wolf," "Le Petit Pas de Souci," and "Les Rapides de la Chanterelle," with imagery of singing water. We ended this trip at the industrial town of Millau, where we sold two of our kayaks and arranged to have one shipped home.

We then drove over the Pyrenees to Portugal. We had heard about Nazaré, on Portugal's Atlantic coast, from a friend who was a writer and photographer, and said that the beauty and variety of the beach was unique. We drove south along the coast and visited Fatima, the Christian Mecca that, if not the most popular, was certainly the most spectacular of all Christian shrines. Then we came to Nazaré, where we stayed at a hotel on the beach, on which hundreds of fishing boats were pulled up. The open boats were about thirty feet long and each held about twenty men. Some had just come in and were being pulled up from the breaking waves by teams of magnificent bullocks.

Fish nets were set right off the beach, and hundreds of fishermen and their wives and companions all pulled on the ropes to draw in the seemingly mile-long nets that contained tons of flopping fish. The men were dressed in Scotch plaid, a tradition that had started a century or so before, when a cloth-laden British ship sank off the coast of Portugal. The women were beautiful, and posed for our camera like professionals. We helped them draw in the nets, and sang with them as they pulled, and Jane and I drank with them in the evenings.

In addition to our films on the Tarn and Nazaré and treasure diving, we had a spectacular hour-long movie that Jane and I had shot in Corsica. Its title was "Bandits, Boars and Breakfast," and it showed a chance encounter that we had in a bar with one of the country's reformed bandits who spent his time between running a saloon and hunting wild boars. He and his companions allowed us to photograph the early morning hunt in the Corsican Macquis, and to share in the toasts and the ample outdoor brunch that later was cooked and served by a couple of stalwart Corsican women. I still view that film with delight.

16

The Start of a New Career

I N THE MEANTIME, I was beginning to write about cancers of the thyroid and breast and to take a controversial position in support of conservative operations. Although at that point few agreed with me, most of the surgeons were interested in listening, with the result that I was lecturing more and more all over the country and abroad too. On top of all this, an event occurred that practically forced Jane and me into writing a book. I met a famous writer. My reputation in the field of breast cancer had become established to the extent that when Rachel Carson, author of *Silent Spring,* had an incurable recurrence of her cancer, she came to see me. I gave her what turned out to be not lifesaving but comfort-sustaining advice, and we became friends. It was Rachel Carson who introduced us to her literary agent, Marie Rodell, with whom Jane and I would work for many years.

After those first experiences in the Ivory Wreck, Jane and I kept trying to write up our underwater adventures. Jane had majored in English at Smith, and I had done the same at Yale. I also had written two medical books and 135 medical papers. In spite of our background, neither of us had the slightest idea of how to go about writing a book. Jane tried a chapter and I didn't like it. I tried a chapter and she didn't like it. If we tried to work together, we just spent our time in arguing about how it should be done. We gave up and went back to school.

A college education may be a great asset in some fields, but I don't think it teaches anyone how to write. Jane's teacher at Smith had been a noted writer and scholar, Mary Ellen Chase. I had, among others, the famous Billy Phelps, as well as a course called Daily Themes, in which I had to write an essay every day. These were graded by graduate students, and the spelling was corrected, but no one ever told me what was wrong with the writing. Moreover there was nothing I could learn from reading Shakespeare or the poems of Keats that would help me much in describing the coral reefs. We decided to try something different. We went to Cleveland State University's night school and took a course in journalism.

The professor was very different from our teachers in college. He was not a degreed teacher, but a professional journalist who wrote for the *Cleveland Plain Dealer*. He told us to write what would be interesting, and advised us not to use complex words when simple ones would do. "Facts, facts, facts," he said. "Gather all the interesting facts that you can and work them all in. People like to read facts." He went on to say that anything to do with sex would always stimulate interest, also of course tension or humor, but mainly "work in the facts—history and geography and anecdotes too. Build your book on facts."

Soon our teacher became our friend. After attending four or five lectures, we met with him and arranged for him to give us private tutoring. We would write up a story and send it to him, then he'd come by our house in the evening, and he would go through it and make suggestions about what we had written, and then we'd all celebrate with a drink. It was about this time that Rachel Carson introduced us to Marie Rodell. We at once sent the first four chapters of *Treasure Diving Holidays* and a summary of the prospective ones to Marie Rodell. Then we held our breath in fear and anticipation. Two days later we received a telegram, "Don't eat, don't sleep, just keep writing. I think we have a book." Needless to say, we went about our work with renewed vigor.

After telling about our learning to dive in San Diego and our adventures in the Bahamas with Captain Joe and the natives, some of whom had never before seen white people, we went on to the accounts of the Ivory Wreck and Looe Key salvage in 1948, then to Corsica, in the Mediterranean, and the Isle of Lavezzi, off whose shores we had found a host of artifacts from an ancient shipwreck. The final chapter was Andros Island revisited, with all the children, including George, now competent divers.

The book would be published in 1954 by Viking and go through four printings. The dedication was:

> To Ann, Joan, Susie and George
> "Come, dear children, let us away;
> Down and away below."
> Matthew Arnold
> "The Forsaken Merman"

Treasure Diving Holidays would be simultaneously published in England by Collins with the subtitle *"The Adventures of a Family under the Sea"* and with line-drawn papers and with the illustrations in color. The book would hit the *New York Herald Tribune's* bestseller list and be translated into Russian, German, and French and be reproduced in condensed form in books and magazines. That is why there was no longer any question about the diagnosis—Jane and I had been bitten by the bug. We would never be able to stop writing. We had a new career.

It was at this time that my ideas about the value of conservative operations in the treatment of breast and thyroid cancers were beginning to crystallize and I was seeing some of the unnecessarily mutilating results of the surgery being done at some of the so-called cancer centers. Opposed to my views were most of the surgeons in the "Cancer Centers" and in the medical schools. The fight was a bitter one, because almost all of my opponents practiced fee for service surgery, in which larger fees were paid for larger and more mutilating operations.

I was in the swing of writing and so I swung on, with Jane's editorial help, into another book. This would be *Cancer and Common Sense*, written not for physicians, but for lay people. It would be published in 1955 and be termed by some critics "Crile's Bombshell," one review beginning, "Violent national controversy on current attitudes toward cancer by the medical profession and laymen has been touched off by Dr. George Crile, Jr."

Cancer and Common Sense was released in the first week of November by Viking Press, but just before then the issue of *LIFE* of October 31 carried the byline on its cover, "A SURGEON DEPLORES BLIND FEAR OF CANCER." The six-page spread inside was a condensation of the book, as well as containing "A Statement Disagreeing with Dr. Crile" in which it was said that my "thesis is contrary to the teaching of the country's 81 medical schools and to the experience of physicians and surgeons." Other "medical authorities" gave their views too.

The book would be printed in England in 1957 by Clarke, Doble & Brenon Ltd. It would be translated into Japanese and other foreign languages. I was delighted to have both the fame and the notoriety and for the next ten years would be kept so busy by my growing practice, the greatly increased requests for participation in medical meetings, and the debates about the treatment of cancer that it would be ten years before I would write another full-length book. In the meantime Jane's and my pleasure in our growing interest in traveling and making and showing moving pictures continued. By now she was a sought-after professional lecturer, using both her slides and our movies.

17

The Postwar Years

THE MEDICAL SIDE

IN GOING through my papers of the postwar period, I came upon the following note, written in my handwriting, *"What is Genius? A genius does not produce a new idea out of the void. A genius is a person who is aware of modern science and technology and whose mind has not been forced into conventional channels by an excess of education. A genius takes someone else's idea, modifies it to make it practicable, and then uses it for a new development."*

I never came near to being a genius, but I did adapt a lot of ideas to useful purposes. I had inherited an interest in diseases of the thyroid gland and had early acquired considerable experience in treating them, but before the war I had believed what I had been taught and I had viewed the diagnosis and treatment of these diseases in the conventional manner. My experience with the treatment of appendicitis and pilonidal disease, however, had made me aware of the fact that what was taught was not always right. I began to look at thyroid disease in a new light.

Between 1935 and my return from the war, I had published twenty-seven medical papers on problems pertaining to the thyroid. These represented summaries of conventional views of how to diagnose or treat thyroid disease or they were case reports or statistical surveys of the results of treatment. Not one of them contained an original idea.

In the postwar period, from 1946 to 1957, I wrote one book and thirty-nine papers about thyroid disease, fourteen of the latter containing new and previously unpublished ideas about diagnosis or treatment, and several others representing uniquely large studies that confirmed someone else's new idea, like the use of radioactive iodine in the treatment of thyroid disease. In the years 1959 through 1987 I wrote fifty-nine more papers about thyroid disease. However, by 1957 most of the major new contributions had been made.

In 1949, Saunders had published my book *Practical Aspects of Thyroid Disease,* in which I reported fifty patients with hyperthyroidism who had been successfully treated by radioactive iodine. Since this therapy had not been discovered until 1941, this was one of the earliest full-length studies confirming its effectiveness. All of this was made possible by my father's foresight. Years before, when radon first came into use, he had employed a biophysicist, Dr. Otto Glasser, who was therefore available in the Department of Radiation Therapy to advise and deal with the storage and dispensing of the radioactive iodine. In addition, the physicians at the Clinic were remunerated by salaries which made them different from those in private practice who had been treating hyperthyroidism medically, controlling it with the administration of thiouracil drugs, whose side effects required close supervision that resulted in considerable income. Private-practice surgeons, some of whose practices were based largely on performing specialized operations on the thyroid, also were reluctant, when referred a patient, to suggest that the patient would do better treated by radioactive iodine. With us, it made no difference. The overall cost of treatment with radioactive iodine was somewhat less than by the old method of preparation followed by operation, but the newness of the method and the fact that locally we had the lead in it, gave us a big enough practice to more than compensate. I am sure that one of the reasons why salaried physicians and surgeons are apt to be the first to adopt simplified methods of treatment is that unlike those in private practice, their income is not directly affected when the treatment is less costly.

In the same year, and again emphasizing the advantages of group practice where physicians work together, Dr. Beach Hazard and I had published a description and gave a new name to a relatively rare cancer of the thyroid which, up to that time, had not been recognized as an entity. It was a tiny one-centimeter type of papillary cancer that rarely is recognized clinically, is found incidentally at autopsy or when the thyroid is removed for other purposes, and does not tend to recur or metastasize. We called it "non-encapsulated sclerosing tumor of the thyroid" and emphasized the fact that its behavior was benign and that it required no treatment.

In 1950 came my declaration of war on the radical head and neck surgeons who were treating papillary cancer of the thyroid and its metastases in the lymph nodes of the neck by the same radical, de-forming neck dissections that were justifiably being used in the treat-ment of extensive metastatic cancers that had arisen in the mouth and tongue and which were highly malignant and difficult to control. Most of these surgeons had been trained as head and neck surgeons and not as general surgeons or thyroid specialists, and although skill-ful and knowledgeable about the treatment of squamous cell cancers, they were inexperienced in and almost ignorant about the treatment of thyroid disease. I, on the other hand, had grown up surrounded by my father's patients with thyroid problems and along with most other surgeons, wrongly considered the metastases of papillary cancer in lymph nodes to be benign congenital anomalies that we called lateral aberrant thyroids and quite rightly treated with extreme conser-vatism.

In 1950, in a paper published in the *American Journal of Surgery,* I had made several clear points:

1. Papillary tumors of the thyroid may grow slowly. I reported one that I followed with metastases untreated for twenty-seven years without enlargement.

2. The involved nodes in the neck do not invade and can eas-ily be removed individually or in groups instead of by radical op-erations that sacrifice nerves and muscle. ("Berry picking" was what the radical surgeons scornfully accused me of advocating.)

3. After simple removal of the involved nodes, prolonged follow-up usually showed no local recurrences.

4. The papillary tumors of patients whose involved nodes were overlooked and not removed for several years remained lo-calized over periods of up to ten years. (These were patients op-erated on by me before the war.)

5. The pattern of metastasis of thyroid nodules is not the same as that of other cancers of the throat, and the removal of the mus-cles and nerves that causes so much deformity in the young women who are so often affected is not necessary. A modified neck dissection preserving nerves and muscles was advised.

These conclusions were tantamount to a declaration of atheism in a chapel dedicated to the pope, because at this time cancer surgery was beginning to be a specialty and most of those who called themselves head and neck surgeons were winning their fame and fortune by do-ing the most radical operations. When I would present my point of view, these surgeons and their followers often discussed my papers with sarcasm and "berry picking" epithets.

It was really great fun and I enjoyed every bit of it. The reaction of the cancer specialists became particularly violent in 1957 when I announced, for the first time, that in people under the age of forty, papillary carcinoma of the thyroid did not behave like a malignant disease. It was more like benign endometriosis because when the endocrine environment was changed, the cells stopped growing and seemed to just shrink and disappear. In the case of endometriosis, it was estrogen that stimulated the growth. Remove the ovaries and the growth stopped. In the case of papillary carcinoma of the thyroid, it was the thyroid-stimulating hormone of the pituitary that caused the growth of the tumor and all you had to do to control it was to give thyroid hormone in doses sufficient to suppress the pituitary. In almost all patients less than forty years of age, papillary cancers would shrink and never grow again as long as the dose of thyroid was adequate.

In spite of the well-documented effects of suppression, which subsequently were confirmed by many sources, treatment by thyroid hormone was not accepted with enthusiasm. The internists had been working with the radiologists to treat the patients with thyroid cancer by radioactive iodine, and the surgeons had been doing total thyroidectomies (for which they were paid much more than for lesser operations) because they wanted not only to remove all possible cancer cells in the thyroid, but also to get rid of all of the thyroid tissue so that the radioactive iodine would be taken up by the metastases rather than by the remnants of the normal gland. This was fine in theory, but impractical from every other standpoint. Not only did total thyroidectomy greatly increase the incidence of damage to the parathyroid glands, often resulting in a permanent lowering of the blood calcium with many resultant side effects, but it also resulted in an increase in the incidence of injury to the laryngeal nerves. The resultant hoarseness often required secondary, sometimes unsuccessful, operations, and sometimes it caused difficulty in breathing necessitating tracheostomy (insertion of a tube) and occasionally resulted in death.

When radical, en-bloc neck dissections were done, removing the jugular vein, the main muscle of the neck, and the nerve that lifts the shoulder, there was much deformity and disability. In addition, the use of large doses of radioactive iodine in the treatment of papillary cancer was not without side effects, including an increase in the incidence of leukemia, the occasional transformation of the low-grade papillary tumors to universally fatal anaplastic cancers, and to damage of the lung, when there was extensive metastasis there that took up the radioactive material.

In the rare papillary cancers in people beyond the age of forty-five that involve both lobes or have metastasized to the nodes on both sides, total thyroidectomy is often indicated. But in papillary tumors, occurring in young people, the same tumors that are treatable by radioactive iodine respond permanently to suppression by thyroid hormone. The thyroid treatment, moreover, has no side effects and costs only one-third as much.

Although I was the first in America to report the regression of papillary cancers in response to thyroid feeding, I was not the first in the world. In 1937, long before anyone had learned that many cancers of the prostate and breast could be made to regress when appropriate endocrine therapy was given, Sir Thomas Dunhill of England had reported a couple of cases in which papillary tumors had disappeared when he gave thyroid hormone. These observations seemed so unlikely that no one paid any attention to them. Then along came World War II and no one had time to worry about the thyroid.

In 1953, Greer and Astwood had reported that some benign goiters grew smaller when treated by giving suppressive doses of thyroid hormone, and in 1954, in England, Balme reported a single case of regression of thyroid metastases. Independently in 1955, I reported several patients whose papillary cancers had grown rapidly when they were made hypothyroid and the output of thyroid-stimulating hormone of the pituitary was stimulated and also five patients in whom papillary carcinomas had regressed in response to treatment with thyroid and had remained controlled for up to four years. The rationale for my having tried large doses of thyroid hormone on patients with thyroid cancer was based on my having observed the rapid growth of the cancers in some of those patients in whom a thyroid deficiency was induced.

In spite of the mounting evidence, the profession was reluctant to switch to this safe and effective therapy, and to this day, in many parts of the country, total thyroidectomies still are done and radioactive iodine still is routinely used in the treatment of papillary cancers in young patients. Fortunately, the head and neck cancer surgeons finally lost their war for the perpetuation of radical neck dissections in the treatment of papillary carcinoma. Since the early 1970s, that operation has been abandoned in favor of the limited procedure that I had advocated.

Even before the advent of radioactive iodine and treatment by suppression, I had noticed that young patients with lung metastases from papillary cancers could live on indefinitely without further enlargement of the metastases. In those days there were no tests to prove why the tumors stopped growing, but in retrospect I believe it must have been because when there was a lot of tumor and when the tumor was differentiated it made thyroid hormone and was able to suppress the output of thyroid stimulating hormone (TSH) and stop the tumor from growing. In any event, in 1953 I called attention for the first time to the striking difference in survival of older and younger patients with differentiated thyroid cancers. (*Annals of Surgery,* 1953, "The Relationship of the Age of the Patient to the Natural History and Prognosis of Patients with Papillary Carcinoma of the Thyroid.") The article, which recounted my experience with 105 patients with thyroid carcinoma, concluded, "Since almost all cancers of the thyroid that occur in patients under 40 years of age are of the lowest grade of malignancy, the prognosis in this age group is almost universally good if an adequate operation is performed."

Long before these observations on cancer were made, I had been using the newly developed Silverman needle to make biopsies of the thyroid. In 1951, for the first time, Dr. Beach Hazard and I had reported the use of needle biopsy in the diagnosis of thyroiditis. By following the patients after needle biopsy, we proved that each of the three types of thyroiditis was distinct and that they did not progress from one type to another. We were also able to show, for the first time, that "subacute thyroiditis" was merely an acute form of the more chronic "pseudotubercular thyroiditis." At the time we began using the Silverman needle to diagnose thyroiditis I was still treating the severe cases of subacute thyroiditis with radiation therapy. The dangers of radiating the thyroid were not then known, but luckily, in these cases, we had no instance of cancer following the radiation.

At about the same time that we began to use thyroid hormone in the treatment of cancer of the thyroid, I began to wonder if its use might not be applicable also to the treatment of the thyroiditis known as struma lymphomatosa. Since we could now diagnose the disease by needle biopsy, we went ahead and tried suppressive doses of thyroid. It worked, and by 1952 we were able to report this new method of controlling, by nonoperative treatment, a goiter that before then usually had to be removed surgically.

At about the same time that I began to treat struma lymphomatosa with subacute thyroid, I went to Europe and attended a thyroid clinic in which patients with subacute thyroiditis were being given injections of adrenocorticotrophic hormone. The work had not been published, but when I got home I found that hydrocortisone had been synthesized and was available in the form of pills. This medicine worked like magic. The hard, exquisitely tender and swollen gland which on swallowing gave pain that shot up to the ears, became pain-less and in a few days felt normal. It was later found that the disease was caused by a mumps-like virus and that although the cortisone did not cure the infection, it resolved the inflammation and made it bear-able until the infection had run its course. Prior to this, many of the af-fected glands had been removed.

In 1955, at the meeting of the American Goiter Association, Dr. Haz-ard and I continued our campaign against the radical cancer surgeons by presenting a series of sixty-five patients with thyroid cancer who had been treated mainly by conservative operations and who had been followed for more than five years. In these patients the results were as good as had been reported by others after mutilating opera-tions. We concluded, "It would appear that radical mutilating surgery is rarely if ever indicated in the treatment of carcinoma of the thyroid."

Soon after our affirmation that total thyroidectomy and radical op-erations were rarely indicated in the treatment of cancer of the thy-roid, Dr. Hazard and I wrote a paper defining and naming a new type of thyroid cancer that Dr. Hazard called "medullary carcinoma." This cancer was very rare but very malignant. It was multifocal, with de-posits all through both lobes so that total thyroidectomy was usually necessary and it metastasized diffusely to lymph nodes and also to lungs. Unfortunately, it was not susceptible to treatment either by ra-dioactive iodine or suppression. It was also associated with a multiple endocrine disorder often involving tumors of the adrenals and parathyroids. From the standpoint of being susceptible to cure it might have been better if we had never defined and reported it!

In many institutions, not only radioactive iodine but also external radiation was being given in the treatment of papillary carcinoma. Since papillary carcinoma is not radiosensitive, practically no cures were effected by external radiation, and when the tumors' uptake of radioactive iodine was small, there was not enough radiation to de-stroy them. The dosage of radiation received, however, was some-times just enough to stimulate the almost benign tumor to change into a highly malignant one. Unfortunately, radiation therapy is still being used in some situations in which I believe it does more harm than good.

In 1962, people were beginning to get so cancer-conscious and pa-thologists were beginning to look so hard for the microscopic cancers that occur in up to 20 percent of the thyroids of normal people, that they began to report a high incidence of microcarcinomas in struma lymphomatosa. In struma there is a deficiency of thyroid hormone and hence an increase in the output of the pituitary's thyroid-stimulating hormone that makes the thyroid cells proliferate and the microcarcinomas grow, so that they are more easily recognized. Because of this the surgeons were beginning to advise total thyroidectomy in the treatment of anyone with struma lymphomatosa, a procedure which of course caused many complications. Since we were not treating struma by surgery but merely diagnosing it by needle biopsy and treating it by thyroid hormone, we were able to report that 222 patients with proven struma lymphomatosa who were treated by thyroid feeding had been followed up for more than one thousand patient years without the development of any carcinomas. We concluded that struma should not be regarded as a premalignant lesion and that it rarely requires surgical treatment.

The connection between radiation treatment of benign disease and the subsequent developments of malignant tumors, like papillary carcinomas of the thyroid, was beginning to be widely appreciated, and as a result many physicians were advising against the use of radioactive iodine in the treatment of hyperthyroidism. We did not believe that there was any danger of its causing cancer if it were used in proper doses, that is to say relatively large doses. That is because if you treat a cell with a large dose of radiation, it is destroyed or at least it is rendered sterile and unable to reproduce itself. If a cell cannot divide it cannot give rise to a cancer. That is why we had seen no cancers of the thyroid after treatment with large doses of radioactive iodine. To encourage the profession to use large destructive doses and not small ones that were consistent with both continued thyroid function and the development of cancer, Dr. Schumacher and I reported our results in thirty-two children treated with radioactive iodine. They had been followed for from five to fourteen years and there had been no recurrence of hyperthyroidism, no nodules, and no carcinomas.

In 1965, Drs. Hazard, Hawk, and I reported a follow-up of 625 patients who had had needle biopsies of the thyroid with excellent accuracy of diagnosis and no significant side effects, but we were still afraid of implanting cancer and advised against its use in nodules that were apt to be malignant. In the next year, still interested in the use of the needle, we reported that thyroid cysts, which constitute about a quarter of all thyroid nodules, could safely be diagnosed, treated, and usually permanently cured by simple aspiration, in the office.

About this time, we began to change our attitude towards the use of needle biopsy in nodules that we thought might be malignant. Our own experience and reports of others had shown that implantation of cancer in needle tracts almost never occurred. All nodules could be biopsied and only the few which were either frankly malignant or possibly so, had to be removed. As a result, the proportion of cancers found in the patients operated on rose from the 3 percent that it had been in my father's day and in the early years of my practice, to between 40 and 50 percent. At the same time, the number of thyroid operations performed at the Cleveland Clinic fell from 2,700 in the year 1927 to less than 50 a year.

As a result of needle biopsy to establish the diagnosis and of the use of suppressive doses of thyroid hormone to treat benign goiters and struma lymphomatosa, and of the use of corticosteroids to treat subacute thyroiditis, we had practically abolished thyroid surgery. I summed it up in a final paper, "Changing End Results in Patients with Papillary Carcinoma of the Thyroid," published in *Surgery, Gynecology & Obstetrics* in 1969. From my standpoint, there was little more in the field of thyroid disease that could be of interest to a surgeon. Fortunately, long before this I had begun looking in other directions.

18

Some New Thoughts about Surgery

☙

P RIOR TO World War II, I had been interested in the ultraradical treatment of breast cancer, and in selected cases I had done not only axillary but also internal-mammary-node dissections, removing the possibly involved nodes that lay behind the ribs and sternum. That was the period in which I was evolving away from my father's conservative views on the treatment of breast cancer and toward or even past the conventional radical mastectomy that was being performed by Dr. Jones. The war interrupted my use of the ultra-radical operation which later, in the hands of others, was proven to be ineffective.

After the war and the death of my father, I had haunting memories of some of the remarks that our prewar pathologist, Dr. Allen Graham, had made. He believed that in terms of cure, there was no difference in the results obtained by my father's modified mastectomies and Dr. Jones's radical ones. For this reason, and because my wartime experiences had made me distrustful of what everyone believed and taught, I suggested to Dr. Aussie Robnett (Robbie), a bright young surgeon who had just finished his training with us and was on the assistant staff, that he might do well to follow up on Dr. Graham's hunch and see if he could demonstrate any difference in the results following the two quite different types of operation. I remember telling him (for this was the early 1950s when to surgeons the Halsted radical mastectomy was as sacred as was the belief in Private Enterprise) that if I were he, I would try to disprove whatever was the most universally accepted surgical doctrine. At that time, and right up to the 1970s, that would be the efficacy of the Halsted radical mastectomy.

Robbie did a splendid piece of clinical research, in which he followed a large number of the patients treated in the two ways and found that there was no difference at all in their survival. Although Dr. Jones did a conservative type of radical mastectomy with relatively thick skin flaps and rarely any necessity for grafting skin, the incidence of swelling of the arm and other unpleasant cosmetic and functional complications was significantly higher than in my father's cases. To my amazement, my father had been right all along!

Although the majority of the breast problems that I was seeing were related to malignancy, there was one very annoying and unsolved one that I encountered in the wife of one of my residents. She had had a sour-smelling cheesy discharge from the nipple and had a chronic draining sinus from an area close to the areola. We put a probe in the sinus and it came out through a duct in the nipple. We then excised the duct, and the pathologist, Dr. Beach Hazard, reported that the duct was affected by "squamous metaplasia," in which the skin had grown down into the duct and was shedding its cells, just as it does on the surface or into a sebaceous cyst or wen, and when that blocks and irritates the duct, it gets infected and drains indefinitely. The patient was cured by the simple excision of the duct. The cause of the problem was reported, and no longer were multiple operations or even mastectomies done to correct it. In 1976, Dr. J. J. Zuska, coauthor of the original article, called my attention to an article in *Lancet* that gave Zuska and me full credit for defining the disease.

In 1949, when Dr. Jones died, I had been overwhelmed with the amount of work I had inherited. This included, in collaboration with Dr. Rupe Turnbull, performing all of Dr. Jones's colorectal surgery. We instituted several innovations, the first of which was primary closure of the gaping posterior wound of the abdominoperineal resection. Before the advent of antibiotics, the incidence of infection had been so high that no one closed the space from which the rectum had been removed. As a result, it took months, in fact sometimes more than a year, for the wound to fill in and close. In 1949, I had reported (with Dr. Robnett) a series of successful closures of this wound using only a tiny catheter to drain it for a couple of days.

By 1950 Dr. Turnbull was doing most of the colorectal surgery and was making some fundamental observations. Most ileostomies, he concluded, functioned imperfectly because the exteriorized segment of the bowel was paralyzed by what he called "peritonitis" of the peritoneal surface. His studies made on reoperated patients showed that the peritonitis extended through the lymphatics even into the adjacent intra-abdominal portion of the bowel. That was what caused the ileus and obstruction that so often made it necessary to reoperate.

At about the same time as Turnbull was studying ileostomy dysfunction, a marvelously original thinker, Dr. Lester Dragstedt, turned his mind from duodenal ulcer and the vagus nerve downward to the ileum and described the "skin-grafted ileostomy." Soon we confirmed the fact that a split thickness skin graft covering the ileostomy from the time of its establishment prevented ileus. It was a great leap forward. However, as time went by, the skin grafts on the ileostomy suffered from irritation and digestion. Then they contracted, causing stenosis and intestinal obstruction. We were back again where we had started, reoperating on most of our patients with ileostomies.

By this time, Turnbull had shown the mechanism by which ileus was produced and Dragstedt had shown that covering the ileostomy prevented the ileus. The conclusion was staring us in the face. Why not graft the ileostomy with mucosa instead of with skin? Perhaps the mucosa, resistant to the digestive action of the succus entericus, would both protect against primary ileus and prevent contracture. Rupe and I discussed it and thought it worth a try. I did the first one, and Turnbull, now with a well-established practice, soon proved that it was a good solution to the problem of ileostomy dysfunction. In the meantime, unknown to us, we had been scooped.

Bryan Brooke, the noted British surgeon, in an article published in England a year before Turnbull's and mine, had described an everted ileostomy. He had buried this landmark in a long article, which discussed all aspects of the management of ileostomies. To read it today, it seems that Bryan had no idea that the suggestion he made, of turning the ileum inside out, would be the century's greatest advance in surgery of the bowel. At the time we published our article we had been unaware of Brooke's contribution. Even after we read it, the notion seemed absurd. Anyone who had been to medical school should know that if you turned the bowel inside out the peristaltic wave of the everted part would go the wrong way and cause obstruction. Only a philosopher like Bryan Brooke could believe that a physician's interpretation of the function of the body is as apt to be wrong as a man's interpretation of the acts of a woman.

Although the everted ileostomy was a great leap forward, still the ileostomy was not quite perfect. If too short, it was difficult to protect the skin. If too long, the thickness and the action of the muscle caused some degree of obstruction. So here comes Turnbull—back into the picture. It was not surprising, because of all of us who were involved in this problem, it was Rupe who had first conceived the notion of what caused ileostomy dysfunction. That was why he next invented the multiple myotomies (incisions through the muscle of the everted part of the bowel) which paralyzed the muscles and allowed a long extruded segment to function normally.

Not content with solving the physicians' problem with ileostomy, Turnbull proceeded to solve the patients' part of the problem. He founded the School of Enterostomal Therapy. At first it was staffed with nurses who had had ileostomies and who, from personal experience and from what Turnbull had taught them, could show new patients how to live comfortably and without embarrassment. The first of the enterostomal therapists was Mrs. Norma Gill, who in person had spread the word through America and many countries of the western world and to some of those behind the iron curtain. The society of degree-holding enterostomal therapists now number one thousand.

In spite of the success of the ileostomy, inflammatory disease of the bowel remained a problem. The incidence of acute toxic colitis was increasing. This was a highly fatal disease, characterized by, but not yet named, toxic megacolon. The problem was that the muscles of the colon, almost devoid of their protecting mucosa, became paralyzed and allowed the colon to dilate. The result was that an area equivalent to about a quarter of the body's surface was a raw ulcer, bathed in fecal poultice. In 1951, a survey of the Cleveland Clinic's experience with toxic megacolon had showed that within a year of diagnosis, 71 percent had died. These patients were desperately ill, yet soon it became obvious that instead of being *too sick to be operated on*, they were, as Ferguson had stated in relation to patients who were bleeding or obstructed, *too sick not to be operated on*. Therefore, I began to do emergency colectomies on patients with toxic megacolon. Prior to this, our mortality rate of emergency ileostomy had been 39 percent with an additional 32 percent of the patients dying of the disease after discharge from the hospital. The mortality rate following colectomy was 14 percent, and the patients who survived operation were well. But that was still too high. Here again it was the genius of Turnbull that solved the problem. He invented the blow hole technique—a term that perhaps he had learned from diving with the whales. In patients with toxic megacolon, colectomy was dangerous because the bowel was so adherent and so friable that it often perforated. "Why not decompress it?" Turnbull thought, and he did. His technique of multiple blow holes has been widely adopted and has reduced the mortality of toxic megacolon to only 6 percent, a more than ten-fold reduction from the original mortality.

During this period, I had inherited not only some of Dr. Tommy Jones's colon surgery, but also almost all of his gastric surgery. I had latched on to the principle of vagotomy for peptic ulcer just as soon as Dr. Dragstedt had enunciated it, because when I had worked in my father's laboratory, I had noticed that stimulation of the sympathetic nervous system stopped the secretion of the acid which caused the ulcers. It seemed entirely logical to produce the same effect by cutting the parasympathetic nerves, whose function it was to stimulate the secretion of acid. The only novel suggestion that I could make to this quickly accepted advance in surgery was to emphasize that if an opening between the stomach and the intestine was to be used to promote drainage of the now paralyzed stomach, it would be most efficient if it were placed close to the pylorus—the place where the food exited to the intestine. As an even simpler and often more effective alternative, I suggested that the pylorus could be widened by cutting it longitudinally and sewing it up transversely. In 1949, I had been able to report in *Annals of Surgery* that Dr. Jones and I had done eighty-seven vagotomies with pyloroplasty or gastroenterostomy and were able to compare the results with eighty-seven gastric resections performed on a similar group of patients. In the patients treated by vagotomy there was a lower mortality rate (1.1 percent compared to 3.4 percent), and a lower incidence of recurrent ulceration, hemorrhage, and pain. I also devised and reported an effective way of identifying the vagus nerves by pulling down on the stomach, palpating them and catching them on a hook.

The advocates of gastric resection were true to their favorite technique and bitterly attacked those of us who tried to simplify and make safer the treatment of duodenal ulcer. I suppose some surgeons still do gastric resections for duodenal ulcers, but if they do they resect much less of the stomach than they used to and they add vagotomy. Dr. Dragstedt made a great contribution.

In 1950 I reported seven patients in whom I had treated bleeding from varicose veins of the esophagus by opening the esophagus and sewing over the veins. The patients were children or young adults who had had thrombosis of the umbilical vein at birth and the portal system had thrombosed forcing the blood to use other channels, including the esophageal veins, to find its way back to the heart. My first patient was one whom I explored, expecting to do a shunt operation between the splenic and the renal veins, but the splenic vein was thrombosed. She gave a history of having had more than 120 transfusions and had been bleeding about every two weeks. Since her veins were thrombosed, there was no way that I could perform a shunt. She was twenty-three years old, a lovely girl, doomed to die if nothing were done. Injection of the huge varices that occur in this kind of blockage had never, in those days, been successful. I decided to take a chance, open the chest, open the esophagus, sew over the veins and go through the diaphragm and do the same with those of the stomach and also remove the spleen, which was draining blood into the blocked system.

The patient did well and had no more bleeding after operation. Then came the big advantage of working in a clinic. I let it be known that I was looking for similar cases and soon I had six more to report. All were greatly improved by the treatment. The same procedure, when applied to those who were bleeding as a result of blockage of the veins from cirrhosis of the liver, was unsuccessful. Those patients died of liver failure.

I think the operation of ligation of esophageal varices might have become popular in this country, if there had continued to be cases of this type in which the blockage was from infection of the umbilical vein. However, along with antibiotics, such infections vanished. As a result the disease vanished. If I had been dependent for my living upon operating on it, I would have starved. The operation is still used in countries where the obstruction of the veins is the result of parasitic infections and the function of the liver is good. In 1974, Dr. L. W. Ottinger from Harvard, writing in *Annals of Surgery*, credited me for being the first in this country to ligate esophageal varices. He concluded, "In the patient with previous surgery in the right upper abdomen or a failed portosystemic shunt, transthoracic ligation would appear to be an effective method of immediate management of variceal hemorrhage."

The only other significant contribution that I made to the science of surgery in the postwar years was an article on the treatment of cancer of the pancreas, in which I was forced to retract the optimism of thirty-two years before, when I had reported the seventh successful resection of a cancer of the head of the pancreas. I had to admit that that patient, and all others that had ever been operated on at the Cleveland Clinic for a clinically apparent cancer of the pancreas, had died of or with pancreatic cancer. This, too, caused a howl of protest, because I said that simple bypass operations relieved the jaundice and resulted in a longer period of survival. I concluded that no one but surgeons with special training that enabled them to have very low mortality rates should perform this dangerous operation and that they should do it only on younger people and in the most highly selected cases. It is interesting that in the past few years, most articles on this subject confirm these views that were so scorned in 1970, when I presented them.

19

Beginning the Battle of the Breast

T HE HEAVY LOAD of clinical practice that I had inherited from Dr. Tom Jones was lifted by the advent of Drs. Hoerr and Turnbull and later by Dr. Robnett. During the first part of this period I was operating every weekday, and my work hours were from 7:30 A.M. to 6:30 P.M. Fortunately, I lived five minutes from the Clinic and usually could get home in time for supper. In those first few years there was a good deal of confusion, not so much in the surgical department, because Dr. Dinsmore was a good administrator and he and I got along together perfectly, but in the management of the Clinic as a whole. Mr. Edward C. Daoust, under the direction of the board of trustees, had managed most of the Clinic's business affairs very ably. When he died in 1947, he had been replaced by Mr. Clarence Taylor, a business executive who had little knowledge of medicine and hence too frequently found himself in conflict with the medical staff.

The founders were now gone and leadership had passed to John Sherwin, president of the board of trustees, under whose management in 1956 a board of governors was elected, and it was the board that then took complete control. I was one of the seven members, and although I have never had any special interest or ability in administration I did enjoy my two terms on the board.

When Dr. Robnett left, almost all of the breast surgery came to me, for by this time Dr. Dinsmore was ailing and losing his interest in operating. Then coincidentally two things happened. Dr. Dinsmore took a trip to Scotland, where he visited the clinic of Dr. Robert McWhirter who was treating cancer of the breast by simple mastectomy and radiation. Dinsmore came home impressed, but not deeply enough to make him change his ways. The other and more important happening was a visit from my friend, Dr. Reginald Murley, an English surgeon who had trained at St. Bartholomew's Hospital in London and had decided to look up the records of the patients who twenty-odd years before had been operated on at Bart's by Sir Geoffrey Keynes.

Reggie, who stayed with us in Cleveland, would later become Sir Reginald Murley, president of the Royal College of Surgeons. He was one of the most amusing, loquacious, and delightful men Jane and I had ever known. Reggie was ambitious and was devoted, as all young and hopeful surgeons are, to the support of the most radical surgery, including even ultraradical mastectomy. Keynes, on the other hand, in the 1930s had treated a large number of patients with breast cancer by wide local excision and irradiation. Murley decided to make a long range follow-up on these patients and to compare their survival with that of a similar group who, at the same time in the same hospital, had been treated by other members of the staff by radical mastectomy. To the astonishment of Reggie and all but the radiotherapist coauthor of the article, it was found that there was no significant difference in the survival of the two groups—in fact, the survival of the patients whose breasts were not removed was slightly better.

It was at about this time that I began to change my mind about the value of the conventional radical mastectomy and to remember the minimum deformity of the patients upon whom my father used to do the modified radical mastectomy. In 1955, I published an essay about my father's work—"The Kinetic System and Its Control—Twenty-Five Years After." In it I mentioned the striking advances that had taken place in some of the diseases like peptic ulcer, hyperthyroidism, and hypertension, but I went on to say, "If all medical treatment were as disheartening as is that for cancer of the breast, we would have little incentive to carry on." I had begun to do some modified radical mastectomies, and when I showed the manuscript to Dr. Dinsmore, he appended a note: "As I read the foregoing I could not help remembering the opinionated viewpoint of the writer as a medical student and resident, and the arguments that took place between father and son. Of course, father knew that in due course the son would look back, realize the folly of arguments and agree with him." Another medical cycle completed!

I did my last radical mastectomy in 1955 and switched over to the modified radical operation. But there were exceptions. A few years before I had had a patient, in her sixties, upon whom I had done an excisional biopsy of a small cancer in the upper outer quadrant of the breast. When I operated I did not know if it was benign or malignant and did not have permission to do anything more than a biopsy. To my horror, the lady stubbornly refused to listen to reason or to allow me to "complete the operation." I warned her of the perils and of the almost certainty of recurrence. That was what I had been taught. She promised me to return if she ever had any further problem with her breast. She never did. I followed her for at least fifteen years, and for the first half of that time I found it almost impossible to believe that she remained well.

By 1955 the above-mentioned experience and Reggie Murley's eloquence had persuaded me that there might be a place for partial mastectomy, with or without radiation, and possibly also for simple mastectomy, in which the regional lymph nodes would not be removed. The latter heresy I acquired in part from another visitor from England, Dr. Deborah Doniach, who could rightly be called "The Mother of Immunology." Deborah was one of the first to apply what was known about resistance to bacteria and infectious diseases to the understanding of the autoimmune diseases like rheumatic fever, arthritis, dermatological conditions, and thyroiditis. It was her reading of my work in treating struma lymphomatosa by suppressive doses of thyroid hormone that prompted her to visit Cleveland, for it was Deborah who first recognized and reported that struma lymphomatosa was an autoimmune disease, produced by a civil war between misinformed lymphocytes and the normal thyroid.

Deborah was beginning to become interested in the role of immunity in cancer, and was wondering about the role that regional lymph nodes were playing in the patient's systemic immunity against cancer. Since McWhirter had set the precedent of not removing the nodes, I wondered whether part of the body's immunity against the systemic spread of cancer did not reside in the regional nodes. I began to wonder if the axillary dissection that was performed routinely in radical and modified radical mastectomies might not increase instead of decrease the likelihood of blood-borne cancer cells, giving rise to metastases. I discussed it with our radiotherapists and they agreed that it was worth a try. For several years, therefore, in patients who showed no palpable evidence of lymph nodal metastasis, I mixed simple mastectomies with modified radicals.

After those two groups of patients had been followed for many years there was no significant difference in their survivals. The ones who did not have axillary dissections did a little better, but not significantly so. Subsequent large, randomized studies have shown that it is just as effective to leave nodes that do not seem to be involved as it is to routinely remove them. If later, in some cases, cancer appears, the nodes can be removed with as good a chance of cure as there would have been if they had been removed at the first operation. In my series also were a few patients (about 15 percent of the total) who had had only wide local excisions of the cancers—partial mastectomy, we named the operation, in order to make it sound more like the conventional treatment. The patients whose breasts were preserved were not only grateful to have been spared disfigurement, but also their survival was the same as was that of patients with similar tumors who had been treated by the modified radical mastectomy.

In 1955, I had no personal experience with long-term follow-up of patients treated by operations less than modified radical mastectomy, but I had been so stimulated by Murley and Doniach, and also by my single experience with wide local excision, that I wrote an article that, to the consternation of all conventionally minded surgeons, was printed in the *Cleveland Clinic Quarterly*. I doubt if any other surgical journal in the United States at that time, when the Halsted radical mastectomy was the Gospel of the Surgical Profession, would even have considered it. The opening sentence read, "Suddenly after 50 years of complacent acceptance of radical mastectomy the surgical world is plunged in doubt. On the one hand, Urban and Baker and Wangensteen advocate extension of the radical operation to include the internal mammary nodes; on the other, there is mounting evidence that simple mastectomy gives better results than the conventional operation." I concluded, "At present there is no basis for advocating any single type of operation for operable cancers of the breast, and there is no basis for employing a general policy, pro or con, regarding irradiation, removal of endocrine glands or endocrine therapy. Surgery, irradiation and endocrine therapy are double-edged swords that may harm as well as help. The challenge to the surgeon is to control the cancer as well as possible and to do so with the least possible harm."

In this same year, my major interest switched over to the field of cancer. In the next year, nine out of ten of my published articles were on the subject of cancer. In November *Cancer and Common Sense* had come out, attacking the radical cancer surgeons who kept advocating the ever larger and more destructive operation. I had had some personal experience when a close friend of mine had gone to a "Cancer Center" and been subjected to an absurdly radical and quite useless operation. In the introduction to the book I had raised the question of whether we had not developed "a technology of overtreatment" that was a step backward into "a primitive philosophy where life is devoted to propitiation of fear." Needless to say, the American Cancer Society and its supportive surgeons did not give a standing ovation to these remarks. A summary of the book which filled six pages of the

October 31, 1955, issue of *LIFE* was accompanied by opinions of a number of experts. All of these except for my old medical school classmate Bert Dunphy, my friend Chuck Mayo, my former chief Dr. Everts Graham, and the Mayo Clinic's medical columnist Walter Alvarez condemned many of my views. The American Cancer Society was not pleased because I had said some things that, rightly or wrongly, they concluded referred to them. An example is my statement, "Those responsible for telling the public about cancer have chosen to use the weapon of fear. They have bred in a sensitive public a fear that is approaching hysteria. They have created a new disease, cancer phobia, a contagious disease that spreads from mouth to ear."

Dr. Elmer Hess, president of the American Medical Association; Dr. Charles Cameron, director of the American Cancer Society; and Dr. J. R. Heller of the National Cancer Institute, wrote that "Dr. Crile offers a dangerous fatalistic philosophy of cancer. His thesis is contrary to the teaching of the country's 81 medical schools and to the experience of Physicians and Surgeons." The sentence that appeared to have precipitated the "experts" adverse reaction was "But there is no clear evidence that immediate treatment is any more effective than treatment given a little later." The sentence had been lifted out of context, for it referred not to a delay of weeks or months but to one of hours or days, as in the period between biopsy and operation.

The American Cancer Society and many others accused me of negating the value of early detection and treatment and of a fatalistic philosophy. What I had said was not that early treatment was useless, but that in some kinds of cancer we had no way of detecting the tumors early and that was why, in spite of larger and larger operations and the increased use of radiation, there had been no lowering of the age-adjusted death rate from cancer. In the treatment of others I said that early detection, as by Pap smear, could save lives. My approach was not negative, it was merely selective and suggested that the ultimate answer lay not in doing ever larger and more deforming operations, but in study of the "chemistry and the very nature of the cancer cell." I even went so far as to commend the American Cancer Society's support of cancer research.

The fee of six thousand dollars that *LIFE* paid me for publication rights I passed on to the Clinic's Research Endowment Fund. After the issue was released with its headline: "A PLEA AGAINST BLIND FEAR. An experienced surgeon says that excessive worry leads to costly tests, undue suffering," there was a warm and understanding exchange of letters between me and *LIFE*'s editor, Ralph Graves. He told me of the many efforts that had been made to stop publication, and said that he had had "a most revealing glimpse of medical politics." He went on to say that of the first eighty-one letters that came in response, fifty-two were very favorable, eleven were critical, five suggested cancer cures, and fifteen offered general comment. I received 136 letters, mostly from physicians, many of whom I knew. All but two of these were favorable. The predominant note was that I had had the courage to say what should have been said years before.

Of the two letters that were not complimentary, one asked why I had "singled out the young man of Britain's air force in World War II as an example of facing instant death without fear." It concluded, "I suggest if you are a real American and not one of those Americans whose pitiable yearning is for the British Empire—that you revise your book to include American Soldiers where you choose to hold up the British as an example par excellence of valor in the face of probable death. You can't do this because your feeling is British." The other noncomplimentary letter contained two large single-spaced pages requesting information about a syndrome that had started in the scalp, "Does the hair grow after death, and if so what causes it to grow?"— etc. etc.

After the publication of *Cancer and Common Sense*, I had many invitations to speak and debate and later, to make known my views on television. In retrospect, most of what I said has been proven to be correct. However, to my knowledge none of my critics ever retracted their statements. Nor was I ever elected to any office in the American Cancer Society, the American Medical Association, or any other self-respecting medical organization. Fortunately, I was at the Cleveland Clinic, where I had access to everything I needed. I decided that neither the people's war against cancer nor mine against the American Cancer Society could be won by words and arguments alone.

In January 1955, with the agreement of my colleagues, we started a policy in which, in patients who showed no evidence of nodal involvement, I would do simple operations, total or partial mastectomy, usually without radiation, and either modified radical or simple mastectomy and radiation when nodes were palpably involved. My colleagues, at the same time, would do radical or modified radical mastectomy on all operable patients. Soon it became obvious that there was going to be no significant difference in the survival of the patients, with the result that in 1957 all of us abandoned radical mastectomy and all the surgeons at the Cleveland Clinic used forms of treatment adapted to the individual tumor and patient.

The results confirmed my suspicions, first aroused by my discovery of the futility of radical surgery in dealing with cancer of the thyroid, that the widely held belief that "the bigger the operation the better the results" was not always true. By 1960, I had accumulated enough knowledge on the subject to write a twenty-two-page article entitled "A Speculative Review of the Etiology, Natural History and Treatment of Cancer" published in *Perspectives of Biology and Medicine,* and concluding, "Our thinking about cancer has come a long way. At least we can view it not as a demon to be exorcised, but in its true biologic perspective—as a phenomenon of growth. Progress comes through understanding the ways of nature rather than from trying to bend them to our will. Not until we understand the factors that control the growth of normal cells will the problems of cancer be solved."

After the review, I went to the laboratory to see what I could discover.

20

The Mouse Lab

𝕏

I N THE LABORATORY, I was interested in the role of the regional
lymph nodes in providing immunity to pulmonary metastases from
tumors implanted on the mice's feet. A young medical student, Bob
Wagar, and a nurse, Margo Kiraly, came in, part-time, to help me.
None of us knew anything about mice or their cancers and all of us
had a wonderful time learning. Bob and Margo were superb helpers.

We found that if the regional nodes were removed in the first two
weeks after the cancer was implanted, the incidence of metastasis was
greatly increased, but later the immunity became systemic and removal of the nodes seemed to have no effect on the incidence or extent
of systemic metastasis.

Clinical studies also were beginning to show that no harm was
done by removing the axillary nodes of patients with breast cancer. In
short, it seemed as if the cancers that we were dealing with in people
were of such long standing that systemic immunity was already established, with the result that removing the nodes did not increase
metastasis.

At the same time, we were studying the effect on distant metastasis
of amputating the tumor-bearing foot of the mouse, as compared to
destroying the tumor by a single massive destructive dose of radiation. We found that:

1. While the tumor was in place another tumor of the same kind
   could not be implanted on another foot.
2. Within a week of amputating the tumor-bearing foot, the
   body had lost much of its resistance to reimplantation.

319

3. If the tumor-bearing foot was destroyed by a single dose of radiation, the immunity to reimplantation persisted for several weeks while the tumor was dying, and
4. Mice with tumor-bearing feet that were treated by amputation had more than twice the incidence and number of pulmonary metastases as those that were treated by radiation.

These results were reported in the journal *Cancer* in March 1971, but to date I have not noticed that the surgical world has heeded the advice. I am sure of one thing, however. If I were ever to have a malignant melanoma, I would not have it removed by surgery. Instead I would have it destroyed by a single large dose of radiation, given just to the tumor. Later, when the area began to slough, I would have it excised and the skin closed. The regional nodes would be removed only if they became palpably involved.

During this period in the Mouse Lab, we also were studying the effects of heat on cancer and of the combinations of heat and radiation. We worked first with mice, heating their tumor-bearing feet in a water bath and then, when necessary, protecting their bodies with lead as they were irradiated.

We worked also with tumors in dogs that were provided to us through the courtesy of local veterinary surgeons who had been given inoperable animals for destruction. One of these, with an extensive cancer of the jaw, we cured. However, when the owner took a look at it, he was so displeased by his pet's deformity that he refused to take it back. We kept it around and it remained well.

We published four articles on these studies. The results were not spectacular, because at that time we were not able to focus the heat accurately enough to selectively destroy internal cancers. We did, however, report the successful control of osteogenic sarcomas accomplished by exposing the tumor-bearing bones, shielding the soft tissues, and then heating by microwaves and radiating the exposed bone. At that time the standard treatment for osteogenic sarcomas was amputation. At about the same time that we started to treat them by heat and radiation, others began to excise the affected bone and put in a graft. This was better than our combination because the heat made the bone susceptible to fracture. But I still believe that shielding the soft tissues and exposing the bone to a single large dose of radiation would be as effective as excision and grafting.

During this period of about ten years, I spent one morning a week in the laboratory and visited it frequently during the other days. Very early I had found that the person in charge of an investigative program should be able to do all of the technical maneuvers himself, and should personally supervise all of the results.

In retrospect, I consider that the time I spent in the Mouse Lab was one of the most pleasant and productive periods of my life.

21

A Time for Decision

I T WAS 1959. At home one night, as we were going to bed, Jane said, "There's something here that stings. What do you suppose it is?" She pointed to the upper outer quadrant of the right breast. I examined her and could feel nothing abnormal. I asked her to sit up and then thought I could feel just a suggestion of a hard area of thickening, nothing definite.

Jane had an engagement for a lecture the next day, but for the day after, I made an appointment for her to see my colleague, Dr. Stanley Hoerr. He confirmed my suspicions. We agreed that Jane, now a couple of years past menopause, had something in the breast that probably was malignant.

The next day, Stan biopsied the tumor which was only one centimeter in diameter, and then, because partial mastectomies for small cancers were not yet standard procedure, he did a simple mastectomy. He felt the nodes and, since they did not seem to be involved, he did not remove them. Stan was one of my best friends, and he knew that at that time I suspected that the regional nodes might confer some immunity against the systemic spread of cancer.

On my pillow that evening, I found a note:

> Barney
> Like wings over waves
> Silent—timeless
> Love glides in ecstasy!
> Jane
> December 5th, 1959

She was out of the hospital in a day and a couple of days later honored another of her lecture engagements. She was fitted with a prosthesis and, because Stan had placed the scar low and transversely, there would be no way of knowing that anything had happened to her unless she was completely undressed. Jane had no false modesty about it. We both were happy. But there was a cloud on the horizon. It wouldn't blow away.

Although I would never have taken on the responsibility of operating on Jane myself, the decision of what kind of operation would be done depended on to whom I would refer her for treatment. Since Stan felt the same way as I did about breast surgery, I knew what he would do and I felt fully responsible for what was done. It also made me decide that since I was getting no younger and Jane might fail to get much older, we had better see what the world looked like and enjoy it while we could. Both of us loved the adventure of travel and the production of our films, and since, from an ancestral standpoint, Jane had a special interest in the Middle East, we decided to visit Israel and Jordan. We had heard much about Petra, "The Rose Red City Half as Old as Time," which is in Jordan, and we wanted to see it. Ann, Susie, and George were with us. Joan had already left the fold, married to Roger Foster, a medical student.

We left the children in Israel with friends, and Jane and I drove to Jordan—eleven hours in all. The road to Petra was along the ancient caravan route between Damascus and Arabia. Before long, we came to the turreted fortress of Kurak, which the Crusaders had built at the site of Moab, of the Bible. We were photographing Kurak's massive ruin when we were stopped by a Jordanian officer, who asked for our passports. We had left them in our bags in the hotel in Jerusalem! We could speak not a word of Arabic. We were incommunicado and scared. We were escorted to the police station and told to sit and not to leave the room.

Before long a smiling young soldier brought each of us black Turkish-type coffee. The cups were tiny—just a swallow in each. "Remember," Jane cautioned, "their custom is to drink three times." We did so, and then waved our fingers to indicate enough. The officers were pleased at our conformity to their customs. Soon a telephone call came through, and from that time on we were guests instead of prisoners. The officers showed us through the spectacular ruins, while we finished our film.

We went on to an oasis where there was a military station protecting the entrance to Petra. The guards wanted us to stay overnight, because it was getting late. "Be careful of the Young Israelis," the soldier told us. "They come over from the Negev and fight our guards. They kill anyone they see." We explained that we wanted to take pictures in the morning sun. Reluctantly they gave us permission and helped us rent what Jane described later as "pint-sized, sharp-backed horses without saddles or bridles." They were led by Moses and Oselman, Arab boys who trotted alongside. A guide on a horse led the party.

There are few horseback rides as dramatic as the approach to Petra. The old caravan route leads through a three-hundred-foot vertical cleft in the one-thousand-foot-high mountain. In places, by putting out our arms, we could touch both walls. In the bottom was a dried-up stream that through the centuries had cut the cleft, which is known as the Siq. It was a mile and a quarter long, and in its side was cut a groove in which a Nabatean tile used to carry water from Moses' Spring. Fragments of the tile still remained.

A ribbon of starlight and the red glow of our guide's lantern guided us through the Siq. Suddenly it ended in a keyhole, overhung with stone. Before us was a canyon, a hundred yards wide, and surrounded by mountains. In its wall, straight ahead and carved into the rock of the cliff, loomed a great temple, ghostly in the starlight, its columns bigger than the Parthenon's, its facade ninety-feet high. We stopped as, through the centuries, all visitors to Petra must have stopped.

Once this ancient city had been on the caravan route, prosperous and made up of merchants, artists, and artisans. Because it was so inaccessible to the West, it had never been heard of in recent times, until 1812, when Burkhart found it and described it as "The Rose Red City Half as Old as Time." The colors of Petra, which is carved out of the soft sandstone, is the result of multicolored layers of sand that were laid down by the sea and then hardened into rock. Many of these deposits were as Burkhart described them "rose red." Others were blue or golden. All of them had designs made by the multicolored layers. In the morning light this City of Caves, carved from the cliffs, was one of the world's most spectacular sights.

Jane and I passed the night in a cave, guarded over by a Jordanian officer. The next day we spent climbing about and exploring and photographing and collecting artifacts. We bought a stone-carved Roman lamp form a veiled Arab woman who inhabited one of the caves. This visit to the ancient world made us feel a sense of timelessness regarding the lives that were ahead of us and we rejoiced.

The next day we returned to join the children in Israel. We visited the historical sites in Jerusalem, rented a car, and drove to the Port of Haifa, where we were to meet Ed and Marion Link. They had crossed the ocean in their new boat, *The Sea Diver,* and had been diving up artifacts off Caesarea, but the heavy swells had damaged the ship and she was being repaired. Instead of cruising with the Links, we made arrangements to have sleeping quarters at the kibbutz and to eat with the Kibbutzniks in the dining hall that everyone shared.

Life on the kibbutz was a pleasant surprise, for we found everyone cooperative and good-natured. No one had any money—there were no wages. Everyone worked. Everything was free. A typical house, such as we were given, had a wash basin, a shower, and toilet, and in each room there were two chairs, a table, two day-beds, a chest, a built-in bookcase, and an electric light hanging from a cord. This was basic living. Anything that a couple could afford to add was their privilege.

We were impressed with the schools, the museum, the library, and the clinic that gave good service to the kibbutz's six hundred people. Our children had no problem with the Israelis, most of whom spoke a little English. They worked with them in the fields harvesting fruit and grapes, while Jane and I with the Links spent our days exploring and photographing the bottom of the harbor which, before the land had settled, had been the site of Roman buildings and walls. These were still standing beneath the sea. Also we gathered many interesting Roman pot shards from the sandy banks; we dug out more shards and a few Roman coins.

After leaving Caesarea, we flew across the Negev desert to Eilat, on the Gulf of Aqaba. To our astonishment, the salty water of this seven-thousand-foot-deep sea was icy cold and crystal clear. The color, through our face plates, was sapphire blue and the bubbles bright silver in the sunlight. We snorkeled along, dodging the jellyfish that trailed ghostly tentacles as they pulsed through the sea. And there were scorpion fish, six-foot "sea snakes," sea cucumbers eighteen-inches long that vomited out their guts when we picked them up, and lion fish that were completely tame, because their porcupine-like spines are tipped with a deadly poison.

On our way back, we passed close to Egypt and saw the site of King Solomon's famous copper mines. Great green hunks of ore still lay on that desert's sand. Next we went to Tel Aviv and to Tiberius on the Sea of Galilee, where we met again with the Links who had discovered a shipwreck and, with an Israeli archaeologist, were busy diving up beautiful intact amphora dating from the time of Christ.

We had a fine stay on beautiful Galilee and we visited the Bedouin camps and bought a goat from them to roast as we had learned to do in San Diego. After the feast, Jane and I sat on Galilee's rocky shore, listening to the tinkle of the tiny waves. We talked of the children and of home. "We've been lucky," Jane said, "to be able to see these places where so many of our traditions and beliefs were born."

I thought of the finite span of human life. Beyond a certain point it could not be prolonged. It seemed to me, on that night by Galilee, that Jane's and my interest in travel and history and archaeology had added length to our lives by projection backward in time. Our experiences might not have been so rich if we had had too much concern about what the future might hold.

22

Back to the Battle of the Breast

I HAD STARTED working in the laboratory before Jane's cancer had appeared. Since she too now had an acute and personal interest in cancer research, she joined me in the Mouse Lab. The scientific side of my studies there has been outlined already, but the lighter side was omitted. First, we had to become accustomed to the ways of the mice, learn how to pick one up, inject it, anaesthetize it, and operate on it. We learned to do autopsies on the mice and examine their lungs for metastases. Most important, we had to keep records of it all—accurate ones with names, dates, and numbers. This was a feat I could never have performed, but here Jane was a master.

We also had to learn about handling and anaesthetizing dogs, for we were heating their bone sarcomas and breast cancers. Often there would be medical students from the university who would come in, part-time, to help. It was a productive period of both Jane's and my lives.

We were busy socially too, for this was a period when many visitors were coming from abroad. The Cleveland Clinic was a high priority on many of their lists. They would watch me operate, then make rounds with me and follow me to the Clinic where they put on white coats and observed the examinations and needle biopsies that we performed in the office. Often I would call Jane and one or more of them would come home for dinner. One of these was Dr. Sem Pringpuangeo from Thailand.

Sem was about my age and a distinguished surgeon. He had successfully separated more Siamese twins than anyone in the world, and he was about to be appointed the head of Surgery at Bangkok's Women's Hospital which had 1,400 beds. His government had sent him to America to observe for three months and most of the time would be spent with us. Sem stayed at the YMCA lodge, but weekends that winter, we took him with us to the country, where together we roamed the woods and fields. Sem was a Buddhist, and Jane and I spent many hours discussing philosophy. I am not sure that Buddhism is a religion, because Buddha was a man, not a god. Among his followers there is a strong sense of spiritualism, but no belief in a supernatural Being. Soon we were converts. Ever since Sem visited us I would remain in close touch with him and often see him in Thailand. He would rise from the head of his hospital to be the minister of health and become a physician to the king.

At about the same time, we had another visitor—Rodney Maingot, a noted British surgeon and medical writer and editor of one of the most widely read English textbooks of surgery. Rodney stayed at our house and on one weekend went hunting with us in the marshes west of Cleveland. As a companion we brought along my sister Peg, who was a good shot. From that time on, Jane and I would have a fruitful relationship with Rodney on both sides of the Atlantic.

Reggie and Daphne Murley and Arthur and Kay Porritt came through Cleveland too during these years, and also became lifelong friends. And there were Drs. Jean and Fany Lacour, from Ville Juif outside Paris. Also Deborah Doniach and her pathologist husband Israel (known as Sonny). Vera Peters, a radiotherapist with a special interest in breast cancer, came to see us from Canada, and from her I learned a lot about the nonoperative treatment of cancer. Robert McWhirter arrived from Edinburgh, the first to back away from radical surgery and substitute simple operations and radiation therapy. He became a friend and once, in the early years, Sir Geoffrey Keynes himself visited the Clinic. That had been before his historic pioneer work on conservative breast surgery had been reviewed and reported by Murley. From France, we also knew Dr. Jean Papillon and Dr. Bernard Pierquin, who was the first to use focused nonpenetrating radiation directed through a proctoscope to destroy rectal cancers. In turn, Jane and I would visit these friends in their own clinics and homes.

My practice was shifting away from the thyroid to the breast, because as a result of our use of needle biopsy, performed in the office, and the modern treatments of hyperthyroidism, thyroiditis, and small nodular goiters, we were operating on less than a tenth as many goiters as we had been. We still saw as many or more than ever in the office, but we now could treat them medically.

During the 1960s, I was kept busy defending my unpopular advocacy of conservative surgery, for in both the field of thyroid and breast the controversy was a favorite subject for lectures and debates. At times, there would be three or four of these a month at medical meetings throughout the country and abroad. By then I had become immune to the diatribe that my surgical colleagues were heaping on my greying head. I knew that in England everything was going my way and that sooner or later in the U.S.A., in spite of the temptation to over-operate that fee-for-service medicine gave, the public would become informed and seek out surgeons who would not unnecessarily mutilate them. Then everyone would have to agree that the radical mastectomy was obsolete.

As for the children, by this time Joan had married Roger Foster, who had graduated from Case Western Reserve Medical School. Ann, not one to stand idly by, had promptly married Roger's medical school roommate, Caldwell B. Esselstyn, Jr., who had gone to Yale and been a member of Skull and Bones. Essy had rowed on the Yale crew and been a member of the U.S.A. team that won the Olympics in Australia. Essy's father had been a well-known surgeon and a pioneer in prepaid medical plans like Kaiser's. Much more important from my standpoint, the senior Esselstyn had been my freshman-year football coach at Yale.

That takes care of the elder children. Susie was growing up and was in Bennington College, majoring in art, in which she had inherited an astonishing skill, not from me, but from Jane who, although she had had no training, was clever at drawing cartoons in pastels. Susie would become a success at her career and in time join the art colony of New York, learning, practicing, and teaching art. George III was still safely in high school. That wouldn't last for long.

23

Some Thoughts
on the Training of Surgeons

🖋

AFTER THE publication of *Cancer and Common Sense* I no longer had any need to change my ways or my remarks to conform with the opinions of the majority. I therefore began to write occasional articles, some of which were published in first-class medical and surgical journals, about such subjects as the training of residents, the fee-for-service remuneration of surgeons, and the positions taken by some of the major surgical boards.

In 1934, when I had started my training at the Cleveland Clinic, the resident did no operations at all, although he did open and close incisions and assist at an enormous number of major operations, the technique of which, by sheer repetition and by working day after day with the same surgeon, he got to know by heart. It was in this way that up until about 1955, one generation of surgeons passed its skill on to the next. Then the American Board of Surgery got in the driver's seat and chaos ensued.

The American Board of Surgery originated with a group of surgical teachers who thought that the American College of Surgeons, which gave no examination and which offered membership to any ethical surgeon who had had an adequate period of training in an approved hospital, did not set high enough standards. The founders of the board wanted to establish a more select group of surgical specialists who had qualified not only by having had an approved training in an approved surgical service, but also by passing written and oral examinations.

On the face of it, one might have anticipated that this would improve the quality of American surgery and at first it did. There was more formal teaching on the surgical services and the residents studied more. Soon, however, the board, composed now largely of surgeons in academic positions, began to wield real power over American surgery. If that small group failed to approve a surgical service, residents would no longer apply for training. This not only downgraded the reputation of a hospital, but also made it difficult to give the patients the surgical care that is normally given by the eager and hard-working house staff.

If the board had judged the services on the basis of their teaching value—in effect, whether or not their residents could pass the examinations—all would have been well. But instead approval was based largely on whether the residents were given "full responsibility" for a specified number of major operations. For a time many excellent teaching services were put on probation, or approval was withdrawn because the residents were not allowed to operate independently and assume "full responsibility." Yet these same professors, who were insisting that residents who had not yet finished their training should have full responsibility for major operations, disapproved of noncertified surgeons operating at all.

The worst of this period was that many of the younger academic surgeons, using "full responsibility of the resident" as an excuse, began to withdraw from the operating room and spend their time in the research laboratories where they could "follow the road to promotion and fame." This was the period in which the government was still heavily subsidizing research, and in which "Publish or Perish" became the watchword of the academic surgeon. As a result, the technique of surgery often became a lost art. The blind were leading the blind. Residents who were largely self-taught were teaching interns and junior residents. Except on the private services, despised because the surgeons didn't often allow residents to operate on their private patients, there was no one to set good technical standards. In many of the university hospitals the mortality rate of standard operations actually rose—this was in spite of all the advances in anesthesia, antibiotics, and the treatment of shock. In one university hospital, the mortality rate of the radical resection of the rectum rose from less than 4 percent in the period when the professor of surgery was personally interested in colorectal cancer and was doing or supervising most of the operations, to 19.5 percent in the period when the responsibility for the operations had been delegated to the residents. This does not mean that 19.5 percent of the patients eventually died of their cancers.

It means that they died in the hospital as a direct result of complications of the operation. This is because in these operations, survival depends very largely on the technique employed and on the skill and experience of the operator.

I do not mean to imply that all university and teaching hospitals abandoned good technique and relegated full responsibility to their residents. But even as late as 1971, a survey by the Professional Activities Study asked the question, "Does university hospital care differ from that in non-university hospitals?" To examine this question the records of 3,583 patients having their gallbladders removed in university hospitals were compared with those of 2,625 patients having the same operations in non-university hospitals. The average age of the patients in the two groups was identical—fifty-one years. The average weight, blood pressure, proportion with gall stones, or with complications such as jaundice were the same in the two groups. It was found that many more complicated tests were done in the university hospitals than in the others. Nearly twice as many transfusions were given. The average hospital stay in the two groups were 14.3 days for the university hospitals and 13.7 days for the others. The incidence of practically all complications was a little higher in the patients of the university hospitals as was also the incidence of postoperative deaths—1.6 percent to 1.5 percent.

The advent of Medicare and Medicaid had a profound effect on the practice of surgery in teaching hospitals. The government, in its ultimate wisdom, stipulated that it would not pay the surgical fee unless a qualified surgeon was in attendance. This resulted in loud screams from academia, when the professors suddenly found that they would have to perform or at least be present at and responsible for the operations done on what used to be the ward or charity patients. The "teaching material" overnight became a source of considerable revenues to the hospital, which quite naturally insisted that its surgeons comply with regulations so that the fees could be collected.

In spite of my unorthodox writings and beliefs, I had friends among those who were leaders in the profession, with the result that in 1950 I was elected to the American Surgical Society—the honor society of American surgeons. To my astonishment, I received about twenty letters and telegrams from my personal friends, like Chuck Mayo, or from my father's friends, like Donald Balfour, or from people like Lester Dragstedt with whom I had shared common interests and for whom I had had the greatest respect. I had also been elected to the Southern Surgical and Central Surgical Associations.

At about the same time that I was being elected to the surgical societies I received a letter from one of my heroes—the person from whom I had learned more about principles of surgery than from anyone else. It was from Allen Graham who, before the war, had been in charge of the Cleveland Clinic Pathology Department:

> I have just read your article on Thyroiditis, *Annals of Surgery,* April 1948:127, 640. So far as I know it is the first article in American Literature that clearly and consistently differentiates subacute (pseudo Tbc), thyroiditis, struma lymphomatosa, and Riedel's Struma. Congratulations. Marvelous! There isn't a single flaw I can find in it.
>
> Would appreciate a reprint if and when they are available.
>
> Best regards.
>
> Allen Graham
>
> P.S. Illustrations perfect.

Dr. Graham was the first in the United States to identify Hashimoto's Thyroiditis (struma lymphomatosa) and to me, a compliment from Graham was a tribute above and beyond belief.

The Surgeons' Club continued to meet, each year in a different city—Boston, New Orleans, New York, Chicago, Detroit. In Cleveland, the junior member of the group would introduce them to his associates, give operative clinics and present and discuss the problems of patients. Then his wife would arrange for all to dine at his home and to fish in the backyard pool, into which, on the day before, a plentiful supply of live trout had been introduced. I don't know about the others, but Jane and I had a wonderful time.

I can't remember just when it was, but in the early years before I lost my professional reputation by advocating less than radical mastectomy, I was one of those who met together with Dr. Glover from Cleveland's St. Luke's Hospital to discuss organizing a Cleveland Surgical Society. This was the only political organization I ever became involved with, and that was not for long, because after the *Cancer and Common Sense* debacle I would never again be on any committee. But before that time I had made one contribution. I suggested, and it was so arranged, that instead of having elections, as most local societies did, we would avoid all local animosities and politics by simply making eligible for membership anyone who was a member of the College of Surgeons or a diplomate of the American Board of Surgery.

24

A New Look at Life

SOON AFTER Mother's death, my sister Elo's son, Crile Crisler, who had been training to be a surgeon, gave me Konrad Lorenz's book, published in 1952, about animal behavior. It was called *King Solomon's Ring* because, according to legend, it was the king's magical ring that enabled him to talk with the animals. Lorenz explained that if you understood animals and knew how to "imprint" them on you, it required no magic to converse with them. Lorenz was the first to define in scientific terms the well-recognized phenomena that patterns of behavior must be established early in life or they can never be learned. Moreover, if they are established early they will never be forgotten.

Jane and I had always enjoyed having dogs and rabbits and the ordinary pets that are readily available, but we had never before appreciated the importance of imprinting. Immediately, we began to acquire more exotic creatures—crows, woodchucks, or any other animal that we could obtain when it was still young. A young naturalist, David McKelvey, was at that time just beginning to work at the Cleveland Museum of Natural History, and he too helped us to obtain young and imprintable animals and educated us about animal behavior and the importance of such things as timing in the process of learning. It is established that people, after the age of sexual maturity, can rarely learn to speak a foreign language without an accent, whereas a baby learns to speak perfectly just by listening and babbling. The host of applications of this point of view fascinated us, and Jane loved having the animals in the backyard and at the Knob.

At this time in the development of our relationship with animals, Jane, who was a trustee of Laurel School for Girls, gave a Hawaiian luau for a new headmistress. We had learned the technique shortly after the war when I had been sent by the Navy on a fact-finding expedition to Japan and on the way home Jane had met me in Hawaii. And so we had a deep pit dug in our back yard, in which we buried red hot rocks, unhusked corn, and a young pig. As the steam rose from the husks, the pig cooked slowly all day long. The luau was a smash, but the next day it rained and we had a pond instead of a pit. "It would be nice to keep it this way," I said. "It's a duck pond," Jane agreed. So we dug it a little bigger, lined it with concrete and had a pond for our ducks and geese and a swan.

Knowledge of Konrad Lorenz's studies had opened a new vista of thought, and we derived great pleasure from exploring it. I was even beginning to consider writing a book on the subject. But Jane's and my interests were by no means confined to our friends and animals. We also had continued to make movies of our journeys throughout Mexico, Hawaii, Europe, the Middle East, and the Orient. Twice, during the next four years, we would go around the world, for since a great deal of North-South travel is allowed free of charge, round-the-world trips are by far the most economical as well as the most interesting way to see the globe.

The pyramids of Egypt were just amazing as everyone had told us they would be. No matter how much one has read about them, they still are unique when, for the first time, they are seen. But far more mysterious to us, and much more exciting, was the Tomb of the Bulls. We had been riding on horseback across the desert, near the site of ancient Memphis. Suddenly there was a flight of stone steps that led down to a gate of stone and a quarter-mile-long tunnel in the solid rock. The light from the guide's flare was dim, but on each side of the wide tunnel we saw great chambers chiseled out of the stone, each one large enough to contain a gigantic granite sarcophagus in which once a bull had been entombed.

Why had the Egyptians spent their meager resources in this interminable task of carving tunnels and burial chambers in the solid rock that lay below the desert? Was this as much of a waste of time and energy as are our present expenditures on atomic armament and the exploration of space? Three thousand years from now, which of the great monuments that we are constructing will appear to our descendants as incomprehensible as the Tomb of the Bulls is to us?

From Egypt, Jane and I went on to explore more of the Middle East. Since both of us had been brought up in the Homeric tradition of the Iliad and the Odyssey, we felt as if we had personally participated in the siege of Troy. We could not lose an opportunity to see for ourselves the ruins of the city where the romances and adventures of our childhood had taken place. We boarded a freighter in Istanbul, which carried us through the Bosporus, the Sea of Marmara, and the Dardanelles, stopping from time to time, to take off or put on freight. The sea was crisp and blue. The distant mountains were purple in the haze. The people on the ship were good-natured and helpful, and most of them spoke some English or French.

It was dark when we arrived at Canakkale, about twenty miles from Troy. Then, with the help of the ship's second officer, we arranged for a taxi to meet us at four in the morning. It would take us to Troy and return us to the freighter by sailing time. That morning we had only a brief impression of Troy. Here nine cities had been uncovered, one on top of another. Six cities had arisen and fallen before Homer's Troy was built. The ruins of all of them were there for us to see. The rising sun gave color to a scarlet flower in a crack between two immense blocks of brown stone. It was as though the blood of the Trojans still flowed on the Walls of Troy. On the plain beneath the mound on which the ruins of Troy VI were exposed was a boy with his bleating sheep. He showed us a handful of coins that he had found in the fields as he grazed his flocks. We bought a few.

On the way back to the boat, we reread Homer's account of the Trojan War and came to the passage that told of the tempest that, on the voyage back to Greece, cut the fleet in two and "brought part of them to Crete where the Cyndonians are settled"—and Homer went on to give details of the area where the Greek fleet was lost. Jane and I decided that we would search for it. The day after our return to Istanbul, with Homer as our guide, we set off for Crete.

In Heraklion we rented a car and told the agent where we wanted to go. "But no one lives there," he told us. "You will have no place to stay." What did we care? Hadn't we slept in the caves of Petra? We drove over winding roads cut in the mountainside, with no banking or railings. Two of Homer's landmarks, Gortyn and Phaistos, were on the way and both had been excavated. Gortyn had once been the capitol of a mighty kingdom that included Libya. Over its Minoan remains were those of Greek, Roman, and Byzantine cities, all now fallen into rubble and dust.

Finally we came to the deep Bay of Matela where a strong wind, like the one Homer had described, was blowing. The waves were breaking against towering cliffs in the face of which were scores of handmade caves, with paths between them, cut in the solid rock. We stopped in amazement. We had never seen or heard of such a thing. Then there was a shout. In a moment the mouths of the caves were filled with people. An old man, with great white mustachios and wearing black baggy Turkish pants, came up to greet us. A crowd of boys gathered and followed us, as we were led to the biggest cave which was the bar-café. Inside a dozen windblown fishermen were sipping little cups of coffee and tall thin glasses of water. No one spoke a word of English.

"Germanicos?" one of them asked.

"Americanos," Jane replied.

The man behind the bar spoke to one of the fishermen, who then left the cave. Soon he returned with a wiry old man, who asked, "Where are you from?"

"Cleveland," Jane replied.

"That was my home for forty years," he said. "You know Lorain?" It was thirty miles from Cleveland and we knew it well. "I built ships in Lorain. I am Stanislas Merikavis, and I welcome you to Matela."

What luck! When Stanislas heard what we were looking for, he introduced us to Elias Fassoulakis, a schoolteacher, who knew much of Homer by heart. He was so learned that we called him "the Professor."

When Stanislas translated the passage of Homer which described where the ships were sunk, the Professor grew excited. "Phaetos, Gordyn, Iardanos," he cried, and each time he pointed and then talked to the fishermen in Greek. When he came to the part about the smooth cliff running down to the sea, the fishermen nodded and gestured. Then came "the little bit of stone that keeps off the great wave" and there was animated discussion. The Professor turned to us. "They know where it is, but today it is too rough. We can try tomorrow. The wreck you are looking for is by Papadoplaka—the Sacred Rock."

Then the Professor showed us the caves in which the peasants were living. They came here on vacation from the hot plains of the interior to enjoy the sea's cool breeze. Some of the caves were half underwater, for this part of the Mediterranean shore, weighted down by the gigantic Delta of the Nile, was slowly sinking into the sea. There was one cave whose entrance was completely underwater and into which we could dive and see the white bones of a skeleton, gleaming in the reflected light. In Roman days these caves had been used for burials. In one of our dives we came up with a flat round black object about the size and shape of a discus. We thought it was a relic from Minoan times, but when the children who had been watching us saw it, they screamed and ran. It was a World War II land mine, one of which a couple of years before had exploded and killed some people.

We drove back, along the cobblestoned Roman road to the area that the Professor called Bouboulia. Here was a vast plain strewn with shards and fragments of artifacts, some of which, including a loom weight, dated from the days of the Minoans. The Professor had known that there were ruins here, and ancient reservoirs—Cisterna Neolithica, he called them—but had not known that they were Minoan. From the summit of the plain, where it plunged down four hundred feet into the sea, we stood on the brink and again read Homer. Every one of the distinguishing features of the landscape were here—the cliff, the sloping rocks, the river, and even Papadoplaka, the "little bit of stone," which stood a hundred yards off shore in the shape of a craggy island a hundred feet high and the same in diameter.

We went back to the cave in which we would spend the night, and spread the blankets that the Professor had arranged for us to borrow. As the sun set, we sipped our ouzo on our stone balcony and then had supper at the bar-café. The next day we would go out with the fishermen and dive for and photograph the wrecks.

We did as we had planned, but instead of finding just Menelaus's shipwreck, we found three of them—great piles of amphora and ballast, and probably many artifacts too, but they were so welded together by salt and coral that it was hard to break anything out. Through the centuries, the wrecks had been undisturbed because there was no sponge diving in this part of Greece, and no one before this had come to Crete with any sort of diving gear. We brought specimens from one of the shipwrecks back to the museum in Heraklion where the amphora were identified as Roman. But the loom weight from the plain of Bouboublia was different. The archaeologist was excited. "You have found a Minoan city," he told us. "No," we said, "it was the Professor who led us to it."

"I knew about the ruins," the Professor said, "but it is they who recognized them as Minoan." And so ended our first adventure in Crete. We planned to return with more knowledge and better equipment.

Again, we were brought up short. Three months after our trip to Crete, Jane and I were returning from a duck-hunting trip when she said her shoulder was stiff and it hurt her to take a deep breath. The next day an X-ray of the chest showed two little metastases in the lungs and a huge mass of lymph nodes in the right central part of the chest—the opposite side from her breast cancer and therefore probably metastases from the lung metastases. It was a fatal combination, but X-ray therapy could shrink the big mass and make life more comfortable. Exposure of the lungs to radiation intensive enough to destroy the pulmonary metastases would cause disastrous damage to the lungs. Dr. Effler, our thoracic surgeon, advised that after the radiation to the nodes, the nodules should be removed.

Two days after that operation, Jane was home and three days later she presided over the dinner that we always gave for the residents before the Christmas Dance. Three weeks after that, when the nodes had shrunk entirely away, Jane and I joyously packed up to fly to Nassau with Susie and George and Jane's sister Ann and her husband, Bob Little. Their boys were the same age as our two and our families were close. Before the trip was over, Jane was padding around with face plate and flippers and photographing the reefs.

Illness, it seems, is often what a patient makes of it. Its duration can be prolonged or considerably contracted. To her illness, Jane reacted with simplicity. She was aware that there was little chance of permanently curing the cancer that had spread to the lungs. Yet she showed no trace of fear. There was sorrow, but not dread. To Jane, faith in those she loved was infinite, "heaven was here and now." Her philosophy was expressed in a note she had written Joan at the time of her operation:

> Take a good look into the heart of the universe, Joan. Somewhere out there you will find that time and space are infinite and beyond our comprehension. That leaves us the alternative of living from day to day.

Jane's philosophy was helpful to me as well as to Joan, for not only was I living with the knowledge that my wife had a fatal disease, but my brother Bob, at this time, also was diagnosed as having an incurable cancer of the lung. Bob had smoked very little, but he had worked for a company that was using beryllium, a radioactive material. Inadvertently, he had had a significant exposure to its dust. His time was to be as short as Jane's. At the end, the two of them would go down the road almost together. It would be the end of an era.

25

The Last Underwater Film

尖

I T WAS 1962. Jane and I had been talking to our friends at the National Geographic Society about our adventures in Crete and had showed them our film on Menelaus's shipwreck. They were enthusiastic and offered to meet us there with an archaeologically oriented photographer who could help us prepare an article for the magazine. Also Jane had never seen the Far East. China was not yet open, but we decided to visit Japan, Hong Kong, Thailand, Indochina, and India on our way to Crete. Thailand was our most important stop, for it was there that we would see our old friend Sem.

By now Jane was as fit as ever. We made only a brief stop in Japan, seeing the sights around Tokyo, and we enjoyed the diversity of Hong Kong before being met in Bangkok by Dr. Sem. We would stay overnight at his spacious house in the outskirts of Bangkok. The next morning we boarded a DC-3 along with Sem and flew north to Chiang Mai on the Burma border, where Sem had grown up. In the teak forest, to which Sem brought us, we watched the elephants pile the logs, each under the control of its personal oozie, who had grown up with that elephant and worked with it since both he and the elephant were children. This was an example of Konrad Lorenz's imprinting of both man and animal.

Back in Bangkok, we visited Sem's huge Women's Hospital—1,400 beds and still growing. There was a sort of assembly line from which an average of forty babies a day were delivered—one about every half hour. When a new baby was added to one end of the line, an older one was taken off the other and given to its parents. It was a model of excellent organization, as was everything else that Dr. Sem was concerned with. He showed us also a pair of Siamese twins that very soon he was planning to separate. They were nine months old, sitting up, crying, and seemed to be fighting with one another.

Dr. Sem took us on a tour of the waterways of Bangkok, for the city has as many canals as Venice, and to the great Buddhist temples, so perfectly constructed and preserved in this land. We saw the Temple of the Golden Buddha, where resided a newly discovered five-ton, life-sized statue of Buddha made of solid gold. It had been covered with plaster to protect it from invaders and had been forgotten and for centuries had lain in a junkyard, before it was dropped by a crane and the plaster cracked open to expose the gold. There was the Porcelain Temple, too, with its facade, walls, and towers all gleaming with cups and saucers that had been taken from a wrecked British ship and set in cement to gleam in the rays of the sun.

At the end of the morning, we visited the Temple of the Emerald Buddha, the most sacred spot in Thailand. I had told Sem about Jane's problem. "I want to take her to the Temple of the Emerald Buddha," he had said. "Things that come also can go." The temple was set in the midst of a shimmering complex of tiled, gold-roofed shrines that surround the Grand Palace. An old priest was telling fortunes by shaking a set of sticks in a cylindrical box. Sem gave Jane a coin for the fortune-teller. She pulled out the stick that was highest up in the box.

"What did you wish for?" I asked her.

"Not much," she said quietly. "I don't want to make it too hard for the Buddha."

We took off our shoes and followed Sem into the temple. High above, in the candlelight of the altar, sat a child-sized figure of the Buddha cut from jasper, emitting a glowing radiance of green. It was still in the temple. The light was dim. There was the faint smell of incense. "It would be easy, with the Buddha glowing there above, to listen to the whispering of the dream," I thought. "Let everything just go on as it is today. But that would be asking too much of the Buddha. We are here to contemplate, not to pray."

After Thailand, our next stop was Vietnam and we were impressed with the strong representation of our military wherever we went. Then we crossed over into Cambodia, which was in a state of turmoil, although its ancient shrines were still inviolate. One of these, Angkor Wat, was huge and derelict and all overgrown with trees. Deep in the rain forest it stood, what was left of it, and as we explored the ruins, we came upon a tiny *sanctum sanctorum*, a room not over ten feet square, in which was a stone image of the Buddha. As we had approached, there had been the smell of incense and we had seen the orange robes of a priest flitting through a doorway. Before the

Buddha, a candle burned. This great shrine had stood for centuries forgotten in the jungle, until in the 1800s a French explorer discovered its ruins.

The vehicle Jane and I were riding in was sort of a cross between a jeep and a truck. The roads were rough and rutted. Jane's back was still sore, because just before we left she had had some palliative radiation to some metastases in her spine. And so both of us were happy when we said good-bye to Cambodia and hello to our favorite island, Crete. There we met all of our old Cretan friends and others from the National Geographic. We finished our own documentary film on Menelaus's shipwreck, and we worked with the National Geographic on what might have been an article for the magazine. However, we didn't see eye to eye with the cameraman, who never seemed to be around when interesting things happened or when the sun was rising on the spectacular views. We didn't care, because Jane's and my film caught them and we had some good, clear-water shots of the wrecks and of our attempts to sample their contents. We thought that in the area that Homer so clearly defined, the wreck of Menelaus's vessel still lay. The archaeologist from Heraklion's museum, who at first had been skeptical of our beliefs, ended up by agreeing. "Everything Homer mentioned is here, just as he described it," Constantine Davaras said. "We will have to make a report to the archaeological journal. I cannot deny now that you may be right." In 1964, Constantine Davaras and I would indeed publish in his archaeological journal an account of our findings. We concluded, "As the spot at which we found the Rhodian wreckage seems to correspond in every topographical detail with the one that Homer described, we believe that the site of Menelaus's shipwrecks could be in this area."

Besides her back hurting her in Cambodia, Jane had other problems. While in Crete, she began to have a nagging headache, a symptom she was quite unaccustomed to. With a lot of wishful thinking, we ascribed it to her having spent so much time diving on the shipwreck. It seemed to get better, as we flew home, where we found to Jane's delight that Joan was about to bear our first grandchild. Jane and I were still deep in our Konrad Lorenz studies of the phenomenon of imprinting, and so on the first Saturday after our return, we went to the country to buy some baby wood ducks for our backyard pond. I was driving and Jane was reading aloud. She asked to change places, saying, "It's hard for me to read on this bumpy road." We traded and Jane, rounding the corner into the duck-farm's drive, drove off the road and into the ditch: "I didn't see it!" That was because she had lost all vision to the left.

Dr. Gardner, the neurosurgeon, knew at once that the problem was a metastasis to the brain. Tests confirmed the diagnosis. Soon her left leg was paralyzed. Radiation therapy had been started. The last thing Jane said to me, before she lapsed into coma was, "Don't worry. There are three pieces of unfinished business. There's Joan's baby. There are those experiments in the lab. And there's the story of Menelaus's shipwreck to write for the archaeological journal. Don't worry. We'll get them done."

We had been working in the Mouse Lab on giving massive single doses of radiation, and in some types of tumors had found them more effective than the usual divided doses spread out over weeks. Here there was no time to spread out the treatments. I consulted the radiotherapists and we decided to give Jane a big blast of cobalt radiation and cover it with the administration of cortisone to reduce the swelling. For six days she continued to lie in coma. My reaction was not so much sorrow as despair. It seemed suddenly that there was no pleasure in living, no possibility of life again containing novelty and warmth and charm.

On the sixth day The Miracle occurred. Jane woke up. At once she recognized me. "I think I'm better," she said.

Jane had no memory of those terrible six days. In another week, her recovery was complete—vision and all. Two weeks after that, she was back in the Mouse Lab. In another week, we had sent off the material to the Cretan archaeological journal *KPHTIKA XPONIKA*. A week later, Joan's son, Roger III, was born. Jane's three predictions had come true. Also we had started to write a book about our travels. We would call it *More than Booty*, the title coming from the Koran: "We had traveled far and wide in the lands under the sun until coming home satisfied us more than booty."

During the next six months, we would look again at some of the films we had made in far-off lands and on the bottom of the sea. We sat in the sunroom overlooking the pond and became better acquainted with the colony of mallards and wood ducks that now inhabited our backyard pond. We spent pleasant weekends at the Knob with the children and our new grandson. Ann gave us the news that she was expecting her baby in a few months, which made Jane happy. We even revisited Andros Island in the Bahamas and attended a meeting of the American Surgical Association in Florida, where my medical school classmate and lifelong friend, Bert Dunphy, had dinner with us in our room. Bert had married a classmate of Jane's at Smith. He was one of the world's most successful and delightful surgeons.

That night, Jane and I talked of perhaps spending a month in Tahiti, where both of us had long wanted to go. Tahiti would be but a dream. For Jane and me, Florida was the last of our travels. By the time we got home, she was losing her muscular coordination. The part of the brain that controls thought and speech was unaffected, but she could not care for herself. She returned to the hospital.

During this period of her terminal illness, Jane wrote in her journal:

> Our life was good. Everything, but never too much of anything. Of course, the secret is our tastes are simple, our resources plentiful and we have been good companions and we have laughed and loved a lot.

On the evening before the day that Jane finally lost consciousness, I had been reading aloud to her from Jack London's short story, "How to Build a Fire." It brought back memories of snowy nights in Canada. "We've got to go moose hunting again," Jane told me. We spent the rest of that evening planning the trip.

The home memorial service, presided over by a Unitarian minister, was short and simple:

> We are gathered together in memory of Jane Crile. If you seek her memorial, look about you—in the hearts of her family, in the faces of her children, in her writings and in her home.
>
> Life has been given and life has been taken away. Life and death are one, even as the River and the Sea are one. Death is only a horizon, and a horizon is but the limit of our sight.

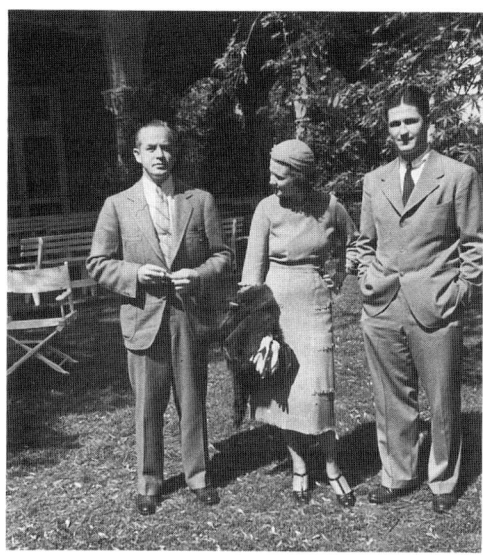

Chuck and Alice Mayo with Barney during one of the Surgeons' Club gatherings, St. Louis, 1938.

Barney Crile's model, Dr. Tom Jones, who was at the peak of his career when Barney joined the staff of the Cleveland Clinic.

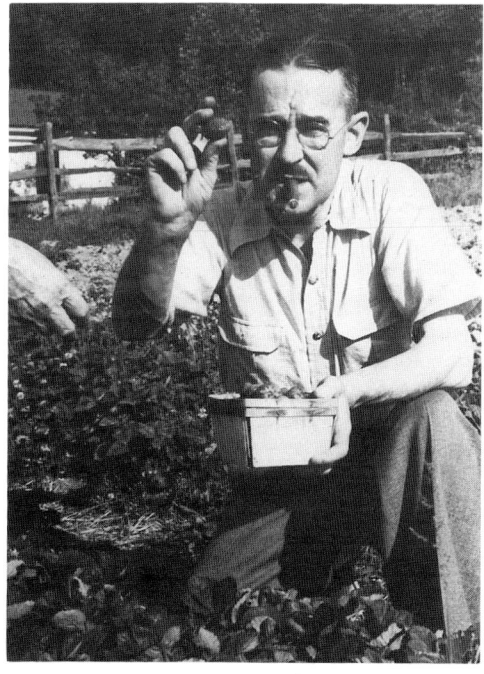

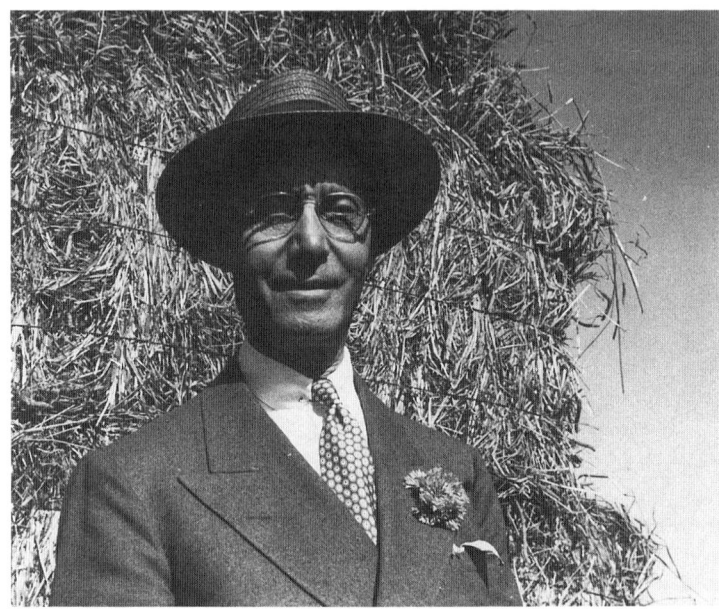

Sam Halle, Jane's father, at the Halle farm circa 1940.

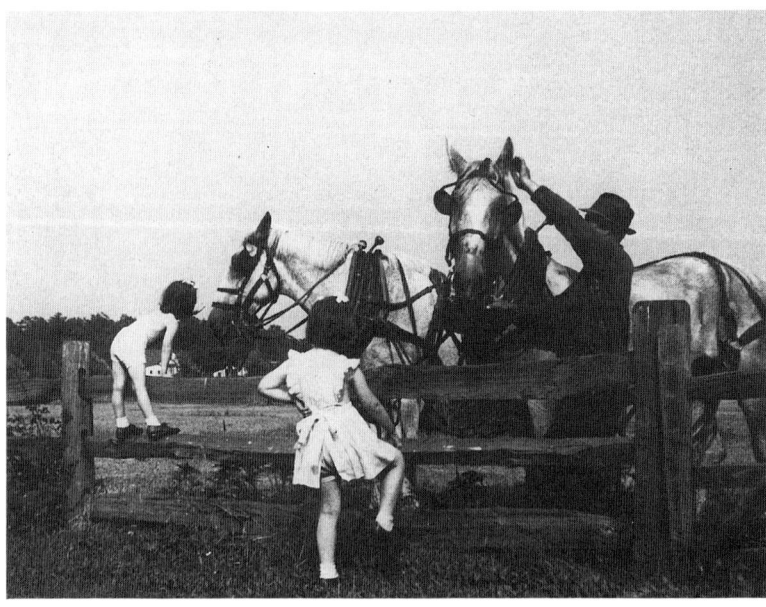

The Crile children spent summers at the Halle farm. Here Joan, left, and Ann help out, circa 1940.

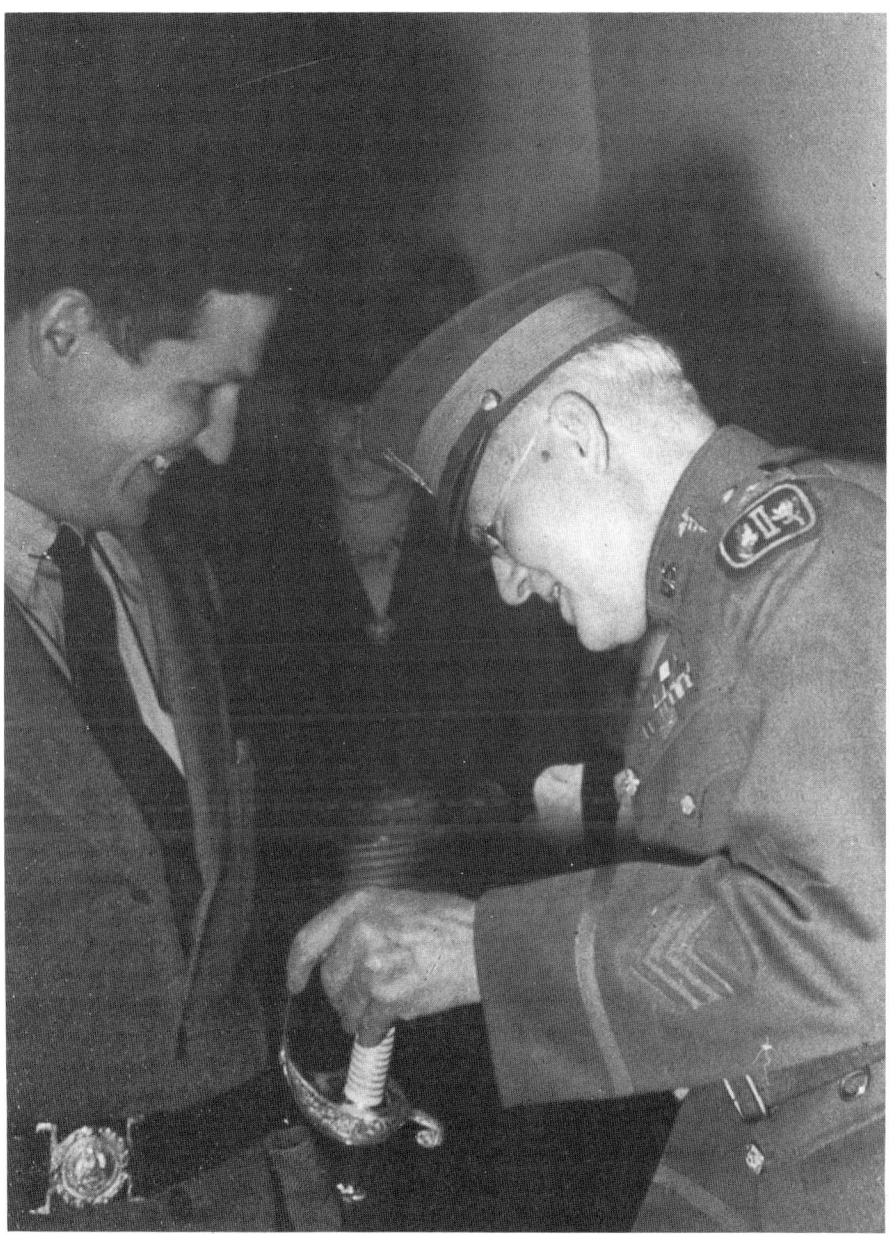

The occasion was Armistice Day, November 11, 1941—the Chief's birthday. It was likely Barney soon would be off to war, so his father gave him a sword he could use to surrender properly.

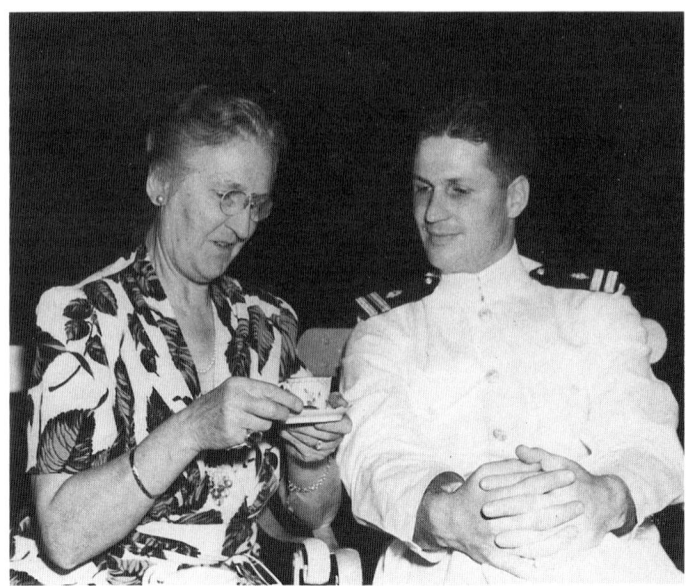

Grace Crile and her son Barney on the eve of his departure for war, 1942.

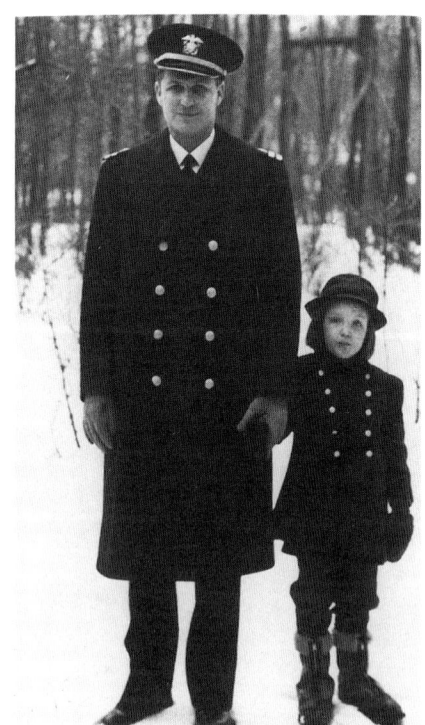

Barney in uniform with daughter Ann, 1942.

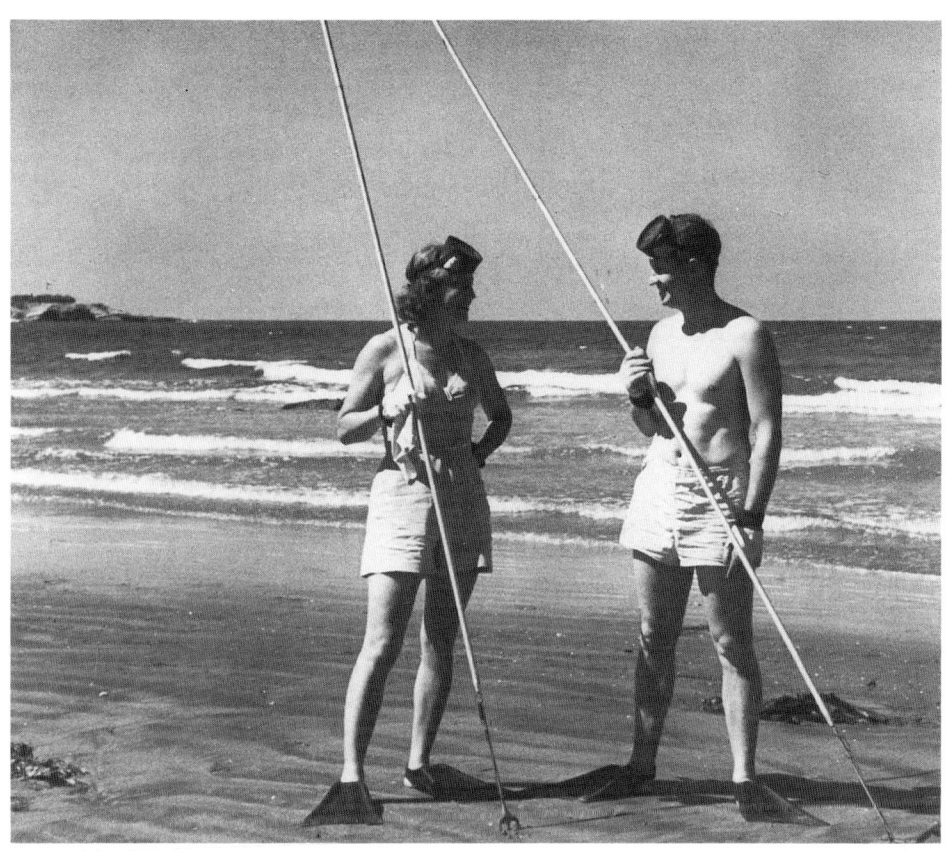

Barney and Jane spearfishing at La Jolla after Barney's return from New Zealand, 1943.

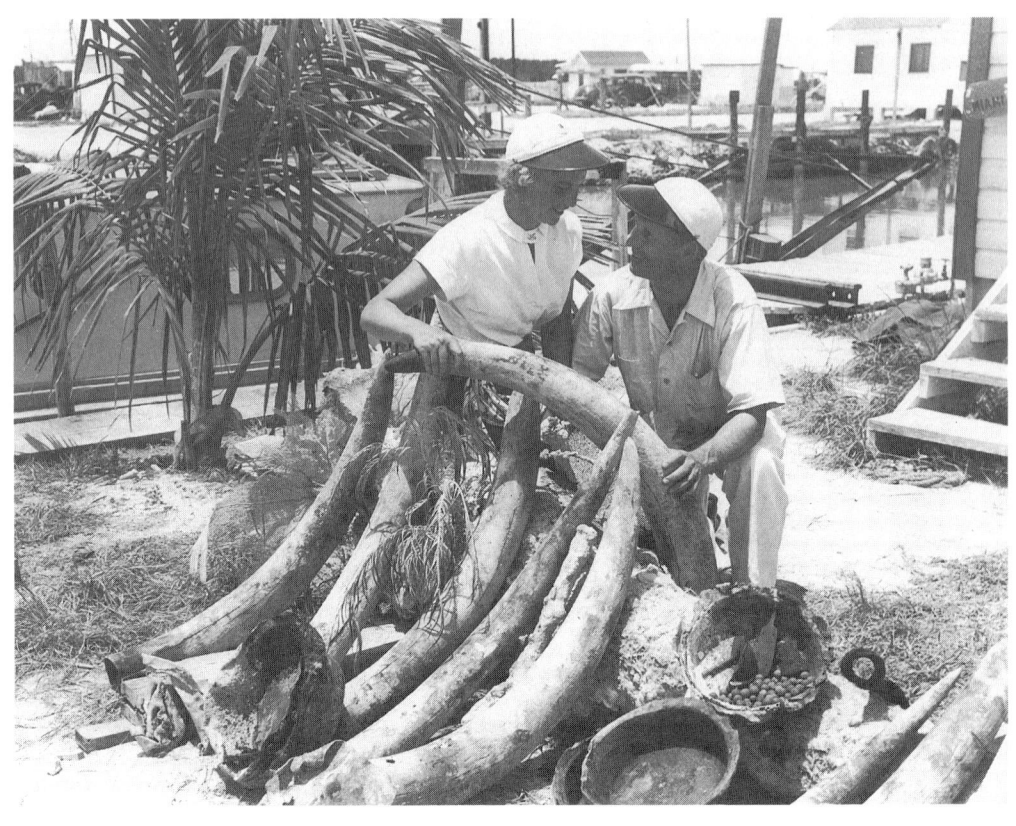

Tusks Barney and Jane salvaged from the Ivory Wreck off the Florida Keys, 1948.

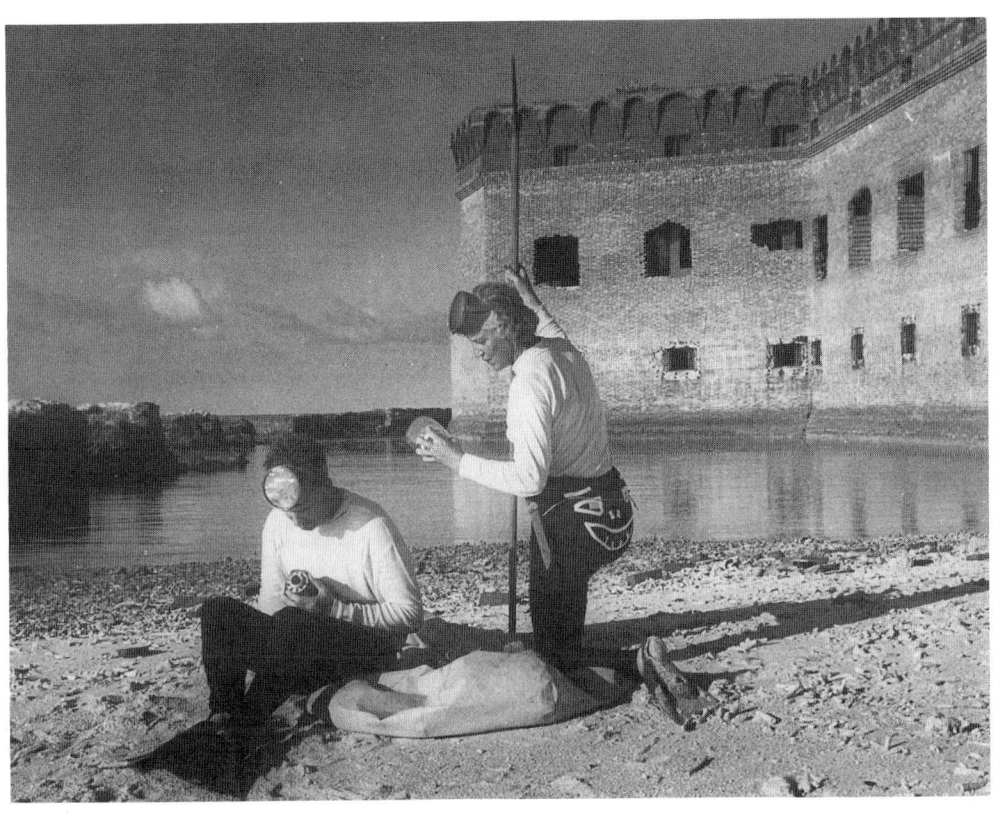

Barney and Jane at Fort Jefferson in the Dry Tortugas, circa 1950. Barney holds the 16-mm camera in a rubber rebreather bag, his solution for underwater photography.

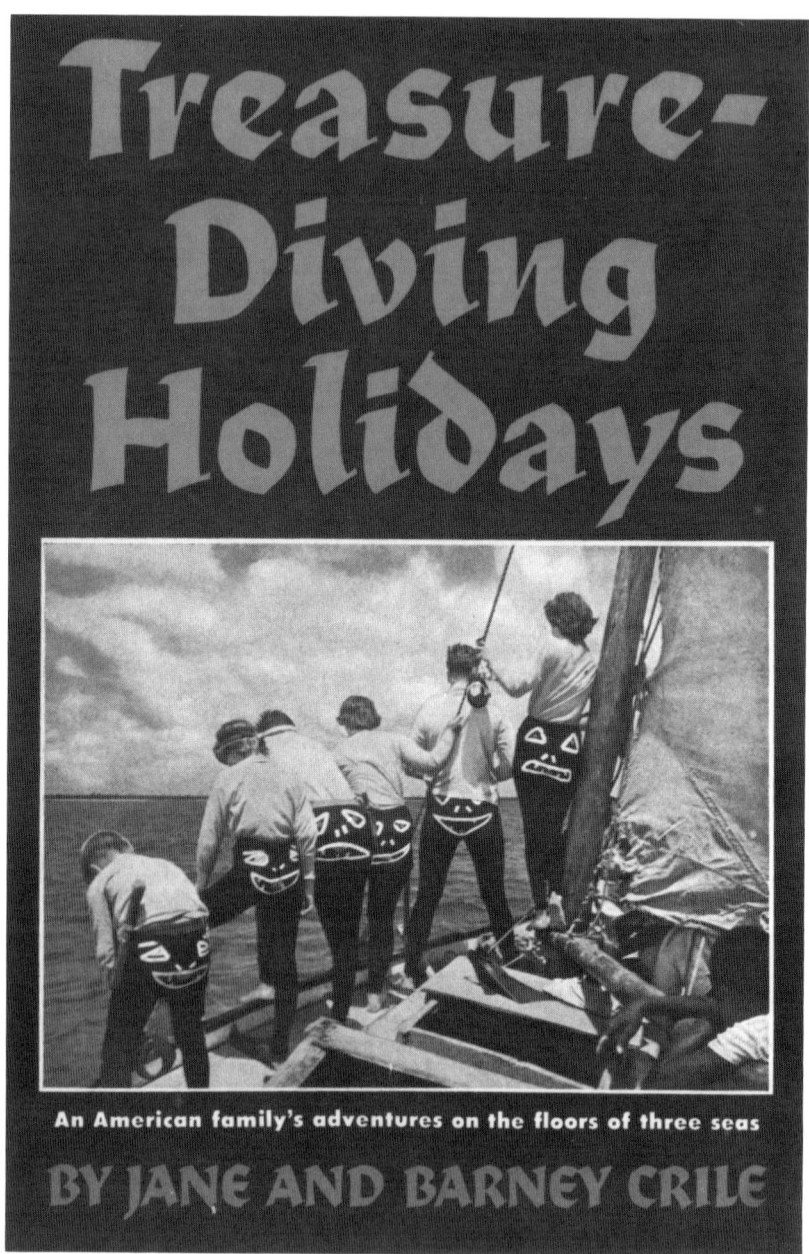

Treasure-Diving Holidays

An American family's adventures on the floors of three seas

BY JANE AND BARNEY CRILE

The Crile family shared treasure diving adventures. Jane and Barney published this chronicle of their experiences in 1954.

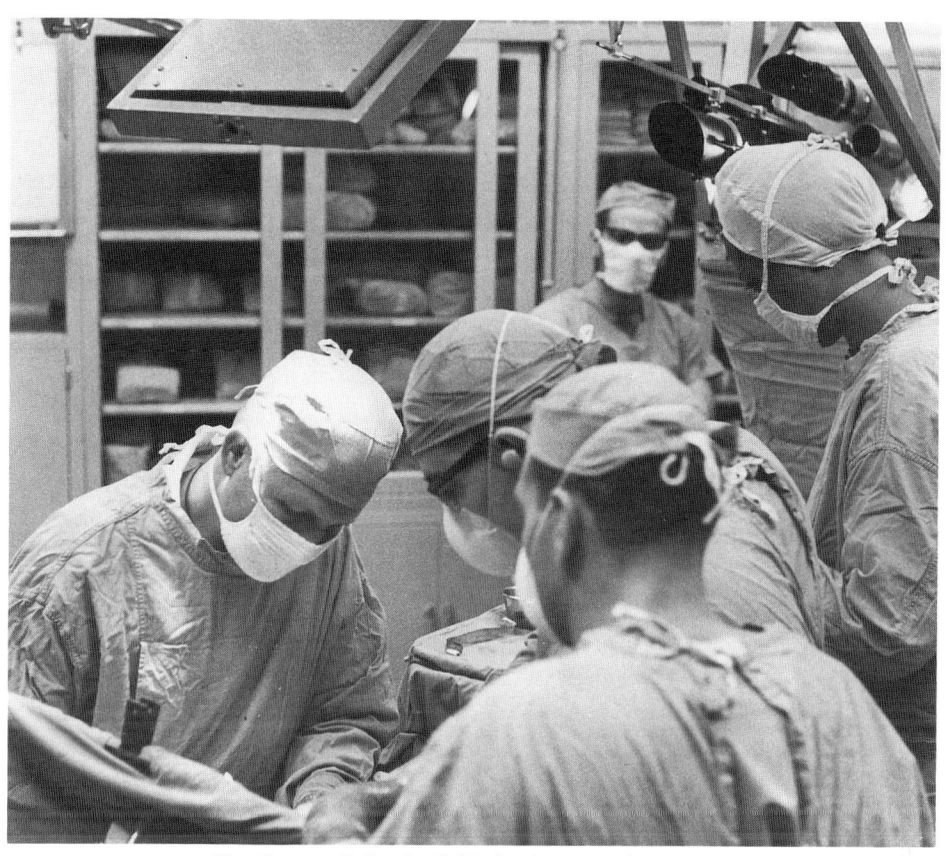

Dr. George Crile, Jr. (left), in the operating room.

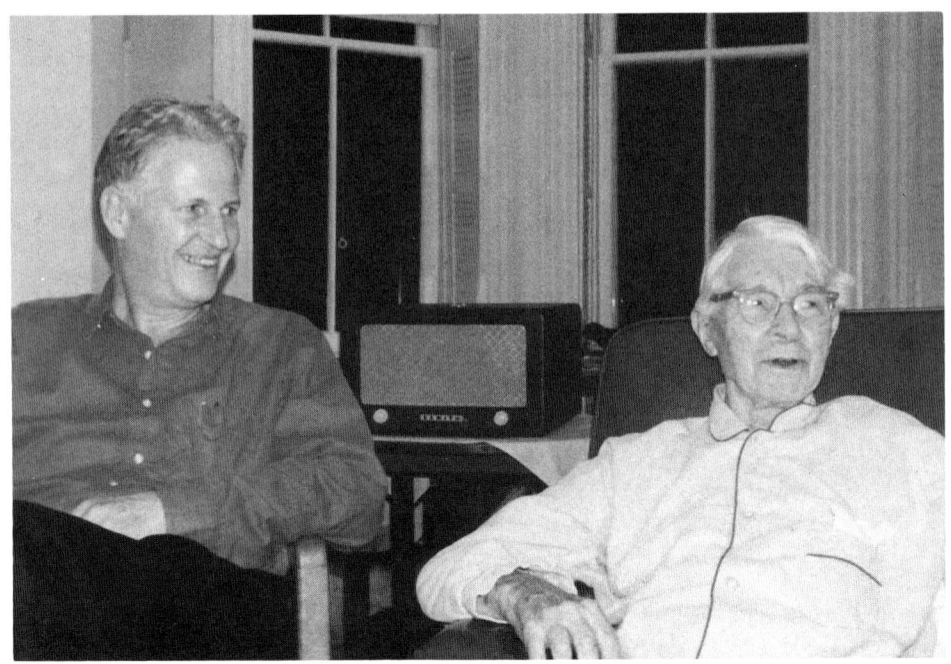

Barney and Helga's father, Carl Sandburg, on a visit to Connemara in North Carolina, 1965.

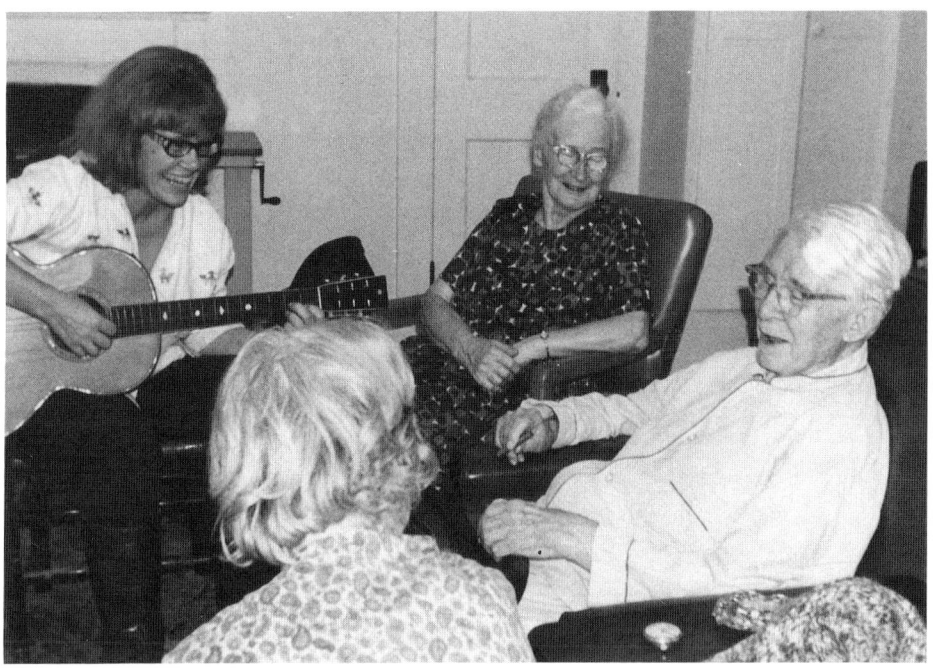

Helga and her parents, Lilian and Carl Sandburg, at Connemara.

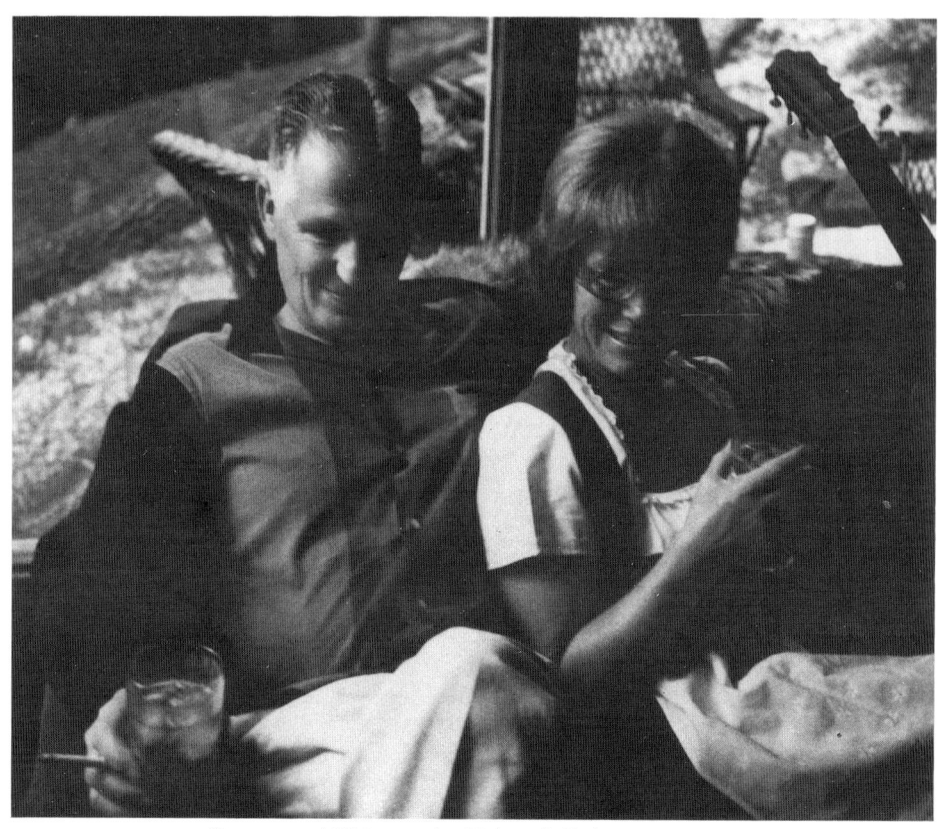

Barney and Helga at the Unicorn's Lair, 1966.

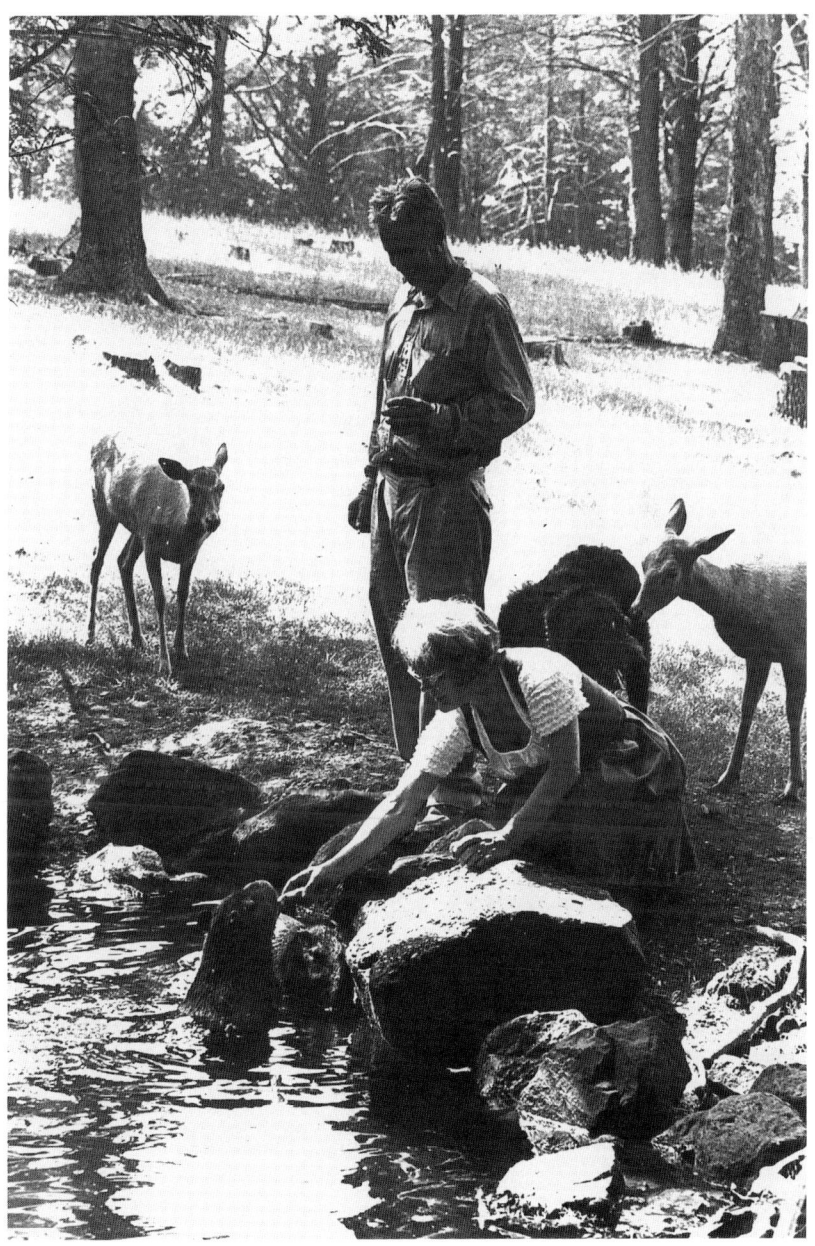

Barney and the two fallow deer watch Helga feed the capybaras at the Lair, 1967.

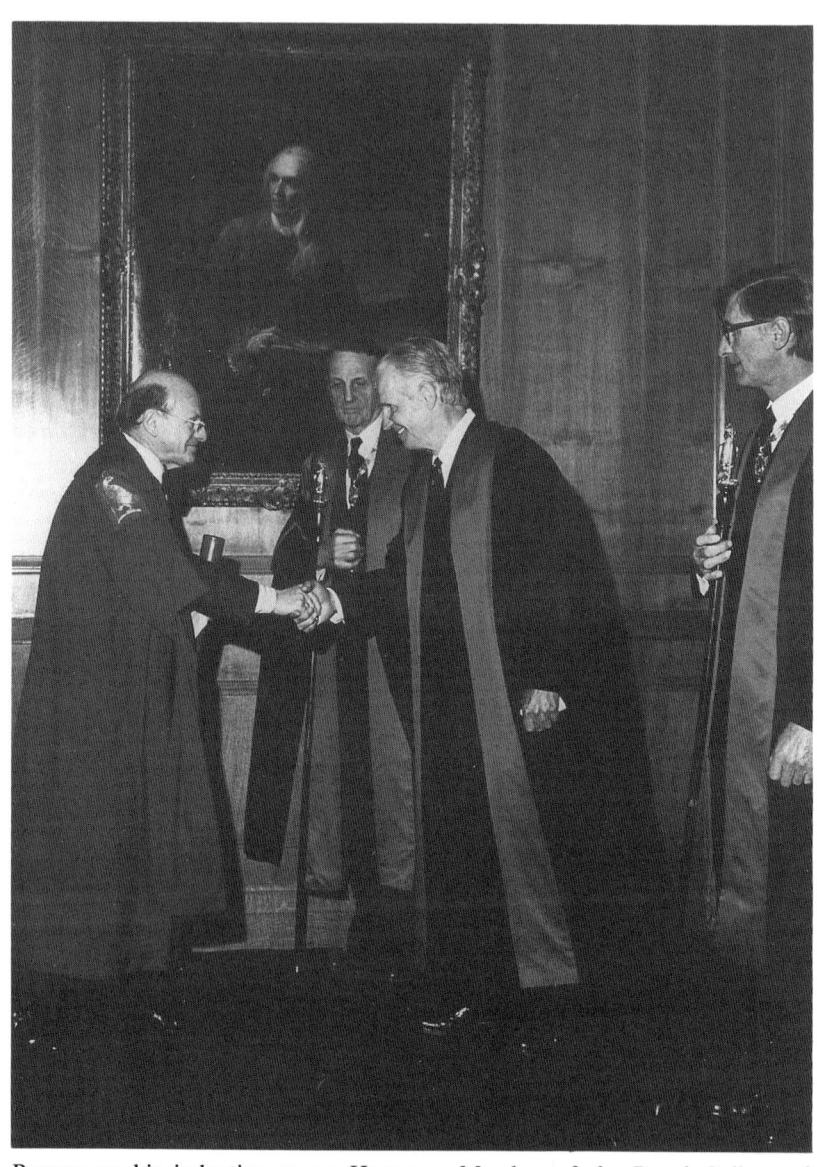

Barney on his induction as an Honorary Member of the Royal College of Surgeons in England, 1978.

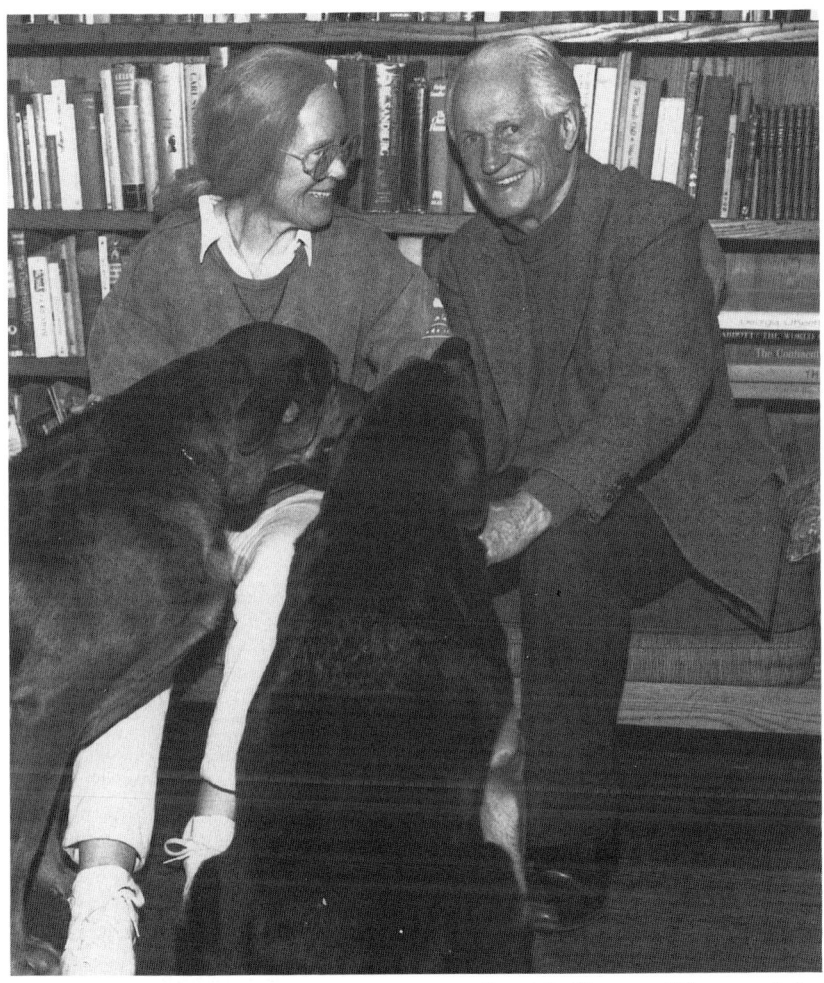

Helga and Barney at home with friends Mowgli and Rolf, 1990. (Photograph by Tom Merce.)

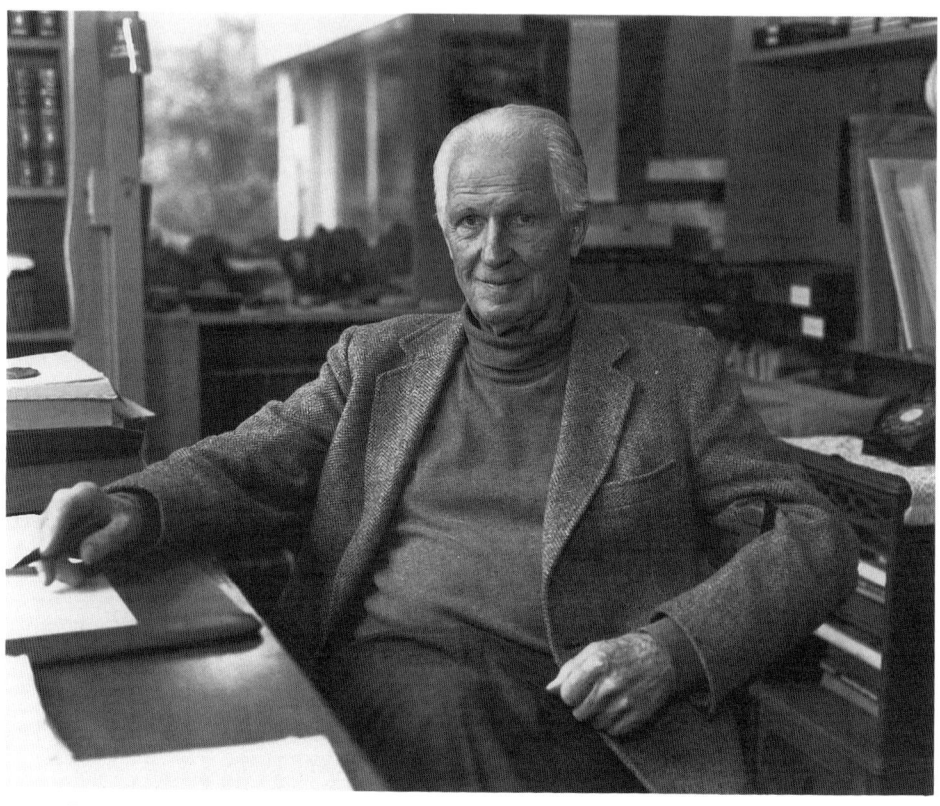

Barney Crile in the "Reminiscence" period of his multifaceted life. (Photograph by Tom Merce.)

26

The Interlude

WITHOUT JANE, my life was empty. Fortunately, about a year before she had died, a lifelong friend of ours who was living in England had heard of Jane's illness and wrote us telling of an au pair Swiss girl who had been doing housework for her and who wanted to come to America. At just this time, when Jane was sick and our housemaid, cook and companion, Barbara Thaine, age eighty, had decided to retire, Marianne Amman arrived from England.

Marianne was twenty years old, red-cheeked, vigorous, and weighed about two hundred pounds. She had a good English vocabulary and a strong Swiss-Deutsche accent. In no time she learned to drive a car, shop, cook, and take care of the house. Then Jane died and I needed someone to take her place, helping me in the laboratory. Marianne was elected.

We were studying the factors that prevented the spread of cancer that were implanted on the feet of mice. On the first day Marianne tried to pick up a mouse and of course was bitten. She didn't scream or drop the mouse. She just asked, "Do they always do that?" I knew that she was going to be a success.

To learn the language of science, which to the uninitiated is a foreign tongue, I had Marianne take a night course in biology. The first time around, she couldn't understand enough English or science to make much sense of it, but then she repeated the course and got straight A's. Now she could converse with scientists. She became invaluable in the Mouse Lab, for she was not only a skillful technician but an original thinker who came up with many helpful suggestions.

The weekdays were tolerable for me. I was busy seeing patients, operating, writing medical papers, giving medical talks, and also trying to finish Jane's and my book, *More than Booty*, which was the tale of our adventures together both above and below the sea. Its dedication would be:

To the memory of
JANE CRILE
Who wrote part of this book
And inspired all of it
—Barney Crile

In 1965, it would be published by McGraw-Hill. I think of it as a memorial to Jane. On the cover, under the title, was the explanation: "A naturalistic account of certain adventures shared in marriage and encountered in travels throughout the world."

A month before the release of *More than Booty,* a shortened version called *The Feather of a Dove* would be published in *Redbook* magazine. That title came from an experience that Jane and I had had in the Great Mosque of Omyad, in Damascus. We had heard the haunting call of the muezzin summoning the faithful to prayer. Silently, they knelt on the rugs, in attitudes of supplication. As Jane and I had sat in the blue shadows of the open mosque, a feather from the wing of a dove floated down from the dome and fell between us. "The mosque had seemed open to all of nature, quite willing to embrace either the birds of the air or men of various faiths," we had written.

All of these occupations were lifesaving, for they kept my mind off my loneliness. I could stand it during the week, but Saturday nights were impossible. Ever since I had reached sexual maturity, except for the time on the ship going back and forth to New Zealand, I had been able to find the companionship of a woman. Now there were none. I decided to organize an expedition and search for one. I needed a knowledgeable guide and a volunteer was available in the form of my old friend, André Pacatte, who by now was living outside Washington and was practically in charge of the whole Berlitz Language School. We decided to accept an invitation from Jane's sister, Margaret Sherwin, and take a cruise with the Sherwins in the Bahamas. On our Bahamian adventure we would encounter many tourists and many cruise ships and many wealthy widows who were wandering about looking for something or other, but not for André or me. After a while, we gave up and came home.

Before we had left I had told Margaret about the problem of Saturday nights. I told her also about my problem with the ladies around the Clinic and my hang-up because of my father's early teaching about

346

sheepdogs not killing in their own flocks. Soon after I arrived home, I had a call from my next door neighbor and lifelong friend, Betty Moore. Unbeknownst to me, Margaret had called her and told her of my needs. Betty, who knew all the choice available women on the east side of Cleveland, started what was later to be known as the "Widow of the Week" Venture, in which unattached females of suitable age and proportions would come to supper with the Moores and me—a different one every Wednesday night.

It would be very impolite for a bachelor, who had been honored by having a lady come to supper with him, if during the next week he did not ask her out. Having been properly brought up by my well-mannered parents, I made it a point to do so. At first it worked perfectly, but gradually a problem developed. You couldn't just drop a friend after the first Saturday night, you had to ask her out again. But there was a new one every week, and there were only seven days in the week!

Soon I found that I was out *every* night. I found myself nodding and dozing off at 7:30 in the morning, as I was scrubbing my hands in preparation for the eight o'clock operation. I was in an almost desperate situation, when I was saved by the advent of spring and of a basic change. I met Helga.

Helga Sandburg was the youngest daughter of the poet and in her own right the author of four novels, four children's books, and two books of poetry as well as a songbook and many articles and published poems. She was on the lecture circuit. She delighted her audiences with her songs and her guitar. She had been twice married and had two grown children who were no longer living with her. During the early 1960s, I went to Washington regularly to give surgical clinics and lectures for the Armed Services Medical Corps. On these trips, I usually stayed with Jane's sister, Kay Halle, who lived in a charming house in Georgetown. On the memorable evening of May 31, 1963, Kay gave a little party for me. Among the guests was Helga Sandburg, picked by Kay for me. I have a vivid memory of where I was and what I said when we met.

We were on Kay's patio, with five or six of Kay's friends, for she was a veritable matriarch of Washington's high society. I was sitting on the porch, when there appeared a golden-haired young woman, unescorted. They told me she was Helga Sandburg, and introduced me to her, but the name "Sandburg" made little impression. In my English course at Yale the poets were Keats, Shelley, Tennyson, and Browning. No one had ever heard of a Socialist named Carl Sandburg, who came from Chicago. I had vague recollections about something to do with

Lincoln, but I'd never seen the book. The first question I asked Helga was what she was interested in and what was her occupation. She said she wrote poetry.

"But you can't make a living out of that!" I exclaimed. Oddly enough she didn't turn and stalk out of the room.

Helga and I at once found ourselves deeply engaged in discussing literature. We ate a hasty supper, bid adieu to our astonished hostess, and hand-in-hand tripped down the hill under the blooming magnolia trees. We were on our way to Helga's favorite nightclub where her friend, Charlie Byrd, played. I whispered in her ear during the performance and the manager scowled and hushed me.

Helga's apartment was filled with memorabilia. There were paintings, some of them by herself, some collected on her trips abroad for the State Department and others by famous friends of hers, for Helga knew everyone in Washington's world of arts and letters. There were comfortable couches, a pleasant view of the broad avenue, and a spacious double bed. In the early morning hours, I began to worry that Kay would be wondering what had become of me, so I made arrangements to pick up Helga in the forenoon and take her with me for the weekend to André and Connie Pacatte's farm in Marshall, Virginia.

I have a vivid memory of Helga, dressed in country clothes and something like a bonnet that made her look as demure as an Amish girl. She slid into the car beside me, guitar in hand as we were off for a glorious weekend—walking through the fields, riding André's horses, rollicking and reveling in the first happy time that I had had for two years.

Helga had been brought up on a farm in Michigan and then had moved to another in North Carolina, where her parents had a vast pre–Civil War estate on which they had a few horses and pastured and milked a large herd of dairy goats. There was nothing about the outdoor life in which Helga was not an expert. In fact, I soon came to the conclusion that "What any woman can do Helga can do better." (Twenty-five years later, I still stick to that story.) When we parted, I said, "Good-bye, darling, it's been great fun." Helga picked up the phrase and made it into a song which she sent to me in her next letter.

> We parted at the station and he turned to me,
> The whistle stared blowing, he got ready to run,
> He kissed me on the cheek rather hastily
> And said, "Good-bye, darling, it was great fun!"
>
> Good-bye, darling, it was great fun,
> Great fun, but I've got to run,

I'll call you from Chicago or from New Orleans,
I'll send you a postcard from Washington.

First I got an airmail from Penobscot Bay,
Then it was a letter stamped at Willow Run,
And each of them was ended in the same old way,
Saying, "Good-bye, darling, it was great fun!"

Helga composed a sweet tune that went with the song and sang it on her tours and would publish it, music and all, in her second poetry book, *To a New Husband* (1970).

She also sent me a poem she had written that night after I left her apartment. It would be the lead and title poem in the book she would be putting out in 1965:

The Unicorns
(For B.C.)

Why my dear, almost at dawn now, when the light
Is a little like twilight, does a mourning dove
Mourn through the stone branches of the buildings
Of this town? Why, in the streets below, do the hooves sound,
Of a snow-white unicorn stepping by, he who is
Love And Disaster, hoping to be seen and known?
Why, my darling, is this the hour of births of children
And goings of lovers and prayers of disciples?
Why, in the countryside now does there ring a noise
Like bells tolled from farm to farm, as the roosters,
The red-capped dawn boys, stand strained
On scaléd legs, and in strange unholy voices proclaim
All the unicorns walking in the lanes and ways?
Why, when I run from you, my dear, and down the stair
And follow him to announce that I see and recognize,
Does he turn his pale blue eyes on me and frown
And leap and clatter away as the dove's cry mourns
And dawn breaks red over the old buildings of the street?

I was overwhelmed. Here was a woman who made no promises, made no demands, had a marvelous sense of humor and who was completely independent. I'd never seen anything like it. I tried my best to respond to her unicorn poem:

You ask me why, my love, why just before the time of dawn
Did my hooves clatter in the streets below?
Why did I look at you that once, the whole of you

349

Standing in the hallway, unabashed?
And then, my white coat pinkening in the break of day,
Run sobbing down the stairs and through the streets away?
Why did I leave you and the softness of your arms
And flee away to distant dread alarms?

Why? It was dawn, my love,
The dawn that breaks the night-cast spell,
And sends all of us, we unicorns
Back to our special daytime hell,
Sends us clattering down stairways and through the streets
Out into the furtive unsubstantial world of light,
Where dreams become reality.
But dreams must always wait for night.

There was no question that Helga and I were drawn together by forces beyond our control. Nevertheless, both of us had commitments for the summer. Helga was on her way west for a lecture tour and to stay for a couple of months with her longtime friend, Douglas Riseborough, the noted Renaissance-style painter, who had a cabin at Kootenay Bay in Canada. I was committed to go to France with André Pacatte, and to meet there my son George and a lady with whom André and I expected to travel through Switzerland. Then on to Norway, where I was going to speak at an international surgical meeting. It was all very complicated, but Helga promised, on her way west, to stop and spend a weekend with me in Cleveland.

The weekend was perfect. Helga was delighted with the Cleveland Heights house, its duck pond and rabbits, the nicely imprinted golden pheasant that roamed the fenced-in yard and the lovely big white mute swan, Jupiter. We had a big Saturday night party on the top of the Knob with all my family and the most musical of my friends. There was a barbecued unicorn (actually a goat), in honor of our poems, and also Helga's songs and guitar as we sat around the bonfire. The whole world seemed bright and warm again. That night there was thunder and lightening and a storm that shook our little cabin.

Then, on Monday, Helga was off.

Dearest Helga,

It seems very lonely here.

Somehow we never did get to the atlas that night to plan out your trip—and mine—but this is what I would like to do. We could be at the most eastern spot that the State Department would send you to, and fly from there on east stopping in Athens or Istanbul or Beirut, as you wish, or Cairo. Then on to India (brief—as it is very unpleasant) and Ceylon where I would like to spend about a week. Then Bali, Formosa, Hong Kong, Tokyo, Hawaii and home. We could do it easily in a month. The cost of round the world passage would be little more than that of a one-way flight to Europe, if you tossed in the return fare that is provided for you by the U.S.A. [Helga had been lecturing for the State Department in Europe and in Scandinavia.] That expense I could easily manage, but it would be well to have them send you as far to the east as possible.

I will miss you on horseback and in the porch of my cabin this weekend—so get to work on our "engagement." (Did you see Susie's eyes when I spoke of it? I of course was referring to our "engagement" to go around the world together. Susie loves you dearly.) And tell me how you like the Great Mountains and the Misty Sea.

> Vive l'Unicorn et l'affaire
> My love
> Barney

And again:

> Saturday
> The Knob

Helga darling,

It is an exciting afternoon. I am in the little "summer house" on the edge of the cliff and a great wind is stirring the trees and moving the paper. I just reread your letter for the third time and there is a great wind blowing within me too. For the first time I feel that you have talked to me from the deep reaches of what is really you. That kind of talk leaves me restless as the gusting wind. I need to curl myself up in a little whirlwind and engulf you and carry you off.

You put your pen on what disturbed me, Helga, and made me scold you a week ago tonight. You wrote that you set your work apart and never shared it with those you have loved. Thus it never occurred to you to share or rather to enter into the things that are important to those who love you. That, I felt, was true until Monday night in the kitchen when we drank beer and got engaged for a trip. That was when we became each a part of the other. Then I knew we could work together.

You and I have one thing in common, Helga. It is the urge for creativity. Once one has felt it there is nothing but emptiness in a life that does not fulfill that urge. I am not a good writer but I love to write, I love to rewrite, and eventually I can say what I want to say. It is all so much simpler and quicker, though, if I have someone to work with. We will try it.

I can make no long-range plans and I cannot talk of marriage. I can love you and I do love you but it is still a compartmented type of love. Perhaps I will never again be able to love completely because Jane and I grew up together from the time I was 13 and our lives were so inseparably intertwined in community of interests and in a passionate physical love that I am not certain whether anything but fragments of that old life can ever be made to live again. It is strange, though, that since you left me I have wept more for Jane than I have in many months. Perhaps our parting was like an echo of the other.

I knew a number of women before I married Jane and I knew several in New Zealand during the war, and I have known several since Jane's death. Physically speaking I find little to choose between the women I have known. Love-making, the act of it— seems to be a common denominator—a sine qua non—but not the essence of love. Jane and I shared the essence and you and I have come closer to it than anyone else I have known. I feel a promise in you, Helga dear, and I think that when we travel together that promise will be fulfilled.

In the meantime I will not attempt to be faithful to anything but our promise. I am still wandering, fascinated, through a world of new experiences and interests. I will be travelling this fall with interesting people—a writer—an artist—a musician. None of these people stir me but each of them awakens an interest in things that otherwise my life might not touch. It would be so much better if it would be you, for the whole trip, and you alone.

It took me seven years to marry Jane—seven years after we first became very close. Things move faster these days because the span of life does not afford the luxury of time. So we will love one another from a distance, see one another when we can, travel together next year for sure and we will watch together with spellbound fascination to see what the evolutionary process of fate holds in store for our still separate lives.

I am glad that you love me, Helga, because I love you too. For suddenly there seems to be something again to write for.

I will send you "King Solomon's Ring" and what clippings I can find on Imprintation. Also I will send you the manuscript that Jane and I tried to write. [*More than Booty* had not yet been published.] Don't try to read it in detail, but I would like you to see what my difficulties are. There is a chapter in it on imprintation. I am going to write a speech on the same subject, starting now.

Thank you for bringing me back to life—

Love

B.

Then I was off, too, and soon met up with my son. George, who was of draft age, had been in Germany doing some sort of CIA work which our neighbor Dan Moore had been able to get him into. It was good to see him again, but André and I had a hard time when we got to Switzerland. We were visiting the mother of a young man who had been a classmate of George's. The problem was that George and I found ourselves sometimes competing for time and space. George was courting his friend's sister and I had taken off after her mother. The evening ended with nothing accomplished. George and I decided that we might do better if I took my friend and went to Norway and he returned to Germany.

In Norway, at the meeting to which I had gone alone, I found myself in the twilight of a long northern day in a bar and bowling alley in the basement of a hotel. A beautiful, forty-odd-year-old woman was there with a rather inattentive man. I found out that he was her brother, that she lived in a nearby baronial estate, and that she was very much interested in talking to an American surgeon, for her father had been a doctor. She was here just for the weekend visiting the family estate. Her husband lived in Oslo.

By this time Vivi, for that was her name, and I had had a couple of drinks and her brother seemed agreeable to anything we decided to do. We all piled into his chauffeur-driven car (for no one in Norway dares both drive and drink) and set out for the castle. It was too dark to see the details of the wooded park, in which the old stone building stood, but the interior was furnished just as it should have been with bear skins on the floor and horned heads on the wall, and a great stone fireplace. The brother went to bed and Vivi and I lit the fire to keep off the chill and spent a totally satisfactory night. At the break of dawn she called a taxi for me and we made arrangements to meet again for dinner in Oslo. She would be with her husband and I with the lady whom I had left there when I went to the meeting.

After an uneventful dinner with Vivi and family, André met me again and we went on together to Istanbul, where we knew a local leader of society named Buran Serif Saru. Her father had been treasurer for the last sultan and her present husband was the editor of the country's largest newspaper. I had known Buran after World War II, when she had been between marriages and was a reporter for a newspaper. She had met my neighbor Dan Moore when he was in the CIA in Turkey, and after the war had come to Cleveland and lived in Dan and Betty's attic. In Istanbul, Buran was very kind to André and me and arranged dates for us.

We met Buran and our girls at a famous dance hall and restaurant, located in a beautiful setting on the banks of the Bosporus. Since André was younger, to him was allotted the eighteen-year-old professional dancer, who was lithesome and dark-eyed and beautiful and spoke not a word of English. We relied on André, as head of the Berlitz system, to work that one out. My companion was a golden-haired, amply endowed actress. Everyone in Istanbul knew Belkes. When she entered a room, all the men clapped or stood up, and cried, "Belkes, Belkes!" She was the Zsa Zsa Gabor of Turkey and the ultimate authority on matters of Love and/or Marriage. Whenever anything pertaining to sex arose, Belkes would be on the front page with her interpretation of the event. She was a lot of fun.

Belkes had been married three or four times, but at present was single. She lived in a hotel with her mother, but she had a friend who was a radiologist. She said that he kept X-raying her because he thought she had gallstones. "Do these stones need a treatment—an operation?" Belkes asked me. We discussed the pros and cons at some length and in doing so consumed two or three drinks. Buran's husband had arrived, and was looking restless. "Perhaps I could examine you, Belkes, and then I could better tell if you need an operation. Could we perhaps go to your hotel?"

"No, no, we could not do that," Belkes said, "My mother is there. She would not allow it." Then she turned and spoke in Turkish to André's friend. "She says she has an apartment not far away," Belkes told me. "We will go there."

André and I had a rented car, so we said good-night to Buran and set off over the hills and vales of Istanbul, heading inland toward the center of the town. We stopped at an apartment building, and André's friend let us in. The apartment had two bedrooms and a living room and a bathroom. The only furniture was a bed in each bedroom. There was no other furniture. The place had just been rented and was not yet settled. I took Belkes to the examining room. The examination lasted much longer than I had anticipated. Sunrise was illuminating the hills, when I knocked on what I thought was André's door. There was no one there. André, petrified by the thought of being left alone with an eighteen-year-old, had driven her home.

André hadn't known there was no telephone in the apartment. We had no way to call a taxi. Belkes had on a sparkling, extremely décolleté evening dress, with no sign of a bra to control the bumping, as we jogged through the empty streets of Istanbul, up and down over the hills, heading for what we hoped was the Bosporus or a place where we could find a taxi. She was a wonderfully good sport about it. Hand-in-hand we were hop-skip-and-jumping when up drove a car and a man got out. Belkes ran up to him.

"I am Belkes," she said.

"Of course," he replied, for everyone knew Belkes.

"I have with me Dr. Crile from Cleveland. We have to get to our hotel. Could you call a taxi for us?"

"You say it is Dr. Crile?" the man asked in English.

"Yes, the surgeon."

Then came the coincidence that one would not have dared to put into fiction, because it would sound too absurd, "I am Dr.——" [I'm ashamed to say I do not remember his name]. He turned to me, "I just finished reading your article about the new treatment of breast cancer! I have been on a house call—an emergency—and I have just gotten home. Please let me take you where you wish to go."

We were thunderstruck with wonder and gratitude. The good doctor took Belkes safely home to her mother and left me at my hotel. I am forever grateful to him.

That's the way travel with André was—fun, but pretty exhausting. I was glad to get home, to Cleveland. I had no idea what had happened to Helga. It was toward the end of September now. Had she settled down with her friend in Canada? What were her plans? I called her to find out. Helga had had a lovely summer with Douglas, had written a children's book called *Gingerbread*. There never was a time when Helga wasn't at work on something. Yes, she had a speaking engagement in Columbus on the first of November and would stop off then and spend a few days.

At home, I was as busy as ever with surgery and lectures. I was working from 7:00 to 7:00, and my schedule was completely filled. I didn't renew my relationships with the widows of the week, because soon Helga would be coming by. I still didn't know how things stood between herself and Douglas. Every night I worked on the book that Jane and I had started. Most of it was done—at least I thought it was.

Then Helga came back. She settled down to do some writing of her own and to give me some superlative editorial advice about *More than Booty.*

By now Helga had become a part of the household and all of our animals were as firmly imprinted on her as on me. Before long, we began to talk together of the other book that I had in mind, *A Naturalistic View of Man.* In this book, I hoped to put emphasis on Lorenz's views of imprinting and their significance in people when applied to the importance of timing in the process of learning, and of the factors that related sexuality as well as emotional stability and the organization of society. Helga was as interested in the subject as I was, for her personal experience with the rearing of animals had been greater than mine.

It was becoming more and more obvious that we two should be working together. Every night, as soon as I returned from work, we would go over the suggestions she had made during the day. I remember one evening when I came in and she was typing. She is the fastest and one of the most accurate typists I have ever known. I walked across the room to her. She looked up at me and gave me a lovely long kiss, and kept right on typing and never missed a word. It was then and there that I decided that this woman was both unique and indispensable.

For example, it was on a weekend during this period when our neighbor, Dr. Perry McCullagh, looking at the leaves of a willow tree against the red and gold background of the maple forest, happened to ask, "What makes the willow stay so green?" Helga reached for a pencil and made a note. As a result came one of my favorite poems.

Dear Love I Said to You
(For B.C.)

Dear love, I said to you from in the dream,
Say what makes the willow tree so green,
Say what makes the light on pale skin gleam,
Say while we lie together in the dream.

Your mouth on mine I hear your heart repeat,
The willow's roots are long and dark and sweet,
The pale light is the space where voices meet.
Then where is love? I heard my quick heart beat.

Love, you said, is of its own self wove,
It is not us; there is no act to prove
In its green time this thing will choose to move,
And then into the dream stood love.

356

It would be the last poem in her book, *The Unicorns*, that would come out in a couple of years.

There was no decision to make. It was inevitable. "We'll wait till Christmas when John and Paula [Helga's children] can be with us," we said. In the meantime, we were making arrangements to move Helga's things from her Washington apartment to our home and to the Knob. She wrote to her mother and father:

22 October, 1963

Dear Mama and Buppong,

This is the poem I wrote for Barney when I decided to marry him [about the willow tree]. Anyway, as the poem says, I don't want to hurry things. I love living, curious, from day to day. He has given me a burro and if we DO marry, I'll string daisy chains for the burro and the goose in his back yard. And maybe Buppong will come and give me away. Anyway, meantime, I want you to meet Barney, here at my flat, before he takes the night plane on the 18th of November. He is handsome and noble and gentle and wears me out tramping over the hills after him or riding the horse at his knee. I told you he is a biologist and scientist aside from a surgeon and a writer. He thinks I am beautiful, but he fell for me because I'm a good editor. Such is life.

Your loving child
Helga

If Helga wasn't a good editor, she ought to be because for years she had typed and edited her father's manuscripts, then had worked for several years in the Manuscripts Division and as secretary to the Keeper of the Collections of the Library of Congress and on the Woodrow Wilson Papers. More recently, she had published several books and many poems and articles on her own.

Mrs. Sandburg replied to her daughter's letter saying among other things, "He must be a very sensible man. And you know I never did approve of your bachelor-girl life." In reply, Helga said that at the wedding, at which she hoped her father would give her away, "I'll start the swan on champagne."

Helga too was beginning to feel that our relationship was too good to pass up. Both of us were deeply in love, but had been bitten by that bug too often to again admit it. So I proposed that it would be more convenient for all concerned if she would take her things from Washington and move in with me. At Christmas, when her son who was in Germany studying physical chemistry would return, we would get married. To my astonishment, Helga assented.

I truly was astonished, for Helga was so well set up in the East where she had her lecture and literary agents and all of her friends. I thought it would be a hard decision for her to make and I was overjoyed that she instantly accepted. We began at once to make changes in the house and to redo and rearrange things according to Helga's tastes. This was not easy, because Jane and I had accumulated a small museum of artifacts from the bottom of the sea and from all over the world, and Helga too had a good supply of similar symbols in Washington. Somehow it was all straightened out and everything was put in order.

The adjustments that Helga and I had to make seemed minimal. To me there was no adjustment and it seemed that she and I had always been living together. But at first some of my family were a bit resentful. There was no reason for it, because Helga and I were truly married. On November 9, 1963, we had gone down to Flat Rock, North Carolina, to visit the Sandburgs, and Helga's sister Janet had questioned our right to share a room without being married. Mr. Sandburg, eighty-five years old at the time, had solved the problem by standing up at the head of the table and solemnly marrying us in the presence of witnesses (Helga's mother and sisters). The press got wind of it and it was widely publicized in papers and periodicals (headline: "SANDBURG BLESSES CRILES").

My attorney assured me that we were legally married. However, my daughter Joan broke into tears and asked me how I could be a trustee of University School when I was living with a woman without a marriage certificate. The next time we were in Washington together, which happened to be four days before President Kennedy was shot, Helga and I spent the night in her apartment. When Helga got up she took off her wedding ring and we went to the justice of the peace. My daughter Susie was our witness.

"Do you want the regular service or the special one?" the black justice inquired.

"Judge, you'd better give us the best you've got," I told him. "She's had two husbands already and I want this marriage to last." The service was worth the extra five dollars, because so far, at least, it has lasted.

27

A New Start

AT LAST all of Helga's belongings had been moved to Cleveland and we had settled down to what would never be a routine, but always an exciting way of life. Helga was busy writing her books or thinking up new ideas for films, for she too had taken up motion-picture photography, and I remained as busy as ever in my surgical practice and in preaching the new doctrine of the breast. In 1963, the debate between the supporters of radical mastectomy and those who thought less destructive treatments gave just as good results was beginning to be the hot subject, not only at medical meetings but also on television talk shows. In this country, the medical profession still supported the use of the radical operation, but abroad it had been largely abandoned. In the next few years I would appear several times both on the "Donahue" show and on the "Today" show as well as on many local programs.

In this period, two very good things happened. The first was that Helga's daughter Paula, who was now twenty and had been in Florida working, decided to join us in Cleveland and go to college. At the same time Marianne, inspired by Helga, decided to go on a biblical-type fast, and for forty days and forty nights she ate practically nothing. The pounds rolled off and the aroma or something so pervaded the atmosphere that the men started to flock around her. It was very exciting at Kent Road for those few years, because both Marianne and Paula had extremely active social lives. Marianne continued to work with me in the Mouse Lab and to take care of the house, though Helga, being a cordon bleu chef, did most of the cooking. Those were happy years.

It wasn't long after Helga and I were married that Helga's son John Carl, who was studying in Germany and heading for a Ph.D. in physical chemistry, wrote to say that he had fallen in love and was contemplating marriage. Helga and I were in Mexico when his letter was forwarded to us, and we wrote enthusiastically in support and gave the letter and the money for stamps to a man in the hotel. The letter was never mailed. A month later came a second letter from John, saying that he didn't care what we thought, he was going to marry Liz anyway. We cabled him and wrote him, and he and Liz came to Cleveland and were married here at our house, but the good Catholic parents wouldn't recognize that and remarried them properly in a church as soon as they got back to Germany. John is now one of the Dupont Company's leading chemical engineers, and Liz, after rearing three sons, is in charge of an office that employs about thirty people. Liz is an extraordinary woman—trilingual, for she grew up in Bavaria, worked in her late teens on a French yacht in the Mediterranean, and then did office work in the Houston Medical Center while John was finishing up his doctorate. She and John are both scholarly and delightful.

Paula, after finishing her college work, became a writer, published an excellent and successful book about the Sandburgs, *My Connemara,* and then, before marrying and going back to North Carolina, she taught at Laurel, a private school for girls, and was adored by faculty and students alike.

All of my children but George had left the fold. Each of the older girls would have four children in time and they and their surgeon-husbands would do well. Ann's husband, Dr. C. B. Esselstyn, was in general surgery at the Cleveland Clinic, and Joan's husband, Dr. Roger Foster, was in the same at the University of Vermont, where he later would become the director of the Vermont Regional Cancer Center. Ann, as soon as her children were grown, would go back to teaching at Laurel and be a favorite with her pupils. Joan and Roger had always run a big business with their kennel of huge Newfoundland dogs that they took to all the big shows where they won ribbons and cups. Our Susie would always remain head over heels into art. By the time she was forty, she would choose a husband, marrying free-thinking Joe Murphy, chancellor of the City University of New York. As for George, we went through some exciting times with him in this period.

In addition to my children, Helga had inherited from Jane a backyard full of pets—a mute swan, a Canada goose, wood ducks, and rabbits. To these soon were added two baby fallow deer, a woodchuck, a pair of silver pheasants, and any other creature that didn't make a loud noise and that couldn't climb over the six-foot fence. Our naturalist friend, David McKelvey, in charge of birds and living animals at the Natural History Museum, helped us find appropriate baby creatures.

David was more Lorenzian than Korad Lorenz had ever been, for he literally did talk with animals—especially the birds—and could make himself understood. Through our connections with the people on the "Today" show, we were able to have David and his creatures aired and soon he was a regular guest.

Cleveland Heights is a populous neighborhood in which there are many children. These kept coming by to see the strange animals in our back yard, which by now included a couple of capybaras from Brazil—amphibious, web-footed mammals that often weighed more than one hundred pounds. They were gentle and loving and totally herbivorous, so that we never had to mow the lawn. They swam together in our pond and were a delight to the crowds of children, who on the two afternoons a week in which the garden was open to them, came in and played with the birds and animals. We had a crow too and a large black buzzard that ate out of our hands.

Helga and I made notes and read and took pictures and consulted with David McKelvey. I had that book in my mind—*A Naturalistic View of Man*. The subtitle would be, "The importance of early training in learning, living, and the organization of society." Among the chapters would be "Time, the Determiner of Development," which emphasized the importance of early training, particularly in the acquisition of language; "Instinct and Memory," in which the parts of our behavior that are innate are compared with those parts that are acquired; "Imprintation and Associative Learning"; "Higher Education"; "Emotional Stability"; "Sexuality"; "Health and Superstition"; and "The Organization of Society." It would really be a book on human psychology, and I believe its conclusions are sound and valuable, particularly those pertaining to the teaching of foreign languages early in life when the child is still a genius at learning to speak and pronounce.

Pretty soon I had a publisher interested—World, who had an office in Cleveland. Prior to publication, Isaac Asimov, the science writer, would send in comments to be used on the jacket, saying that it was "an extremely good and important book... an excellent popular introduction to the new psychology. It is the new method of approaching the human being as a member of the animal kingdom and not as an object in a class all by itself. I have never seen a more entertaining and comprehensive and keep-your-cool expression of it."

Helga was so fascinated with *A Naturalistic View of Man* during the writing that she occasionally overdid her editing a little. However, I stayed stubborn and finally she let me have my way. (If she had written the book, it might have been a best-seller when later it was published.)

A little after our marriage, Helga and I had gone on a somewhat belated honeymoon to Andros Island, taking with us, as chaperone, Helga's old friend John Henry Faulk. He was the hero of the famous trial, with Louis Nizer defending him, in which McCarthy was defeated and freedom of speech restored. Johnny was one of the most amusing men I have ever known, as well as being a great philosopher. We lived in Captain Joe's house at Stanyard Creek, and Joe took us out in his little outboard to the Great Barrier Reef of Andros, from which New York's Museum of Natural History collected its coral specimens.

Helga was enchanted with the underwater world and quickly learned to snorkel like an expert. In the next few years we would visit most of the national underwater parks, including those in the Florida Keys, the Dry Tortugas, the Virgin Islands, the Channel Islands off the California coast, and Padre Island in Texas. Most of these visits were planned in connection with my medical meetings. You guessed it, not one to miss an opportunity, Helga began at once to get involved in her own book, *Above and Below: A Journey Through Our National Underwater Parks*. She was commissioned to write it for McGraw-Hill as part of Justice William O. Douglas's American Wilderness Series. I would be coauthor, which meant that Helga worked on the book during the day when I was at the Clinic and read it to me at night, when I would make suggestions that she would or would not accept. *Above and Below* and *A Naturalistic View of Man* would both be published in 1969, six years after our marriage.

Two years before the publication of these books, I would write another medical book—*A Biological Consideration of the Treatment of Breast Cancer* (Thomas, 1967). It was dedicated to Sir Geoffrey Keynes who, in the 1930s at St. Bartholomew's Hospital in London, had begun treating breast cancer by wide local excision and radiation. The book contained a summary of the development of thought about the treatment of breast cancer and the support for the statement made by the British surgeon, D. C. L. Fitzwilliams, that the surgeons who favored radical mastectomy were those who were "repeating dogma and not speaking from formed judgment." Needless to say, my book was not acclaimed by American surgeons, for in it I reported a comparison of the survival of patients at the Cleveland Clinic in 1955, 1956, and 1957 by simple mastectomy or local excision with that of patients in the same years treated by radical or modified radical mastectomy. At eight years, the survival rate of the patients treated by simple operations was 12 percent higher than that of the ones subjected to radical operations. Although the difference was significant, the trial was not randomized and the difference in survival probably was partly the result of selection of the more favorable cases for the lesser operation.

During this period, my son George had been having an exciting time. After having been given an award for leadership in his freshman year at Trinity College, he got into some absurd infraction of rules that involved having a girl in the dormitory and was suspended for a year. His classmates marched and waved flags and demanded George's reinstatement. The president of Trinity remained firm. This was the best thing that ever happened to George because he went to college in Washington for a year and stayed with his aunt Kay Halle, through whom he met many of the important people in the town, including Joe Alsop, the writer, and his attractive seventeen-year-old step-daugher, Anne Emily, who in due time George would marry.

George had at first had a hard time accepting Helga, and he and his fellow Cleveland students had swung some wild and slightly devastating parties at our house. This would not be tolerated by Helga, and that was when George moved to Washington and when his career began, because after returning to Trinity and finishing school he was able, with the help of Mr. Alsop, to get a job with the newspaper of Gary, Indiana, and start doing investigational reporting. He did such a good job that he discovered that one of the town's chief officials had been cheating at taxes. This resulted in a lawsuit that George won, but also in his being dismissed by the owners of the newspaper, who, apparently, were not completely free of similar tax sins.

After an exciting career on the Gary paper, George married Anne Emily and also was drafted into the army. He was sent to the West Coast to a school where he was to learn Russian, but before he could become proficient, the military emergency subsided and George returned to start again as a reporter, this time as the Washington editor for *Harpers Magazine*. This lasted for a couple of years until he was offered a job by CBS to produce documentaries. Out of this came the famous suit by General Westmoreland against CBS and Crile. Eventually the general dropped the suit, but it was not until the name *George Crile* had become a household word, and I, as *George Crile, Jr.*, had become widely mistaken for George's son.

Two relics of this era survive in Helga's files. One is an excerpt from a long letter she wrote to George soon after our marriage. The other is an essay on matrimony that I wrote in 1968 at Helga's request.

14 November, 1963

Dear George 006,

[George was in Germany with the OSS at that time.] I thought you might worry about my role in your household and

life in relation to your mother. I mean, that I might want Jane forgotten or her image altered. You simply can't worry about that
because you are what you are and so is the spirit of your wonderful home and even Roger III and Rip are great—and of course
Barney—because of her. I know a good deal of Jane because of
the book, you know.

And I am not like her—I'm me. I'm not in conflict with and
I'm not replacing. What I'm doing is starting to live the second
part of my life with Barney, who is doing the same with me. We
both know what we want, and what we'll do with it. Which is extraordinary. I left a life I loved, marrying Barney. I didn't marry
for loneliness. I think it's healthy. I'm moving into a life I love. I
adore your father absolutely and completely, and I want him fulfilled and in his own way. I won't interfere or hover or protect. I
might follow now and then. And we have no time to waste. . . .

I am glad to go to the Midwest, where my roots are. I like being a Buckeye. No one seems to know Ohio's State Song, but I
intend, patriotic, to find it.

Come home soon. I'm marrying Barney partly because of the
quality of his daughters, whom I love. I have no question of my
affection for his son.

Yours—
Helga

Then comes the essay. It is heavily laden with the verbiage of Konrad
Lorenz and observations on the imprinting of animals. The reference
to the elephant's tusk was provoked by a letter from George in which
Helga was implored not to remove the Ivory Wreck tusk that hung in
our living room over the mantle. Needless to say Helga at once moved
it to a place of honor in the sunroom. My essay was to head a collection of letters and memorabilia that Helga had assembled into an album which she named "The Elephant's Tusk."

This record has been assembled for the benefit of any of
Helga's and my descendants who may happen to lose a spouse.
By referring to it, the unfortunate one may find that the problems that beset him are not unique, but have been shared by everyone who falls into a similar situation.

When the bereaved remarries, the emotional reactions of relatives are based on two factors. One is territoriality, symbolized
by the elephant's tusk. The other is the principle that painful
memories are soon forgotten.

When a woman moves into a man's home she immediately changes it to denote that it is now her territory. This offends all relatives of the man because it means that the home is no longer their territory. Had I known this at the time I remarried I could have viewed with humor many of the actions and words that I then found quite inexplicable.

The second principle, the necessity of forgetting a painful experience in order to be able to live in equanimity, is of course applicable primarily to the one who is bereaved because he is the one who has suffered the most. It is imperative, for his peace of mind, to forget his memories as soon as possible. In the case of the relatives, however, there is lesser incentive to forget, for they have their own lives and are therefore not as strongly affected by the loss. Because of this difference the bereaved one forgets or at least puts from his mind any thought of his former spouse much more rapidly than do the relatives. This enables him to adapt to his new way of life and find happiness in remarriage. To those who view these mysterious manifestations of the mind, the bereaved one is perceived as callous, thoughtless and crude. Instead of being happy for him because he was sensible enough to be able to readjust so quickly, they criticize him for the very things that enable him to go on living happily.

The lesson in all this is a simple one. Do not judge the actions of others from your point of view but from theirs. And from your standpoint, if you are so unfortunate as to lose a spouse, do not be angry at those who criticize your remarriage. "Forgive them for they know not what they do."

G. Crile, Jr.
January 1968

And also, in Helga's files, is a copy of a memo to Susie and George who, in 1963 and 1964, were spending some time with us in Cleveland. It starts with Kipling's verse:

> Now this is the Law of the Jungle—
> As old and as true as the sky,
> And the Wolf that shall keep it may prosper,
> But the Wolf that shall break it must die.

USE THE BEIGE TOWELS LIKE THE ONES IN YOUR BATH NOW, WHILE YOU ARE AT HOME...THEY BELONG IN THERE.
DO NOT BORROW THE YELLOW COMFORTERS OR ANYTHING AT ALL FROM THE GUEST ROOM, OR THE GUEST BATH CABINETS.

DO NOT BORROW ANY SUPPLY FROM THE BATHROOM, BUT CHARGE
WHAT YOU NEED AT MILLERS AND KEEP IN YOUR OWN.

STATIONERY OR OFFICE SUPPLIES MAY BE USED FROM THE LITTLE
ROOM WHICH IS VIOLA'S TERRITORY, BUT NEVER FROM MINE,
WHICH IS A SPECIAL TAX EXEMPT ACCOUNT. I DO NOT SUPPLY
STAMPS.

And the instructions go on a full page. Since Helga had once worked
for the Library of Congress, it concluded:

THE BOOKS IN THE HOUSE ARE NOW IN ESTABLISHED PLACES. BE-
CAUSE I ALWAYS WANT INFORMATION HURRIEDLY, NO BOOKS ARE
REMOVED FROM THEIR PLACES OF REST UNLESS THEY ARE RETURNED
AT ONCE.

THIS REFERS ALSO TO THE BASEMENT LIBRARY. LET ME KNOW IF THERE
IS A BOOK YOU WISH TO KEEP.

Incredible as it may seem, these children would grow up and it
would be a delight to have them visit us.

28

The Unicorn's Lair

F IVE MONTHS after our wedding, we had recovered enough from
our brief honeymoon with John Henry to plan a true one of our
own. I had not yet met Helga's son, John Carl Steichen, who had been
studying chemistry in Munich. Helga also had relatives, on her mother's side of the family, in Luxembourg. So we flew to Frankfurt, rented
a car, and drove through Belgium to Luxembourg where a host of
Helga's relatives threw a huge party for us. I was better off than Helga
because few of the Luxembourgers spoke English but most of them
knew French.

We traveled on to Munich, where I was deeply impressed by the
university, the beer halls, and by John Carl. I remember that John was
driving us along a thruway, when I tossed an empty cigarette pack out
of the window. John stopped the car, went back and picked it up. "You
could be fined one hundred dollars for that," he told us.

We drove through Germany and Austria with John and then into
Yugoslavia to Split, on the Adriatic Coast. Here we visited the restored
palace that was built by the Roman emperor Diocletian, and then we
left John, whose scientific and chemically oriented mind had impressed me, and took a ferry across to Italy. Both Helga and I had been
to Italy before, so we drove up through the Alps to France and then
south again to Spain. There were bullfights in Madrid, and encounters with surgeons to whom we had been introduced by Dr. Tony
Autunez, who had come originally from Spain but in 1964 was the
head of the Cleveland Clinic's Department of Radiation Therapy. We
thoroughly enjoyed Spain and then moved on to revisit Nazaré, on
the coast of Portugal, where Jane and I had photographed the oxen
pulling the boats up the beach and the people drawing the nets.

Nazaré was as unique and lovely as ever, and we stayed there for two days before going on to the magnificent shrine at Fatima, and then to crowded Lisbon. Next there were medical meetings in England, at which I had been asked to speak and which gave the excuse for the journey. In England, I introduced Helga to my old friends Reggie Murley, Deborah Doniach, and Arthur Porritt, who had done so much to direct my thought about the treatment of breast cancer, and also to Rodney Maingot, the surgeon and author with whom I had kept in touch ever since he had visited us in Cleveland and we had gone duck shooting together.

At the time of this European journey, Helga and I had just started making films. I had given her a small 8-mm Kodak movie camera much more portable and convenient than the bulky old 16-mm one. We came home with three films, "Europe 1964," "Nazaré 1964," and "The Spanish Heritage." The latter was an interpretation of the bullfight we had seen in Madrid. Helga's and my career together as director and producer of films was off to a good beginning. She brought to the screen much of the beauty and excitement that characterized the photographic work of her uncle, Edward Steichen. That was the end of our second honeymoon, but later in the year, again in conjunction with a medical meeting, we would stay three days in Andros Island with Captain Joe.

On that leisurely European journey, Helga and I had spent a lot of time discussing the future of the Knob. There were two hundred acres, one hundred of them in Lake County on the hill of the Knob. The other one hundred were in Geauga County and flat and contained two ponds, two barns, and the house in which my parents' groom and his family used to live and which now was occupied, rent-free, by Mr. and Mrs. Konick whose job was to keep off people who might do damage. The period was beginning in which teenagers would break into any empty house, take what they could use, and bust up anything they couldn't.

Helga had lived on a farm with her family's famous dairy goats. Her tastes were firmly rooted in the land. Neither she nor I had any desire to live in solitary splendor at the top where there was nothing to do but look at distant Lake Erie. Instead we decided to build a little weekend resort down near the barn which had been the stable for my father's horses. There was a sweet water spring there—"White Stone Spring" we named it, because it welled up from the sandstone in which were thousands of white quartz pebbles. Below this we would build a dam and make a small lake for fish, ducks, and geese.

Through our local friends, Don Farinacci, the lumberman, and attorney Mark Sperry, we found a builder. We had no need for an architect, because Helga had clear ideas. The building would be supported by the huge hand-hewn beams that in generations past had been used to build a neighbor's barn. Since the beams were thirty feet long, our "architect" ordained that our house would be thirty feet square. In order to keep it warm in winter and cool in summer, we would fit it into the hillside, half underground. There would be one large room with a king-size bed, a kitchen space, a living space, and off the kitchen, a little bathroom with a Japanese-style double bathtub, a toilet, a bidet, and a washstand. There also was a small coat closet. Above the kitchen was a second story area through which the house was entered from the driveway and where there was Helga's desk, a couple of bureaus, and twin beds for guests. All of this, both floors, looked down and out through great double-glassed picture windows onto the field where deer and cows and horses and a donkey and geese grazed, and on the pond where the ducks swam and beyond to the distant hills of Chardon.

There wasn't a visible trace of civilization. Helga and I loved it. Because Helga had just finished writing her poetry book, *The Unicorns,* we named our new house the "Unicorn's Lair." It had a French-tile floor with drains that could be hosed down when necessary. It was heated centrally by oil, but we depended mainly on our wood stove. There was hot water, a dishwasher, a clothes dryer, a fridge and a freezer, radio and television. What more could anyone want? Helga drew up all the plans. The builder, Mr. Zakany, who was a genius, inserted details and got the government's approval. A hundred yards away, we fenced in and plowed up an area where once a pigpen had been and made it into a vegetable garden. What we couldn't eat we would freeze. At the garden, there is a little shed that houses the tools and cultivators which Helga runs herself and won't let me touch. Each year we can hardly wait for spring to come and planting to begin.

In 1965, we were so busy with the Lair that the only vacation we took was ten days in Mexico with Helga's daughter Paula and my son George. Traveling by bus and by car we visited the spectacular pyramids, tombs, and ruins of Chichen Itza and Tulum, and did some skin diving and exploration of the water off the Isla Mujeres. Again, of course, it ended up with a medical meeting, this one in New Orleans.

It's a wonderful thing to live in the city and to have a country place to which you can go for weekends. The change is so complete, the activities and interests are so different! There are the birds and the bees and the flowers and the snowdrifts and the raccoons and the foxes and the fish and the frogs. Back in the early days when we built the Unicorn's Lair, there were whippoorwills. By now, the evenings are silent. Even the songs of the tree toads have been dimmed, as a result of acid rain. But the garden grows and there is wood to cut and split and always a dozen things that need to be done. As I drive past the huge high-rise apartment buildings that are beginning to surround our cities, or when I travel in the communist countries and see that almost all of their housing is in the form of high-rise towers, I wonder how the marriages of people can last when couples are condemned to live in lifelong, near-solitary confinement, with no gardens, no pets, no place for their children to romp and play. I would like to see the results of a study that compared the divorce rate of couples who lived in high rises as compared to that of the ones who had gardens.

Helga and I kept adopting not only ducklings, baby crows, vultures, and all sorts of wild birds, but also lambs and baby pigs. We had a great grey-bearded dog called Gustav, a cross between a giant poodle and a German shepherd. It was beautiful to watch him race with our white fallow deer through the wooded glades and around the ponds. And it was fascinating to hear the legendary tales that David had to tell about his discoveries in the field of animal behavior. When he left the Natural History Museum to take a position in the West we mourned, and so did our creatures that he was so good at talking with.

We had friends near us in the country. One was the attorney Mark Sperry, who had grown up in the Chardon area and practiced there all his life. He had been in the CIA and in the Pacific in World War II. He had a classical education and knew every myth the mind of man had ever conceived of and had read any book you might mention. Our other friend was the lumberman and entrepreneur, Don Farinacci, who did not read books, but had bought up thousands of acres of forest land, timbered it, and then sold it to real estate companies. These two knew everything about the area and the land and from them, we would continually learn much.

Helga would invite in her literary friends, whom I would proceed to challenge and insult, to her horror. One of them was the famous poet Stephen Spender, to whom I insisted on reading one of my poems, which he seemed to enjoy. I gradually got used to those she brought into my life that were nonmedical. It was a change to have someone besides doctors to talk to, because when one is busy in his profession, he is apt to end up with most of his friends being doctors too—a situation that does not always lead to the most open and interesting intellectual encounters.

In spite of the fact that Helga was single-handedly caring for two houses and a working husband, she found time to write a lovely book for children, *Anna and the Baby Buzzard,* which Dutton would publish in 1970. Helga was also busy lecturing, although she had left her New York bureau when we married, as she wanted to confine her activities to Cleveland. Those were busy years for both of us and good fun. We loved it and so did our assorted imprinted offspring, including the capybaras.

29

The Start of a Long Journey

IT WAS the twelfth of January 1966, and Helga and I had gone to Washington where I was giving lectures to the doctors in the Armed Services Training courses, and Helga was seeing old friends. On the way home from dinner with Connie and André Pacatte, our taxi was struck sideways by a car and all of us were injured. I was sitting on the left side of the back seat and took the full force of the blow. Ten ribs were fractured, one lung was pierced letting air into my chest cavity, and my spleen was ruptured. I did not regain consciousness until some time later when I was in the emergency room of the Washington Hospital Center. Helga incurred a bad fracture of the wrist and her face and legs were filled with fragments of shattered glass. The Pacattes were bumped and bruised. The driver of the car that crossed the dividing line and sideswiped us was on medication and also had been drinking whiskey. He had passed out at the wheel and drove on for six blocks before a policeman, who had witnessed the accident and called the ambulance, caught him.

I had what is called "retroactive amnesia"—no recollection of the accident or of anything that occurred for the ten or fifteen minutes before it. This was a result of concussion from a severe blow on the head. The ambulance came promptly and took us to the Washington Hospital Center where Helga made it clear that I was a distinguished surgeon, who must have special treatment. She made her point, and it was given to me. I remember clearly lying on the table in the emergency room and watching the bottles of blood that were running into me. My blood pressure was 72/40 and my pulse rate 60. Soon it became apparent that I was bleeding internally. I felt my abdomen becoming distended and watched the blood running into my veins. I remember trying to say, as best I could with no breath, that the blood they were putting in was all bleeding into my belly. I have always thought that transfusions were dangerous and always have tried, when possible, to avoid giving them. Here I was getting them—lots of them. There were nine in all.

Fortunately, the emergency room attendant was able to reach Dr. Harold Hawfield, a highly competent general surgeon, who immediately made the diagnosis of ruptured spleen and had me prepared for operation. The spleen and about three liters of blood were removed from my abdomen. Since there was no evidence of other injuries, the abdomen was closed and all went well. I was fortunate also in having, as a consultant regarding my chest injuries, the expert thoracic surgeon, Brian Blades, who had been a resident at Barnes Hospital when I was interning there. Later, several of my colleagues at the Clinic came on from Cleveland, but by that time I was on my way to a painful, but uncomplicated, recovery, from which I drew only one conclusion. The spleen is not an essential organ.

I stayed in the hospital only eight days, during most of which time Helga stayed with Kay Halle. With Helga's painful arm still in a cast and my chest still too sore for a deep breath, we were flown home in the private (industrial) plane of a friend. The pleasure of being back again, with Helga, in our own bed was one of the sweetest memories of my life. But the pleasure was replaced by agony when Gustav, our shaggy 150-pound Bouvier dog, welcomed me by leaping onto my chest.

I am eternally grateful to Washington Hospital Center and its staff for the prompt and expert service that saved my life. The physicians refused to send me bills—professional courtesy, they called it—until I insisted and said that I would take all they charged me from the insurance company's $25,000 settlement and give it to "The Needy Sick Fund," which was the charity of their choice. These physicians were not only skillful, but also charitable and considerate.

The accident had made the front page of the Washington and Cleveland newspapers, and there had been many criticisms of the light fine and sentence given to the driver, who was not only drunk but who also had left the scene of the accident. As a result of the publicity, my room had been completely filled with flowers from old friends and patients and from some people whose names I had a hard time remembering. There were literally hundreds of letters from all over the country and from abroad. Helga too had her share of them and then, true to form, while she was in the hospital, Helga had written a poem:

Lines To a Husband in Washington Hospital
Center After an Accident

Now that you lie down the cold corridor from me,
Your ribs shattered, not mine, and me with a broken arm,
I consider the thin thread that binds
The great fleshy monuments of ourselves to the earth.

This is so fine a filament, its strength in superstition almost
   lies,
For it has to do with the aim of each small splintered piece
   of glass
And the speed of the ambulance and how far it must run
And then finally whether it is or is not time for the thread
   to break.

That is the mystery: The time and place and movement of
   each still and whirling thing,
Then the controlled tweezers and needles and blades and
   white-coated men,
And how within the wounded, the disbelieving blood and
   spirit stirs,
And sometimes, as with us, the thread the white-columned
   bodies to the earth still holds.

"It's an ill wind that blows no good." The Washington accident
didn't help my professional career, but it did make me come to some
valuable conclusions.

At the time of the accident, I was fifty-nine years old. Until then,
my view of time had stretched on and on into infinity. Suddenly I realized how short my remaining time might be. I thought also of Jane's
death, and I realized that it is rare for solidly married couples to reach,
together and in good health, the designated retirement age of sixty-
five years. I thought of my friends, many of whom or whose wives already were either dead or incapacitated. I decided that now was the
time to travel. If Helga and I were to see the world together and to forever after have the interest of hearing about and reading about the remote places that we had visited, this was the time to do it. Five years
from now, when I would have retired, might be too late. Moreover we
would have missed five years of enjoyment in reading and hearing
about the exotic places we had been. There was only one problem.
How should we go about selecting the places to visit?

The other good that the ill wind of the accident blew to me, was to
make me realize that to go on smoking cigarettes was absolutely stu-

pid. This accident, plus the scars to my lungs that had resulted from my long-before encounter with pneumonia, made me aware, when I exercised, that my lungs were not fully competent. I stopped smoking cigarettes, but as a token of independence and out of deference to my wife, whose father had been a cigar smoker and who therefore liked the smell of them, I would continue to smoke a single Marsh-Wheeling stogie every Saturday night.

Having made the decision that now was the time to travel, I applied for and received a three-month leave of absence from the Clinic which, with the allotted month of vacation, would enable Helga and me to take all the time we needed for a four-month round-the-world journey. We planned it with Jerry Howard of Round The World Travel. He gave us open tickets and we never got over being amazed at how well it all worked out. I would keep a journal that was bound into a 458-page book titled *A Slanted View of Some of the World's Customs, Traditions and Beliefs*. The "slant" of *A Slanted View* is from the viewpoint of a surgeon who had just finished writing the book, *A Naturalistic View of Man*. I now wanted to go to the world's remote places and see how the principles I had been writing about applied to cultures other than our own.

In planning the trip, which began in August, I took a cue from Darwin, who had found that the study of animals on isolated islands gave him the greatest insight into the principles of evolution. Helga and I decided, therefore, to view human societies and customs as they existed on islands or in isolated lands. Throughout this trip, on which Helga would turn fifty and I sixty-one, we traveled with little or no knowledge of the places we were to visit. We viewed each new land through the eyes of innocents, recording our own conclusions before reading what others had said. We were like the mythical bird that flew backwards because it was more interested in where it had been than in where it was going.

Two factors influenced our planning, both of them economic. One was that I had been invited to speak at a meeting of the Royal College of Surgeons of Australia, all expenses paid. Melbourne, incidentally, is exactly opposite Cleveland on the globe and is as far south of the equator as Cleveland is north of it. I had also been invited to speak in South America. The other consideration was that the travel agent told us that if we went around the world much, if not all, of the north or south deviations that we made would cost us no extra.

The first stop on our itinerary was Rome. Helga had been there a few years before traveling for the State Department and had loved the city, and a male companion she had met there. In fact, she had been dragging her feet about starting on this trip to the antipodes, until I promised her a day in Rome. We arrived breakfastless and weary and with no hotel reservations. On this trip we had made none in advance. Helga remembered the Terminus Hotel where once she had enjoyed herself, but it was full, and we were referred to a small and ancient hotel that was just what we were looking for. It was clean and had good service.

We spent a busy day revisiting the ancient ruins and the modern buildings, and we walked through the forum with a portable tape recorder as our guide. History came to life. After dinner in a streetside cafe we took a bus to go to a movie entitled *Helga,* and were astounded at how helpful the driver and passengers were in instructing us where to get off. That was not the kind of treatment that people who didn't speak English could expect if they boarded a bus in New York. The movie was all about sex life in the army and seemed to us funnier because we couldn't understand the language. Afterward, it was the hour of the promenade, and although we were in a shabby part of town we felt completely secure. Everywhere around us we saw nothing but love. On the way home we stopped at the Trevi Fountain to watch by moonlight the smooth flow of the water over the bowl's even rim. Then to sleep with Helga in a big soft bed. The total cost of our two-day stay in Rome had been about the same as that of our farewell dinner for four in New York.

We flew on to Athens and then to Crete, where we rented a car from the same man from whom, seven years earlier, Jane and I had rented one. He remembered me, because he had been so astonished at the remote area we had wanted to visit and that we were using Homer as our guide. We saw all of my old friends and visited all of Homer's landmarks, but now Matela had a tourist hotel in which we slept instead of a cave. The cave-dwellers now were no longer farmers, taking seaside vacations to escape the heat, they were hippies—hundreds of couples cohabitating without a trace of wedding rings. It was a gentle culture, and we saw no open use of drugs.

Elias, the Professor, and our old friend Nicolas were in nearby Pitsidia. We had a fine banquet one night, with chickens and wine and toasts and songs, and we listened as Elias recited Homer in Greek. I even found Radamanthus, the fisherman, who had worked with Jane and me on the wrecks. It was a good reunion, and now Helga too was a little in love with my Crete. On the drive back to Heraklion, we subsisted on half of a roasted suckling pig that we had purchased from a roadside vendor.

We flew back to Athens where we were met by Pan Michas, a Greek surgeon who had visited the Clinic a couple of years before and had stayed in our home for several days including a visit to the Unicorn's Lair. Returning our courtesy, Pan invited us to stay with him and his wife, Iris, in their charming summer home—a mini palace with marble floors and walls of multicolored granite that was set in a miniature garden of Eden, replete with olive and fruit trees. There were pomegranates, oranges, lemons, limes, and peaches all ripe and fresh and ready to eat. And there were the largest, loudest, and most vicious mosquitoes that we had ever seen.

Pan was professor of surgery at the University Hospital, which we visited with him the next day to watch some operations. The technique was excellent, based on the English—but some of the treatments seemed to me to be a decade or so out-of-date—at least by my standards. The Greeks were still in the period of hoping to improve the survival of patients with cancer by performing ultraradical operations. Pan said that one of the troubles with Greek medicine was too much training. After seven years in the university, the doctor had to work three years in some remote community, then two years in the army. Only then can he return to the hospital to begin training in a specialty. After several years of that, he had to go abroad for two years to get a foreign degree, such as that of England's Royal College of Surgeons. After this he could work as a "registrar"—a sort of super-resident, under the direction of the chief of the Service. In this system a forty-year-old surgeon would still be in training, with the result that by the time that he became independent he would have passed the age when he could easily develop new ideas and techniques.

After a delightful stay with Dr. and Mrs. Michas, during which Helga was able to see all the historical monuments, we heard of a Russian ship, *The Latvia*, that was leaving for Odessa by way of Istanbul. It was a huge combined freighter-and-passenger vessel, into which cranes were loading freight and up whose gangplanks hundreds of Arab and Negro students from the Sudan were climbing aboard. We were stopped by an officer who didn't think we looked like Sudanese students, but when we showed him our passports and first-class tickets he waved us aboard, indicating that we had to leave our luggage on the dock to be brought on later. Needless to say, we sat on the deck where we could watch it until it was loaded. Finally, everything was aboard and we were shown a clean and comfortable two-bed cabin that shared a bath with the one next door. The bar, where for fifty cents we bought an ice cold drink of Vodka and a bottle of beer, was filled with dark-skinned Arabs and blacks who had a blaring record player to the music of which they danced wildly, spilling whiskey all over the floor. The Russian barkeeper looked disgusted.

After a hearty and well-cooked supper there was a dance. We attended, but no one danced except the ship's engineer, who danced one after another with all the waitresses. Meanwhile, on the top deck, all hell was breaking loose. The Arabs were drinking and dancing to the music of their Japanese recorder. When the Sudanese saw Helga and me they were interested and settled down to talk. They were twenty-one to thirty years old. All were men, and none of them were married. With them was an attractive black American girl, having the time of her life dancing. Some of the students were headed for medicine and tried their best, in French or English, to question us. It was a great night, and we came to like the Sudanese.

In the morning we were in the Sea of Marmara, and then we had traversed the Dardanelles and landed in Istanbul. I wanted first to show Helga the Blue Mosque, now a museum, for Islam is no longer taken seriously by the Turks. We sat in the darkened silence and watched the pigeons fly through the vast and once holy space. Most of Istanbul has been westernized. The main market, "the Covered Bazaar," is the world's greatest supermarket. It covers a square mile and you can buy anything, and all smuggled in from all over the world. It was there, in the bazaar, that I met my first disaster. When Helga was in the jewelry area, looking at opals, I was stricken with the "Tourista." By the time I had walked a quarter of a mile to the nearest facility and found that there was no toilet paper and that in Istanbul one wipes oneself with a water-moistened left hand and then washes the hand and never uses it to touch food—by this time, I had learned all that and made my way back to the jewelry department, Helga had bought about a drawer-full of beautiful stones. I couldn't complain, because I was too weak and dizzy and because opals are my favorite jewels, and these were absolute bargains.

From Istanbul we flew on to Beirut, which at that time was inhabited by people with fascinating mixtures of races and religions. Tension was beginning to build up. An American-educated Saudi Arabian told us that the United States, through the CIA and against all good sense, was supporting the fanatically religious Arab minority. We also noticed that everywhere were small children working as apprentices instead of being in school.

We rented a car and drove to Biblos, the world's oldest continuously inhabited town. Its name means book, because it was there that papyrus was first used to make paper. The nearby Crusader's Castle is built of marble and pink granite taken from Roman temples. Here too, beside the sea, were found the shaft tombs built by the Phoenicians and filled with golden treasures. In my journal I wrote:

Why dig a shaft 20-feet square through 60 or 70 feet of solid rock in order to bury a king? Yet today we still do the same sort of thing. We spend $100,000 on a heart transplant and usually, from the standpoint of the Welfare of Society, it is just about as productive as the shaft tombs were.

In Lebanon we also visited the Great Grotto of Jeita, famous for the intricacy of its stalactites and stalagmites, and also the ruins of the famed cities, Tyre and Sidon. We concluded that Lebanon was the dead center and the meeting place of Western and Middle Eastern cultures. Before leaving Lebanon we did some skin diving and saw many underwater ruins and roads and the rusting anchors of ancient ships. Helga even found a murex—the famous snail from which the Tyronean purple dye was made, "the dye of kings." Looking at the ruins, I wrote in my notes: "One senses the destructiveness that has characterized man. Succeeding cultures have been completely destroyed every two or three centuries. Is it good or bad?" I went on to wonder if, with the advent of science and technology, it was any longer necessary to have the wars that in the past had destroyed the old civilizations to make way for the new. Continuing, I wrote:

I am not sure that the archaeologists are always correct in their interpretation of their findings. Maurice Dunand, for example, who for some 30 years, has had 300 men employed in excavating Biblos, says that the finding of pots with provisions in the graves proves the belief in an afterworld. I cannot accept this. I was brought up with no religious belief, and am sure there is no afterworld. Yet if someone in my family were to die I would want him to be dressed when cremated. This would not be done in expectation of a future, but out of respect for the past.

I wonder about all the human sacrifices that the Ancients are alleged to have made. Helga and I have visited the Mayan ruins in Yucatan and have heard the stories of the virgins flung into Chichen Itza's sacred pool. It is a sunken lake with cliffs 50-feet high. Any child who fell in would never get out. The people lived there for centuries yet only a few bones were found in the pool and almost all of them were children's. Maybe no one ever was thrown in. Certainly not as many as we have electrocuted or hanged for crimes. Poaching, only a few centuries ago, was a capital offense, and if the English had thrown all dead poachers into a pool, the size of the one at Chichen Itza, there would have been no room left for the water.

379

While in Lebanon we also visited Baalbek, the world's greatest pagan ruin. Some of its stones are incredibly large. "The Stone of the Pregnant Woman" is 21.36 meters long by 4.60 wide by 4.33 high. It weighs more than 250 tons. It was wedged out of its bed by putting dry beams in holes in the stone and wetting them, but how was it transported? Baalbek is magnificent, well worth the journey to its isolated location, away from easy access by land or by sea. The situation is reminiscent of the Mayo Clinic, the world's largest and most famous health complex. Perhaps it is only in isolated communities that such institutions as the Mayo Clinic or Baalbek can develop to fulfill their own personalities without intervention from the outside and before the establishment is aware of what is going on. Perhaps there were two brothers, named Baal and Bek who, like the Mayo brothers, operated a spa at the site of these ruins. Once they had it successfully started, the world beat a path to their door.

In this center of Middle East disagreements, we encountered people with divergent views of both the present and the future. A fifty-seven-year-old Lebanese man said that the Arab-Israeli dispute could be settled only by a world war and the establishment of new boundaries. A younger Lebanese said that the hope of Lebanon lay in trade with Israel. All agreed that the Syrians were the most rigid of the Arabs in respect to religious beliefs. (This, of course, was before the coming of Khomeni.)

In Lebanon there was no hospital insurance, but there were free medical clinics. A hospital room cost ten dollars a day. Family and friends chipped in to help any sick person who could not afford to pay. My notes on Lebanon conclude with the following observation: "There must be two standards of honesty here—one for Arabs, which includes bribery, and another for outsiders, for they never tried to cheat us. Probably that's why Beirut has a good international reputation as a center of trade." (In view of subsequent events, there is bitter irony in my impressions. But, twenty years ago, that was the way I viewed Lebanon.)

From Lebanon we flew to Egypt and were met at the airport by Dr. Mohiy El Kharadly, the head of the Egyptian Institute for Medical Research. With him was his twenty-one-year-old daughter, Afkar, who had a recurrent papillary carcinoma of the thyroid and upon whom I would later operate. (I am glad to say that Afkar, who now is married to the editor of one of Egypt's most important newspapers, has had no recurrence.)

Dr. Kharadly put us up in a palatial room in the Semiramus Hotel, which had a ceiling three stories high and a bathtub big enough for a giant to fit in or for Helga and me to lie in side by side. Our windows looked out on the Nile, where the boats were lowering their lateen sails to pass under the bridge. We dined with the Kharadlys in the roof garden, where a belly dancer performed. Her only clothing was a sort of mosquito netting, required by law. Sadly this was the only such netting that we saw in our hotel, for our windows were unscreened and our room was filled with flies.

Unfortunately, the research institute was closed for a three-week summer vacation. However, the museums and the displays of mummies all were open, although, as a result of the recent war with Israel, many of the most important relics had been removed for safekeeping. Perhaps this was just as well, because when Helga visited the "Salle aux Mommies" and saw Queen Nefertiti's, she related to it and had to beat a hasty retreat and sit on the bench in the hall. The queen looks just like her portrait, the contour of her face perfectly preserved.

Dr. Kharadly had been a classmate of Colonel Nasser and was his personal physician, and as a result he wielded influence. He was able to get us admitted to a newly discovered passage in Chephren's pyramid. Led by Dr. Kharadly we crawled through the tunnel, only four feet high and sloping downward at twenty-five degrees. It was hot and the air was thin. Soon the tunnel leveled off and then went upward. It was then that, simultaneously, Helga and I were overcome with claustrophobia and shortness of breath. It may not have been a psychological reaction, because later we learned that when the tunnel first was cleared many of the workers lost consciousness from lack of oxygen and the air was so depleted that candles wouldn't burn. Panic-stricken and air-hungry, Helga and I retreated, while Dr. Kharadly climbed on up to a gallery in the center of the pyramid.

At lunch, Dr. Kharadly told us of the reforms that were taking place in Egypt. Formerly 0.5 percent of the people owned 90 percent of the land. Now no one can own more than one hundred acres. There are four kinds of rich now: (1) the army, (2) the politicians, (3) the landowners, and (4) the entertainers. As yet there was no economic acknowledgement of science or technology. Dr. Kharadly himself does well, not because of his salary but because he has a large private practice in five different hospitals. The one thing that is improving most rapidly is public health.

On leaving the Middle East, I concluded, "There was something in the Arabs that makes them peculiarly stubborn about clinging to their beliefs. They seem to be like geniuses or idealists who overdevelop a single narrow point of view and are, therefore, unable to adopt any other. Thus, the Arab way of life is the result of tradition. That makes it almost as hard to change as a genetic code."

We were warned in a tourist agency about the dangers and discomforts of flying with East Africa Airlines, but my past experience with such warnings had always been that they were nonsense. It was no surprise then to find that the flight from Cairo to Nairobi was the most efficient, courteous, and well-appointed one yet. When the Comet landed in Kenya, neither Helga nor I felt any jolt to let us know that we were on the ground. In Nairobi we rented a Volkswagen and drove through the game preserves. We saw great herds of zebras and antelope, watched the lions, the rhinos, warthogs, and buzzards and stopped to wait as an elephant, twice as big as our car, slowly crossed the road in front of us, waving his ears. We spent a night at the famous "Tree-Tops" and saw troops of elephants at the watering hole as baboons and birds played around us on the porch. We visited several famous lodges including the one at Ngorongoro and the Great Rift that contains Lake Victoria, the Red Sea, the Jordan Valley and the Dead Sea. This was a land filled with history, both in the surviving animals and in the remains of man that Leaky was excavating.

From Africa we flew on to Bombay, where we were appalled to find, just as described, the streets filled with beggars and people for whom, like the sacred cows, the street was home. The stench of the bay, on whose shore the city was built, was that of a latrine. We were met by the father of one of the doctors at the Clinic, who showed us the city and introduced us to his family, all of whom were strict vegetarians.

Our schedule called for spending about a week in India, but we decided that we had seen enough of it and would like, instead, to visit Ceylon—now known as Sri Lanka—which in 1968 was a land of peace. The hospital ship *Hope* was at anchor off Colombo and we visited her and also the main hospital in Colombo. The *Hope* was well staffed, with fully qualified physicians and surgeons, but of course the physicians didn't know half as much about the tropical diseases that predominated here as did the native doctors. The local surgeons had been well-trained in England and seemed to me to be just as competent in treating ordinary problems as those from the *Hope*. There were some specialists on the *Hope*, but the ship was not equipped to perform major cardiac or other specialized and complicated types of surgery and hence they wisely did not attempt it. As a result, there was a sort of competitive stand-off between the medical staff of the ship and that of the hospital. Since we knew a surgeon from the hospital and got to know one from the ship, we heard both sides. It added up to the fact that in countries where the surgeons were Western (British) trained the *Hope* could not bring much help. What it could do, however, was to teach the pharmaceutical staff and the nurses how to obtain, prepare and administer certain medicines and treatments. This aspect of the *Hope*'s mission was a success.

In the name of surgical cure, absurd things were being done both on the ship and ashore. A sixteen-year-old girl who had had a single attack of pancreatitis had been treated on the *Hope* by subtotal pancreatectomy. Ashore a fifty-five-year-old woman who had just had a part of her stomach and esophagus removed for cancer, and who had not more than a 5 percent chance of being cured, was now being operated on for an asymptomatic nodule in the thyroid.

The fascinating part of Sri Lanka was not its hospitals or its cities, but its ancient monuments and temples, its forests and the elephants, and the clear water for diving and the cliffs to climb to ancient shrines. We had an English-speaking guide and driver named Wije, who knew all of the history and all the people along the way. We made a circuit of the island. We saw the Temple of the Tooth, where one of the Buddha's teeth is still enshrined and where three hundred trained elephants make their annual parade to exhibit the tooth in an emerald-studded gold casket. We saw the crystal Buddhas and we climbed to the caves of Siguriya, where frescoes of the famous barebreasted ladies adorn the walls. A thousand feet below us, through the monsoon's rain, we looked down on the remnants of the ancient civilization.

On our return we walked through an area where thousands of monarch-like butterflies congregated, and where we saw the thumb-sized Sisyphus beetles named for the king who was doomed in Hades to roll uphill forever a great stone, which always rolled down the hill again. A beetle was busy shaping cow dung into a golf ball-sized mass that it could roll to its den.

Along the way, by the side of the "tanks" (huge artificial lakes built long ago for irrigation), we saw herds of wild elephants. Further on we visited Ella Gap where there was a cave and a passage fifteen miles long that had been dug into the mountain and where bats filled the air. At the far end, to which we later drove, was a temple where a huge cobra lived and was worshipped. Nearby a statue of Buddha forty feet high had been carved into the rock. Beside the streams in Ella Gap are mines dug in the soft sediment of the valley's bottom. In these sapphires, rubies, garnets, and topazes were being found. I searched the stream beds for them, but not knowing what they looked like, found only a lovely clear rock crystal with a rainbow in it, which Helga would take back to Cleveland. Back at the hotel, we played with the wild monkeys that swung from the trees and decided that Sri Lanka is the world's most varied, interesting, and delightful island.

Our next stop was Bangkok, where we were met and entertained by Jane's and my old friend, Dr. Sem Pringpuangeo, who was glad to meet Helga and, along with his wife Chalam and some of his family, welcomed her. First, we were taken to a huge feast they had ordered in a Chinese restaurant. Then, they presented a silver bowl to Helga, engraved with our names, that they had prepared for us. Helga was touched, knowing what Sem had meant to Jane. (In later years, Sem and Chalam would come to Cleveland and stay with us while Sem visited the Clinic.) Bangkok has as many canals as Venice and Sem showed us all of them by boat. Then we were taken to his lavish home in a fenced-in compound on the outskirts of the city. We visited his hospital the next day and then went to the temples where the Buddha is revered, including the one where the tiny jade Buddha looked down on Jane and me so long ago.

Then it was to Bali to visit Prince Agung and stay in his palace. At least so we hoped, because a girl I had met in Africa had told me that anyone who was recommended could stay with the prince because he had three or four rooms in the palace that he rented out to people with whom he was acquainted, "and he charges practically nothing," the girl had told me. We landed and in the lounge ran into a young man who asked us where we were going. "To Prince Agung," we told him and he said that he was too. The prince's driver was there and took our baggage and drove us through the rice fields and past the streams, where bare-breasted women were bathing, and to the palace. Prince Agung met us and was at first bewildered. Finally, however, he remembered the girl, and then he found that Carl Sandburg, whose multi-volume Life of Lincoln he cherished (Bobby Kennedy had given him his set), was Helga's father, and finally that one of his best friends, Helen Costello, who had stayed there with him for months, was also one of Helga's Washington friends. So the palace and the driver and everything in Bali was ours. For several days we lived in the splendor of the royal court, constantly attended by a servant who carried to us refreshments and hot water for our baths and did Helga's washing and hung it out to dry on the bushes of the palace compound.

Before leaving, we visited the local hospital where three operations were scheduled—a radical mastectomy and two radical amputations of the penis for cancer. This type of cancer is almost unknown in America, but is one of the commonest cancers here, because a carcinogenic herb, placed beneath the foreskin of the penis, is used as an aphrodisiac. If, in the United States, so many people didn't persist in smoking cigarettes, we could say the Balinese men were stupid or out of their minds to engage in this dangerous custom.

From Bali, we flew to Java where Jakarta's three million people live on the banks of a canal into which people defecated and urinated, publicly, and from which they drew their water for washing and drinking. It reminded us so much of Bombay that we left as soon as we could for Singapore.

In contrast, Singapore was a model of how a city should be run. There was not a shred of paper or a cigarette butt on the streets (there's a heavy fine for littering). We stayed at the ancient and elegant Raffles Hotel, where old English settlers still gather to drink and smoke and talk of bygone times. We were enormously impressed with the organization of the society, whose per capita income is exceeded in the Orient only by that of Hong Kong. The food was bizarre and delicious and the people were predominantly Chinese and highly intelligent. Religion was a cause for celebration, but not to be taken seriously. Two million people lived in Singapore and it was growing.

Our next stop was Darwin in the north of Australia, where it is almost as hot as at the equator and where Chinese and aborigines feel more comfortable than do Europeans. We went down through central Australia to Mount Isa, then west to Townsville and took a short flight over to Magnetic Island, where we saw wild koala bears in the backcountry, then by helicopter to Heron Island on the Great Barrier Reef, where we spent a few days skin diving and watching the wild life. Then, we returned to the mainland by helicopter and went south to Sydney and Melbourne where there were medical meetings and lectures to give, and marvelous museums and zoos to visit where we saw our first duckbilled platypus. Before flying on to New Zealand, I should mention the Walter and Elija Hall Institute of Medical Research in Melbourne where Sir Macfarland Burnet, the pioneer in virology and immunology, did so much of his work. This institute is one of the world's finest scientific institutions.

Then we were off to Wellington, New Zealand, where we stayed with my old friend, Sir Arthur Porritt, by now the governor general of New Zealand. His wife, Lady Kay, and I had some great games of croquet on the lawn of the royal mansion. After a day or two of breakfasts in bed and toasts to the Queen in the evenings, we left Wellington for Auckland in the north of the island. Here Helga insisted that I stop dashing in and out of phone booths, and head for our hotel. There I called my old Saturday-night date, Jean Milson (now Mrs. Ray Emory and looking very beautiful and a happy grandmother), who said she could not meet with us because her husband, who ran the airport, was busy that night. Helga took over the phone and soon it was arranged that Jean would come to the top floor of our hotel, where Ray would join us later, and we would have a huge party to which I would ask any and all of my friends from the war days.

From Auckland, we flew to Fiji where we rented a car and were supposed to have a reservation in a seaside hotel. There was no room for us. We sat down and sulked. The manager came and gave us the key to a cottage a mile away, right on the shore with a marvelous coral reef only a hundred feet seaward. A sign that read "Hideaway" hung over the door. Inside were comfortable beds, a living room, and all kitchen facilities plus running water and a toilet. In the garden were fruit trees and coconuts. We had with us all we needed to dive and snorkel. Around the corner was a Chinaman who sold groceries. This was as close as Helga and I ever would get to heaven. Moreover, we were charged just half of what we would have paid for a room. We stayed there nearly a week before driving on around this varied and beautiful island. Before leaving, we spent a day visiting the hospital in Suva, where we were impressed by the high quality of the British type surgery and by the excellent medicine practiced by the nonphysician medical officers who had been trained there in the hospital.

After Fiji, Pago Pago in American Samoa was a disappointment. Rising prices and American economic interventions had brought practically all activity to a halt. The island subsisted on imports. But the scenery was lovely.

It was midnight when we arrived in Tahiti, and there wasn't a hotel bed available. I had learned French as a child and could converse with the taxi driver who ended up by bringing us to his home where he gave us bed and breakfast and then took us to the car-rental place. That hospitality and the genial, half-naked father of the driver would never be forgotten.

We drove out of the city to the end of the island where there was a restaurant, "Chez Pepe." Pepe also had a couple of grass shacks on the beach that were for rent. We settled in a comfortable one, were given a dug-out canoe to take us to the offshore reef, and we had all of our meals at "Chez Pepe," which offered a Tahitian French cuisine. We became fast friends of Pepe, who took us on boat tours of the island. The city part of Tahiti was like Miami Beach. Pepe's part was paradise. We enjoyed three days of it.

Once a week there is a flight to Chile with a ten-hour stopover at Easter Island. There were twenty of us on the plane. We got horses and rode all over the island, viewing the ancient statues, the Fallen Heads, and the places from which they were carved. It was a great study in archaeology. And then, late in the evening, we were back in the plane and early the next morning we landed in Chile.

We were very tired and thirsty when we checked into the hotel, so we went to the crowded bar for breakfast. When we entered, the men whistled and made what sounded like snide remarks. I was offended, because I thought their mirth was directed at Helga's femaleness. Not at all—it was my Darwin shorts that were causing the mirth. Chileans are more European and custom-bound than are true Europeans and all wore dark suits and ties.

We spent a few days driving around Chile in a most ancient French Citroën that had a profile like a nineteenth-century four-seater hack. But we saw the country, spent a night at a comfortable seaside resort, and went to a party given by the parents of one of my friends at the Clinic.

In Bueno Aires, population three million, we spent two days and that was enough. We visited the Alvera Hospital with an old friend, Dr. Alvera, and found that the medical care was first class. We admired the balance in Argentina between socialism and private enterprise. There also was a good school system.

In Brazil, it was a two-hour bus ride from the San Paulo Airport to the center of that city of seven million. Building was going on at a deafening rate, the sound of the air hammer everywhere. The drivers in Brazil were madmen. It was like a bullfight, and the language, of course, was Portuguese—to us unintelligible. One friend, whom we visited, had a wife and two live-in servants. "You can't do anything yourself," he explained, "If you did you would lose face." Finally, I spent a day in the hospital as "Professor pro tem." About 20 percent of the students were women—many of them Japanese. We found the life in Brazil gentle and pleasant, but we worried about the uncontrolled growth of the population.

In Lima, Peru, we ran out of money and in spite of the fact that the city is filled with huge banks and that we had American Express credit cards we couldn't cash a check. Finally, at a 2 percent discount it was arranged. We rented a car and drove south from crowded Lima, with its incredible hillside shantytowns and also its statues and cathedrals and parks, and went down along the coast, past marvelous archaeological areas, grazing llamas, huge mountainside remains of the pre-Incan civilization, and past partially excavated graves in which we found scattered bones and mummies' hair. We continued on south through the seacoast desert, until at last we came to Pisco where the fishing fleets bring their countless tons of anchovies to be dried, ground into fish meal, and exported. Here we settled down for a couple of days. We took a boat trip to the offshore "Guano Islands," where the bird droppings are piled so high that they are collected by the ton and exported for fertilizer. The bird and sea life off these islands is certainly the greatest in the world, and in the water there were hundreds of big brown seals and tiny penguins.

We flew on to Cuzco, high in the Andes, and there took the train down the valley to Machu Picchu, the greatest and best preserved ruin of antiquity. The reason it is so great is that it is so remote and so high that no one can get there to plunder or destroy it.

Helga had friends in Trinidad—Helen Costello and her husband, Bill, who was the American ambassador, and we wanted to visit them. On the way we spent one day in Guayaquil, Ecuador, where we had friends. But we thought the city was crowded, dirty, and unattractive. We were happy to fly off to the islands again.

On the way to Trinidad, we stayed at the ambassador's mansion, swam in the pool, and were cared for and fed by Helen and the servants. It was a luxurious stay that included a visit to the well-appointed-and-staffed hospital and a formal wedding reception to which the Costellos had arranged for us to be asked. It was a mixed party. The chief justice, who was giving it, was black, the governor general was Chinese, and he had a wife who did not seem to be Chinese but was surely of Asian origin. Half the guests were blacks or mulattoes and the rest were from India. All were highly educated and spoke English with a British accent. It was delightful.

At Helen's insistence, we took a twenty-minute flight to the Island of Tobago, where we were met and guided by a friend of Helen's—"Tall Boy Hercules"—a six-foot-five, jet-black Negro. He took us to skin dive in a reef populated with an extraordinary number and variety of large colorful fish.

It would not have been possible on our way home to overfly Andros Island in the Bahamas, where Helga and I had spent our honeymoon. There we stopped and again our friend, Captain Joseph Johnson, who was born and had spent his life on Andros Island, took us out to the Great Red Reef once more. We greeted our old friends, both underwater and ashore, and then flew to Nassau, where we spent a night at the Royal Victoria Hotel, built in the days of the Queen and after whom it was named. This hotel had bedded down Helga and me on our honeymoon, my late wife Jane and myself on several occasions in the 1940s and 1950s, and back at or before the turn of the century, Jane's parents had stayed there soon after their honeymoon. That was our last night away from home. The next day we would be back in Cleveland.

The four months of around-the-world travel was planned first by Helga and myself, then worked out with Jerry Howard of the Round The World Travel Agency. We had no hotel reservations and no guided tours. By word of mouth, we found our way from place to place. In countries like China, where it is hard to find accommodations unless they have been reserved, it is wise to travel with a guided tour. But the fun of a vacation is finding your own way. There is nothing more satisfactory than deciding where you want to go, going there, and then finding all the things you want to do and see. For four months on this trip we did just that and we loved it.

In 1977, we would spend three and a half months going around the world again—adding Japan, where I had been invited to speak, and Taiwan, Hong Kong, Macao, Burma, Nepal, Afghanistan, and Finland to the countries previously visited. Again in 1980 we rounded the world, visiting, among many others, Morocco, Tunisia, Sicily, Malta, Italy, Macao, and China.

But you don't have to go all the way around the world to have fun. In 1978, we went to London and then to the Balkan countries—Czechoslovakia, Poland, Hungary, Bulgaria, Romania, as well as Turkey, Iran, Kuwait, Egypt, and Jordan. On other occasions, we have visited Cuba and seen its splendid hospitals and medical facilities. On the same trip, we stopped in Jamaica and Puerto Rico. We also have taken a special medical tour with general surgeons through Russia—visiting Moscow, the Caucasus, and Leningrad. We have been to Mexico nine times in the last twenty years and we have been six times to the Bahamas, mainly in Andros Island. In all, we visited ninety different countries.

I am now over eighty years old and my days of long-distance travel are coming to a close. As they do, I have but one regret. Always I have wanted to visit Timbuctu, but something like a strike or unrest always prevented my going. Then I found that the wife of one of my best friends had been there. "It's nothing special," she said, "cement roads and dust." And so for now I am dissuaded from going to Timbuctu. Perhaps, on my way to heaven, I will pass through it and see if my friend was really right. Until then, I think I'll just go south to Mexico and spend the winters there with Helga, who now has mastered the language and is the best guide I know.

Lastly, I present this classic offering, which Helga and I wrote and sang during the 1968 Round The World Journey:

Her shoes wore out in Kenya
On the Serengeti plain,
Her stockings tore in Thailand
And were never worn again;

She lost her bra in Bali
And her slip in Singapore.
Her panties fell in Fiji
On Suva's sunny shore;

She came to Easter Island
With a Polynesian air,
Wearing just a muumuu
And a flower in her hair!

30

Cancer Again

B ACK HOME again, I was increasingly busy with surgery of the breast, for the swing was now towards breast-saving operations and the more I was cursed by the profession for doing them, the more patients heard about the possibility of saving the breast and came to see me. What with this and the increase of my writing, which now was not limited to the technical but included also the socioeconomic aspects of surgery, I was nearly as busy as Helga. Since our marriage Helga had published her book of song and reminiscence, *Sweet Music*, as well as a novel, *The Wizard's Child*, in which one of her characters is based on our experiences with the turkey vultures we had imprinted. And she was writing and publishing her short stories, which would in time be collected in *Children and Lovers: 15 Stories* (Harcourt Brace Jovanovich, 1976). During these years Helga was getting her materials and the files in order to begin writing a book on her family that would in time be published, *A Great And Glorious Romance: The Story of Carl Sandburg and Lilian Steichen* (1978). It was not just the writing that kept Helga busy. She was concerned also with the band of baby birds and animals that inhabited our backyard, all of which were convinced that we were their parents and kept both of us fascinated and enthralled.

In the midst of all this activity, Helga and I joined my old friends, Ed and Marion Link, in February of 1969 on a Caribbean cruise that would wind up on the island of Cozumel. The trip proved to be exciting. We saw thousands of porpoises in a line that extended for miles, all migrating from somewhere to somewhere, and we ran aground on reefs that were uncharted. Then Helga was seasick and began to bleed and have cramps. She was miserable, but was better when we got ashore. As soon as possible, we flew home where the D & C showed endometrial cancer. Cobalt radiation was started.

Before entering the hospital in April for her hysterectomy, Helga's chest X-ray was taken. The radiologist called me up to his office. A thoracic surgeon was there too. They looked grim. The X-ray showed several areas that were typical of metastasis. "They can't be from the endometrial cancer," I protested. "She has had symptoms for only two weeks and the curettings showed a superficial cancer. I've never heard of an early endometrial cancer metastasizing like that. You know she had a cold about a week ago."

"There it is," was all my friends could say. But everyone agreed to go along with the hysterectomy anyway.

The pathologist could find no cancer. It had disappeared, destroyed by the radiation. Another X-ray was taken and this time the chest was perfectly clear. The radiologists saw several more patients that month, who had what appeared to be pulmonary metastases but which cleared spontaneously. I've never heard of such an infection before or since. We were ecstatic, but I had told Helga everything, including my doubts, and there had been a few sad days for both of us.

I continued to be busy in clinical work and began to write more and more. I published the first paper that I know of that recommended aspiration as the definitive treatment of thyroid cysts and I demonstrated that the destruction of the carotid artery at its bifurcation, in patients with carotid body tumors, was not the result of invasion by the tumor but of mechanical destruction from the force of the jet stream against the walls of the arteries that had been deviated by the size of the tumor. I also, in the laboratory, demonstrated that in mice the obstruction of lymphatics (as occurs in radical mastectomy) results in more rapid growth of any residual tumor. For this reason a complete axillary dissection of thin skin flaps would tend to stimulate the growth of any cancer cells left in the skin. Thick skin flaps instead of thin ones were advocated, and we noted that when flaps were thick and the circulation was not impaired fulminating local recurrences no longer appeared. I also wrote an article that to me at least was original, showing that parathyroid tumors sometimes could be found in the thymus. I suggested that, when four parathyroids could not be found, the thymus should be removed. And, of course, the war against radical neck dissections for papillary cancer continued.

After a period, early in my surgical career, in which I was quite radical and advised such operations as extended radical mastectomies, I had gradually lost confidence in extended surgery. Guided also by my observations in the laboratory and stimulated by the work of Dr. Deborah Doniach, in London, I went so far as to write, in 1973, an article in which I questioned the value or even wisdom of performing lymphadenectomies in cases in which involvement of the nodes was not palpable. In cancers like melanomas and those of the breast in which the drainage areas are palpable, survival is not increased by prophylactically removing nodes as compared to that when resection of nodes is not done unless they become palpably involved. I coined the term "partial mastectomy" which I thought expressed the wideness of the excision better than lumpectomy or local excision, and I wrote a controversial article that was published in *Surgery, Gynecology and Obstetrics* (1970), that in terms of survival showed the advantages of bypass operations over radical pancreato-duodenectomy in the treatment of pancreatic cancer. To this day, there has not been a single patient operated on at the Cleveland Clinic for adenocarcinoma of the pancreas who has been cured. More and more, when the bizarre types and incidental microcarcinomas occurring in pancreatitis are excluded, it appears that my pessimism is justified. Even the Mayo Clinic published a retraction of its earlier optimistic reports, which they found had been based on misinterpretations by pathologists.

31

More Controversy

꒜

I N NOVEMBER of 1972, I had become sixty-five years old. I had
stopped operating, but still saw patients who wanted my opinion,
and did the necessary office work and referred them to my associates.
I was very busy with my new vocation, for more and more I wanted to
educate the lay public about the treatment of breast cancer. That first
book, published in 1973, *What Women Should Know About the Breast Cancer Controversy*, had been timely. Before long, Betty Ford, wife of the
president, as well as Happy Rockefeller, wife of our vice president,
would be operated on for widely publicized cancers of the breast. I
wrote articles for *Harpers, American Medical News, Hospital Physician,
Medical World News, The Medical Tribune,* and *Modern Medicine.* I would
appear with Barbara Walters on the "Not for Women Only" and the
"Today" shows, as well as the "Donahue" show.

Right in the middle of all this confusion, what should happen? In
April of 1974, I asked Helga (because risk of breast cancer in those who
have had endometrial cancer is increased) to have a mammogram.
She was found to have a tiny cancer about one centimeter in diameter,
that lay deep in the breast and could not be felt. The next day, Dr. Esselstyn removed it by partial mastectomy, and no further treatment
was given.

Helga at once wrote an article called, "Let a Joy Keep You" that was
published in that November's *McCall's* magazine. In the same month
Time magazine printed a piece called "Breast Cancer—Fear and Fact,"
and along with the photos of Betty and Happy and Helga's smiling
face was a picture of the X-ray of Helga's shapely breast. The latter was
also on the covers of the European pictorial magazines, *Paris Match*
and Germany's *Stern.*

All of this publicity has been great for mammography and for the promotion of lesser-than-radical breast surgery. It did what I had hoped it would do. It made women examine themselves, have mammograms, and seek early treatment. Since that time, there has been a drop both in the size of the breast cancers that we saw and in the incidence of nodal involvement.

All of this was good for the health of women, but bad for the professional reputation of Crile. When the *Cleveland Plain Dealer* came out with a quote from one of my interviews, in which I said that radical mastectomy was obsolete and except in extraordinary circumstances should not be done, the Cleveland Academy of Medicine held a special meeting and reprimanded me, saying that I had "an obvious lack of concern for the patients who have had a radical mastectomy performed," and that "my comments already had had a deleterious effect on the relationship patients have with their surgeons."

I replied that I thought the Academy was unethical, because it gave "no consideration to the welfare of the patients who in the future would be treated for breast cancer and who I thought should be entitled to know about recent developments that make radical operations unnecessary."

The Academy did not at that time retract the reprimand, but later, when I was about to go to press again in another book, I challenged their Ethics Committee, threatening not only to expose its actions to the public, but also to start a class-action suit in which any settlement was to go to the American Cancer Society. That was a couple of years after the reprimand, and by then, radical mastectomy had been proven to be unnecessary. A spokesman for the Academy called on me and offered to "expunge the record." Since this proposition was not made in writing and since I have no way of telling what has happened to the record, I feel free to write about it in this final summation of my life and times. My basic opinions have not changed. I think that the central organizations—the AMA and the American College of Surgeons—act with care and with consideration for the welfare of the patient. But the local branches of these organizations, like the Cleveland Academy of Medicine, often act selfishly to protect the reputation and the income of the private physician.

The conflict with the Academy brings me to the end of my medical career. I should mention that regardless of what my Cleveland colleagues in the Academy think of me, I was elected to Honorary Membership in the Royal College of Surgeons in England, an honor that never before had been bestowed on a father *and* son. I have also been elected to membership of the American Surgical Society and all other special societies that I have wanted to join. Except locally, the Cleveland Academy's reprimand has not had a profound effect on my life. It just made me more conscious of the evils of the fee-for-service method of remunerating surgeons.

The last few years of my practice, until my retirement in 1972, had been busy ones professionally, and also in other ways. I not only (with Dr. Alexander Bunts) wrote the book about the history of the Cleveland Clinic, *To Act as a Unit,* and directed a motion picture of the same name that showed the Clinic in action, but I also continued to write about ten scientific papers a year until the total added up to 452.

32

Extracurricular Activities

🙢

I N THE FIELD of moving pictures, Helga and I continued to be busy,
and produced more than 260 films, all edited and with accompany-
ing narration and music tapes. The first few were from Jane's and my
16-mm films, many featuring our underwater adventures. There are
also four or five black-and-white 16-mm films of my father's African
adventures, dating back to the 1920s, that we have edited. The rest are
8-mm or Super-8-mm color films. We show new ones and old ones
every year at our film festival that runs from 4:30 to 7:30 P.M. on the
Friday, Saturday, and Sunday of each of the three weeks before Christmas. There is a self-service bar and great loaves of black pumpernickel
bread with raisins. About a hundred people a night come through,
some leaving early, some arriving late. In the "Theater," which once
was our living room, about seventy people can be seated on chairs, on
benches along the wall, and on desks and chests and the hearth of the
fireplace. Another twenty or so can sit or stand in the hallway or on
the porch and see the screen. Helga runs all the projection equipment
and amplifiers and the guests help themselves at the bar and at the re-
freshment table. A schoolgirl comes in the morning after and cleans
up. Except for that, we do everything ourselves, including the music.
Helga is an expert and has a large collection of tapes and records to select from. Also when we travel, she buys recordings, typical of the
country, to use with the films.

Most of our films are of travel, but we also have a collection of
animal-behavior films, dating from the days when our yard was filled
with creatures. As an example, in 1987, we showed more than five
films every night, and also each night there was a "live act"—dance,
song, or recitation. We also show a few "Foreign Films"—never more

than one a night. These are films made not by the Criles but by their friends and approved by the "Kent Road Film Festival Committee." The 1987 Program begins:

ANNOUNCING THE NINETEENTH ANNUAL
KENT ROAD FILM FESTIVAL
NO RESERVATIONS
ADMISSION IS FREE
FORTY-SIX SCHEDULED FILMS IN FULL LIVING COLOR AND
A FILM FEATURING GOD EVERY SUNDAY
TWO HUNDRED FORTY-EIGHT FILMS AVAILABLE
ON SPECIAL REQUEST
EIGHT LIVE ACTS—EIGHT

Annual Message from our Producer:
In accordance with the spirit of the times [election year] those who have committed plagiarism or adultery or have ever used marijuana will not be eligible for admission to the Festival.

George Crile, Jr.

We send out about five hundred announcements—many serving as Christmas cards to friends far away. Amazingly, except when there is a terrible blizzard, about the right number of people come every night. It is great fun, and by this means we are able to repay indebtedness and do most of our entertaining for the year.

In the years of my retirement, there was one activity that gave me a lot of fun. That was writing the lyrics for country music. Years before, I had had as a patient ten-year-old Diane Leslie, nicknamed "Cee Cee," whose mother, a music teacher, had brought her to me from Pittsburgh because she had been advised to have an operation for a multinodular goiter. "I want you to know that I have taught singing all my life and my daughter has the best voice of any student I have ever had." There was no way that one could guarantee that removal of a goiter like this would not produce a change in the quality and resonance of the voice, even if there were no injury to the laryngeal nerves. There was nothing about the goiter that suggested malignancy. I decided to try suppressive doses of thyroid hormone and to follow the patient along.

Through the years the goiter grew no larger; in fact, it seemed to shrink a little. The ten-year-old matured and grew up and became a well-known singer and recorder of records in New York. She married and had children and always kept in touch with me. One day in the 1970s, she came to Cleveland for a checkup, and I asked her to come home with me so I could hear her sing and play. She sounded great. It so happened that I had just written a song for a party given by a friend of mine, who was just my age, and I needed it put to music. Sitting at the piano, Cee Cee read the lines, fingered the keys and picked out a tune, then she played and sang the song.

The tune that Cee Cee wrote was so catchy and good that I was entranced. I began to send her lyrics and she would make up a tune to go with each one, sing them, put them on a tape and mail them back to me. It was a lot of fun and I couldn't stop writing lyrics. Included in the album were "Mystery in the Memory," "Prelude to My Symphony," "Sunshine Highway," and eight more. Next, Cee Cee got together a group of seven musician friends who played bass, drums, guitar, cello, harmonica-and-bells, country fiddle, and piano, and, with no charge except for the recording studio, put together a flashy album called *Our River of Love* from the title song, which began:

> My love is like a river to the ocean,
> It flows forever, deep and swift and still.
> The river carries all of my devotion,
> And the ocean never seems to get its fill.

A lovely seacoast scene is on the front of the album and on the back is a beautiful photo of Cee Cee and me, taken out by the pond. There is also a "Comment from Helga Sandburg":

> This is the first album for Dr. George Crile, Jr., explorer, author and world-renowned surgeon, who has been writing country lyrics for the last few years to the astonishment of friends in all three fields. When composer-singer-pianist Diane Leslie, whose unique voice spans the range from rock to opera, by chance heard Dr. Crile's lyrics, it seemed inevitable that she should set them to music and interpret them in all their vibrancy, humor, pathos and sensuality. This unique combination of one of the more revered names in the medical profession and one of the most talented young performers in our country today is a first for the contemporary music world.

Our friends loved the album, and Cee Cee and I had many favorable comments, although no commercial offers. Then suddenly, and just as inexplicably as it started, I stopped writing lyrics and, except for special occasions, I haven't written any since.

About then another thing happened to distract my restless mind. I knew a man named John Craig, with whom I had worked on some medical television and radio programs and who ran an organization called Communicorp which got together advertisers, television and radio stations, newspapers, and performers to the advantage of all. John asked me if I would do a short radio program that would be aired twice a day every Wednesday. Since I could tape ten or twelve at a sitting, it wouldn't be much of a bother. He wanted it to be no longer than ninety seconds—that is 250 words—less than one double-spaced typewritten page. I could discuss whatever I wished so long as it was controversial, interesting and not too shocking. I named it "90 Seconds with Dr. George Crile, Jr.," because I remembered what had happened to my son, George Crile, and General Westmoreland on the CBS documentary, and thought that ninety seconds would be legally a lot safer than "60 Minutes," of which my son was now one of the producers.

The advertisement for the show read:

He's charming. He's controversial. He's always surprising. He's bright. He's funny. He's shocking. He's risqué. He's contemporary and informative. He's internationally renowned surgeon and Cleveland Clinic Emeritus Consultant, Dr. George Crile, Jr., and his commentaries are heard on "90 SECONDS," an exciting new radio show at 8:50 A.M. and 5:50 P.M. every Wednesday on WERE 1300 AM. Next week, Dr. Crile's topic will be "Democracy vs. Hypocrisy."

The titles for the programs varied. Some were:

> Pit Bulls, Popes and Ayatollahs
> Let's Legalize Polygamy
> Are We Being Outsmarted by the Commies?

At first, I had great difficulty in limiting my discussion to the required ninety seconds, but as time went on this changed. I always wrote up my pieces and had them typed and then censored by John Craig— who did the latter to quite a few of them. Soon, whenever I wrote anything, it always ended up between 240 or 260 words, exactly ninety seconds. It got so that I thought in ninety-second splurges.

One of the reviewers of the show used the headline: "CRILE OFFERS SHOT IN THE ARM" and said, "It's probably the shortest show on Cleveland radio, which may be why it's the best. . . . While Crile's show hasn't attracted any litigation in the nine months it's been on the air, his views on everything from euthanasia to pit bulls have gotten more than a few listeners riled up."

Needless to say, the show would fall by the wayside. John Craig's letter came:

September 15, 1988

Dear Barney:

I hate to have to say this but, as I think you already know, I simply have not been able to line up the necessary advertisers for another season of your radio program. I wish I could hold out some hope for later in the year but, frankly, even though the station liked the fact that your show was controversial, Cleveland being the conservative town it is, potential advertisers were just too wary.

I think the program was a noble experiment and I really regret not seeing it continued.

Sincerely,
John

In addition to being read on the air, many of my ninety-second pieces, if they were in any way related to medicine, found a new publisher. This was the international *Medical Tribune,* a paper with a large worldwide circulation. The pieces were now known as "Crile's Corner."

While on the subject of these occupations that I found so delightful in the years of my retirement as an Emeritus Consultant at the Cleveland Clinic, in 1980 I privately published a collection of my works called *The Crile Cornball Collection of Fiction, Fact and Fantasy.* On the first page was:

This volume is gratefully
dedicated
To all of those girls
Who refused to
marry me

There were satirical, sentimental, and serious prose pieces and poems alternating in the book. Helga, who had done the selecting and editing, did a preface. There is a poem written in 1917, when I was ten years old and relating to the war. There is a novelette called "Broken Bridges" about five women with breast cancers and how their lives went after the "discovery." There is an article, "Homosexuality, Anita Bryant, God, and the AMA." There is one called "Skonk Measure I" all about Jules Olitsky's work and the situation in art today. There are poems to Helga, to the dog Gustav, to Mycerinus, to the moon, to "A Brother-in-Law with a New Valve," and one to our buzzard, ending:

> That magnificent eagle we all hold so regal
> Will kill any creature alive,
> So give me a vulture with my kind of culture,
> I want to be patient and thrive.

This little book was reviewed for the *Yale Alumni Bulletin* by my friend, Ted Williams:

The Crile Cornball Collection of Fiction, Fact and Fantasy, by George Crile, Jr. (selected and edited by Helga Sandburg), Publix Book Mart, 1310 Huron Road, Cleveland, OH 44115 (216-621-6624), 1980, 156pp, hard cover $15, paperback $5.

This is a compilation of the writings of the world famous surgeon, Dr. George Crile, Jr., over a period of many years. Seldom have so many unrelated subjects been covered in so few pages. Seldom has such varied means of expression been used; matter-of-fact prose, the delicately rhymed poetry, and on to free verse. Seldom does one find a book with rollicking humor on one page and a profoundly serious treatise on the next. No wonder the title had to be stretched to cover all these varied classes. The result could have been a disastrous hodgepodge of confusion were it not for the skillful editing and tasteful arrangement of Helga Sandburg. The reader will wholeheartedly agree with some passages and violently disagree with others. He will never be bored.

33

As Time Goes By

A S I GOT into my mid-seventies, I had already lost a brother and a brother-in-law. My sister Peg, six years older than I and one of the most sensible women I have ever known, decided to waste no time. After the death of her husband, she promptly and successfully remarried. In 1984, my sister Elo died. A beautiful woman, she had had Parkinson's disease and progressive speech and motor disabilities ever since the terrible influenza epidemic during World War I. Her funeral in Memphis was a satisfying and well-attended service. Her husband, Dr. Gus Chrisler, and her four children had all adored her.

And then, in 1986, I had a repetition of the accident that I had had years before in Washington, D.C. This time, however, there were no internal injuries. As for Helga, except for aftershock (she had been driving and I had been reading aloud to her when we were hit) and some whiplash, a headache, and soreness of neck and shoulders, she was untouched. I wrote up some "Revelations" afterwards, going partly:

> There are a few times in life when one views his Maker eye to eye. That is if the person believes that he has a Maker. But even in the life of an atheist, there is at least one time when he suddenly becomes aware of his life as a visible, self-contained unit that can be weighed, measured, conserved or scattered. That was the experience that I lived through.

> I was reading to Helga. The next thing I remember was the agonizing necessity of getting my breath. My shoulder belt had been on. How or when it was removed, I don't know, but my vivid recollection was that I must stand, for only in that position could I breathe. I do not remember thinking, "This is the end."

Nor do I remember thinking, "I will be able to make it." All I remember is a gigantic image of myself, the door of the car open, standing in that door and supporting myself on it.

In fiction, one often reads how in moments of crisis, images of all the past flash across the screen of memory. This experience was not like that, but involved the same principle. Suddenly, as I stood there, I saw myself not as a part of a long string of nearly 79 years of life. Instead the moving stream of life had been condensed into a tiny capsule. Then it was round and white and I saw myself, tall and white-haired, looking at that capsule and trying to decide if it was something that would be broken to powder and scattered or whether it would be planted as a seed. Nothing more happened to this dream. It was just a vision and not a sequence.

My recovery was prompt and complete. By now, I had had a total of nineteen fractured ribs and there was no question that this left me a little short of breath on exertion, for in addition to the bronchiectasis that had followed my college-days bout of pneumonia and the mild emphysema that no doubt was aggravated by even the moderate smoking that I had indulged in until the 1970s, I had had mild seasonal asthma for most of my life. Although I no longer felt like climbing mountains and making deep dives, I remained in better health than most of my male contemporaries. Then just to be stylish and do what all my friends did, I decided to have a transurethral resection of the prostate.

The decision was not a sudden or impulsive one. A couple of years before, when Helga and I were in Russia, we had gone to a party where there was a lot of beer. When we got back to our hotel, I had had acute retention and could not void so much as a drop. Fortunately, I had foreseen such a possibility and had brought along a catheter and appropriate antibiotics to prevent infection.

I didn't have any more trouble for about a year, and then again I had increasing difficulty and again I had to catheterize myself. There were two choices—accept self-catheterization as a way of life or have a transurethral resection. The latter is a relatively minor operation that involves no incision, little discomfort, and only two or three days in the hospital. Ralph Straffon, the head of the Department of Urology, performed the operation, removing about one hundred grams of tissue—an unusually large amount.

Convalescence was uneventful, and I have had a perfect result. This operation is not one to be rushed into unnecessarily, but when the indications are clear it should not be avoided. In the hundred or more sections of the tissue that the pathologist examined, there were, of course, a few (four) that showed cancer. At least 75 percent of people of my age have microscopic cancer of the prostate if it is searched for. There would be differences of opinion in medical circles as to what more, if anything, need be done. My surgeon, being not only skillful but also wise and philosophical, said that no more treatment was necessary and that I probably would have no more trouble with the prostate. He was well aware of the fact that I was eighty!

The treatment of prostatic cancer can be as controversial as that of breast cancer. In the presence of even a trace of cancer, some urologists would advise radical prostatectomy with its attending complications of impotence and often incontinence of urine as well as a far from negligible mortality rate. Others would advise radiation therapy, which sometimes has devastating effects on bladder, rectum, and other organs in the field. Finally there is the endocrine approach that involves either castration or the use of the female hormone estrogen. Particularly in older people this has a good chance of slowing or permanently arresting the growth of prostatic cancer, even when it has invaded surrounding tissues or metastasized. Since this therapy is just as effective when it is used late, after metastases are identified, as it is when used early, there should be no hurry about starting it. That's why I am content to live happily, free of symptoms, and have myself checked once a year to see if there is any evidence of spread.

It is interesting, at this time of life, to be confronted with one of the same kinds of therapeutic choices that I have for so long been making for and with my patients. I intend to walk the conservative path, just as I have in the treatment of cancers of the breast and thyroid.

34

The Way It Is

NOW THE WORLD is no longer looking backward, to ancient times, but living in the present and basing decisions on recent developments. The world as I have known it is rapidly changing. The dynasties of China, the empires of the pharaohs, of Babylon, of Greece, and of Rome lasted for centuries. In those days, communications were by foot or by horseback. Now news travels with the speed of light. That is why the supremacy of the British Empire lasted for years instead of for centuries and why that of the United States has lasted for an even shorter period of time.

When one views the economic supremacy of Japan and the ascendency of Taiwan and Korea, and realizes that the Chinese are developing rapidly in the same direction, it is clear that it will not be long before we will have to either put a high tax on all imports or lower our standard of living so that we will be able to compete with the Orient. That would mean abolition of the high cost of medical care, for which it is said that General Motors pays more in the way of insurance for its employees that it does for steel. We will have to reduce the price of law and the cost of malpractice and personal injury suits and that of all of the other legal actions that result from the contingency fee, that allows the lawyers to share in the judgements awarded to their clients.

I think we have lived through the Days of the American Empire— much of its luxury and splendor has been recorded here. Ahead, I believe, lies inflation, readjustment, and a much lower standard of living. In the future, I do not see how we can support a system that allows part of the population to be so poor that they are homeless and another part to be so rich that in this country there are more than forty billionaires. Remember, a billionaire is a man who has a thousand times a million dollars. I do not believe these changes will come suddenly. At first it will be a slow evolution, as it was during the decline of the British Empire. I fear, however, that America's racial problems may, somewhere along the line, give rise to a civil war between the haves and the have-nots. I hope I am wrong, but I am happy that I lived when I did.

As I look back on the eighty years of my life, I have no regrets. I was born into the lap of luxury, I grew up in high society, I enjoyed my schooling and my professional training and practice. I was fortunate in my first marriage and in the children that ensued. With my family I shared many adventures in treasure hunting and travel and I enjoyed writing about them and about medical and philosophical subjects. I also have enjoyed, always in partnership with a wife, the production of moving pictures that fixed in film what otherwise would have been fleeting memories.

I suffered one major misfortune—the death of Jane. I received one major compensation—the discovery of Helga. Helga and I still live in the house that Jane and I bought in 1935. I drive an ancient and dilapidated Chevrolet back and forth to the Clinic—four minutes away— where on weekdays I have lunch and pick up and answer my mail. Once every two weeks the ninety-year-old seamstress, Mrs. Jones, comes to our house and with incomparable skill, repairs everything that has fallen apart. Once a week Mrs. Brown comes by and does laundry and housekeeping, and from time to time a cleaning company moves in with men, women, and machines and spends an hour scouring the house.

Helga and I rarely go out to dinner. In noisy restaurants or at cocktail parties, I have difficulty in hearing anyone except the person right next to my left ear. Helga, raised in the isolated duneland of Michigan, feels at ease when she is alone with her family. We are not enthusiastic about driving at night, and Helga won't drive if she's had anything to drink and she won't let me drive her even if I haven't, so we prefer to have people visit us rather than to go out. For three weeks every year, there is the Film Festival, and that gives us all the social contacts we need.

We have two large dogs—Mowgli, a Doberman-Shepherd, and Rolf, a Rottweiler-Shepherd. And we have two large black cats named "Sweeter than the Bees Humming" and "Wednesday Evening in the Twilight and the Gloaming." Since all of Helga's creatures are neutered, they don't roam, run away, or give us trouble. Every weekend we go to the country and cut wood or tend the garden, and the dogs come with us, delighted. The cats are glad to see us go and glad to see us return.

Helga and I have loved our travels. Together, we have seen most of the accessible parts of the world and Helga, at the age of sixty-nine, has just returned from a three-week trip to the Xinjiang region of China near the Russian border. Alone, she flew off to Beijing to meet Clara Reece, of the Cyrus Eaton Group in China. From there they flew on to Urumqi, where Clara was engaged in all sorts of agricultural and livestock enterprises.

Helga is the busiest woman I have ever known. She not only takes care of the house, does the shopping, the cooking, the caring for the animals, the feeding of the wild birds and of the fish in our backyard pond, but she also is always writing, and also always editing my papers, essays, and books. Helga is the most talented woman I have ever met. She not only looks fifteen years younger than she is, she also acts that way. "What any woman can do Helga can do better," is still my characterization of her. She writes on her word processor with the speed of lightning. She is master of all the recording and projection equipment that we use at the Film Festival. She is an expert barber and has saved me thousands of dollars by cutting my hair for the last twenty-five years. Helga is an artist in the kitchen and in both preparation and preservation of food. I've never seen anyone as good as she in a garden. She knows all about goats and cows. She is an excellent horseback rider. She is as good at filing and accounting as she is in her library work. She plays the guitar and sings professionally and she is a fearless and helpful traveling companion, talking to everyone she meets and learning all about the countries she travels in. In addition to all these skills, Helga is a devoted mother, a perfect wife, and a person who loves everyone for what he is and not for anything else.

I end my story with this synopsis of Helga, because if I had told it all, this book could go on for volumes. Autumn is here. The leaves are turning. It has been a pleasure to have been a physician and to have had insight into and some understanding of the processes that are involved in life. It has been pleasant to follow the philosophy of my father and to live with women who have been as diversified in their skills and interests as was my mother. "The world goes round and round." The silver spoon that my mother put in my mouth is still there, and Helga has put a gold one beside it.

Perhaps, with all these natural advantages and all of this help I might have become rich and famous, if I had been able to develop a field of interest and stick to it. I was never able to accomplish this. My maximum span of attention seems to have been about five years. It is therefore possible to summarize my biography by dividing it into sixteen five-year periods. Except for the first five, of which I have little memory, and the five that are yet to come, most of which I am apt to forget, all of them have been great fun.

Age	Chief Interest
0–5 years	The Breast
5–10	Fishing
10–15	Hunting
15–20	Athletics
20–25	Women
25–30	Medicine
30–35	Marriage
35–40	Treasure
40–45	Writing
45–50	The Breast Again
50–55	Despair and the Interlude
55–60	Marriage Again
60–65	Movies
65–70	Attacking the Establishment
70–75	Song Writing
75–80	Radio Program
80 +	Reminiscence

THE END

Index

Index

The Way It Was
was composed in 10-point Palatino and leaded 2 points
by Point West, Inc.;
printed by sheet-fed offset on 50-pound Glatfelter Natural
acid-free stock with halftone signatures
printed on 70-pound enamel stock,
Smyth sewn and bound over 88' binder's boards
in Holliston Kingston Natural cloth
with 80-pound Rainbow Antique endpapers,
and wrapped with dustjackets printed in three colors
on 80-pound enamel stock and film laminated
by Braun-Brumfield, Inc.;
designed by Will Underwood;
and published by
The Kent State University Press
KENT, OHIO 44242